Medical and Surgical Management
of Adrenal Diseases

Medical and Surgical Management of Adrenal Diseases

Editor

Joseph C. Cerny, M.D.

Clinical Professor of Urology
University of Michigan Medical School
Ann Arbor, Michigan
Chairman Emeritus
Department of Urology
Henry Ford Hospital
Detroit, Michigan

Medical Illustrator

Jay Knipstein

Medical Arts Division
Henry Ford Hospital
Detroit, Michigan

LIPPINCOTT WILLIAMS & WILKINS
A **Wolters Kluwer** Company
Philadelphia • Baltimore • New York • London
Buenos Aires • Hong Kong • Sydney • Tokyo

Acquisitions Editor: Lisa McAllister
Developmental Editor: Leah Ann Kiehne Hayes
Manufacturing Manager: Kevin Watt
Production Manager: Robert Pancotti
Production Editor: Thomas Boyce
Cover Designer: Karen Quigley
Indexer: Mary and Ron Prottsman
Compositor: Lippincott Williams & Wilkins Desktop Division
Printer: Maple Press

Library of Congress Cataloging-in-Publication Data
Medical and surgical management of adrenal diseases / editor Joseph C. Cerny ; medical illustrator, Jay Knipstein
    p. cm.
   Includes bibliographical references and index.
   ISBN 0-683-30344-9
   1. Adrenal glands—Surgery.   2. Adrenal glands—Diseases.   3. Adrenal glands—Cancer.   I. Cerny, Joseph C.
   [DNLM: 1. Adrenal Gland Diseases—therapy.   WK 700 M487 1999]
RD599.5.A37M44   1999
616.4'5—DC21
DNLM/DLC   96-54024
                                                     CIP
for Library of Congress   Rev.

*This book is dedicated to
Reed M. Nesbit, Jerome W. Conn, Raymond Mellinger,
William H. Beierwaltes, and Bruce H. Stewart,
pioneers and outstanding contributors in their fields
to the advancement of knowledge in the diagnosis and treatment
of adrenal disease.*

*I have been privileged to work and study with these
distinguished physicians and surgeons,
and their inspiration has made this book possible.*

Contents

Contributing Authors

Mahul B. Amin, M.D.
Department of Pathology and Laboratory Medicine
Emory University Hospital
Director of Surgical Pathology
Department of Anatomic Pathology
Emory University Hospital
Atlanta, Georgia

Robert A. Bonzani, M.D.
Chief Resident in Urology
Henry Ford Hospital
Detroit, Michigan

Joseph C. Cerny, M.D.
Clinical Professor of Urology
University of Michigan Medical School
Ann Arbor, Michigan
Chairman Emeritus
Henry Ford Hospital
Detroit, Michigan

Michel Gagner, M.D.
Professor of Surgery
The Mount Sinai School of Medicine
Chief, Division of Laparoscopic Surgery
The Mount Sinai Medical Center
New York, New York

Ricardo González, M.D., F.A.A.P.
Professor and Chief of Pediatric Urology
Children's Hospital of Michigan
Wayne State University
Detroit, Michigan

B. Todd Heniford, M.D.
Chief, Minimal Access Surgery
Co-Director, Carolinas Laproscopic and Advanced
Surgery Programs
Department of General Surgery
Carolinas Medical Center
Charlotte, North Carolina

David A. Iannitti, M.D.
Assistant Professor of Surgery
Brown University School of Medicine
Providence, Rhode Island

Terri L. Johnson, M.D.
Staff Pathologist
Department of Pathology
St. Joseph Mercy Hospital
Ann Arbor, Michigan

Charles M. Keoleian, M.D.
Senior Staff Urologist
Department of Urology
Henry Ford Hospital
Detroit, Michigan

J. G. Kim, M.D.
Senior Staff Anesthesiologist
Department of Anesthesiology
Henry Ford Hospital
Detroit, Michigan

David C. Leach, M.D.
Associate Professor of Medicine
Loyola University of Chicago Stritch School of
Medicine
Executive Director
Accreditation Council for Graduate Medical
Education
Chicago, Illinois

H. Michael Marsh, M.B., B.S.
Professor and Chair
Department of Anesthesiology
Wayne State University School of Medicine
Specialist-in-Chief
Department of Anesthesiology
Detroit Medical Center
Detroit, Michigan

Milan V. Pantelic, M.D., M.S.E.
Senior Staff Radiologist
Department of Diagnostic Radiology and Medical
Imaging
Henry Ford Hospital
Detroit, Michigan

James O. Peabody, M.D., F.A.C.S.
Senior Staff Urologist
Department of Urology
Henry Ford Hospital
Detroit, Michigan

Orlin Sergev, M.D.
Fellow in Endocrinology and Metabolism
Henry Ford Hospital
Detroit, Michigan

Sugandh D. Shetty, M.D., F.R.C.S.
Senior Staff Urologist
Department of Urology
Henry Ford Hospital
Detroit, Michigan

Craig A. Smith, M.D.
Clinical Assistant Professor
Department of Surgery
University of Illinois at Chicago
College of Medicine at Peoria
Peoria, Illinois

Norman W. Thompson, M.D.
Henry King Ransom Professor of Surgery
University of Michigan Medical School
Chief, Division of Endocrine Surgery
University Hospitals
Ann Arbor, Michigan

Max Wisgerhof, M.D.
Senior Staff Physician
Division of Endocrinology and Metabolism
Henry Ford Hospital
Detroit, Michigan

M. Saeed Zafar, M.D.
Senior Endocrinologist
Division of Endocrinology and Metabolism
Henry Ford Hospital
Detroit, Michigan

Preface

More than 30 years have elapsed since the landmark contributions of Jerome W. Conn and Reed M. Nesbit of the University of Michigan firmly established parameters for the practical clinical diagnosis of primary aldosteronism and described surgical techniques for adrenal exploration, identification of the causative adenoma, adrenalectomy, and, in most cases, cure of the hypertension and electrolyte abnormalities characteristic of Conn's syndrome.

Since that time, our knowledge of the basic mechanisms underlying adrenal diseases and our ability to diagnose and treat these diseases have undergone dramatic improvement. Advances in adrenal imaging now allow precise preoperative localization of adrenal masses, permitting targeted operative procedures and minimizing need for exploration. Improvements in preoperative preparation, anesthesia, and perioperative care have greatly reduced the morbidity and mortality of adrenal surgery. Efficient diagnostic algorithms permit early and accurate diagnosis of adrenal endocrinopathies. Laparoscopic adrenalectomy has evolved and, with reduced morbidity and other advantages, is applicable for most adrenal tumors.

This book is written for clinicians responsible for the diagnosis, treatment, and care of patients with adrenal disease. We believe that internists and surgeons alike will find the elucidation of contemporary principles of adrenal disorders, ranging from basic mechanisms of disease to practical clinical management, useful in their practice. Likewise, together with relevant bibliographies, the book is structured to be of use and interest to residents in urology, surgery, and internal medicine. The organization and indexing of *Medical and Surgical Management of Adrenal Diseases*, with chapters ranging from anatomy, pathology, imaging, and description of the individual disease entities to anesthesia and adrenal surgery, allows for the selective identification and retrieval of information as needed.

The editor and authors hope that *Medical and Surgical Management of Adrenal Diseases* will be a useful text and a welcome addition to the armamentarium of clinicians treating patients with adrenal disease.

Acknowledgments

The editor expresses his deep appreciation to each of the authors for their excellent contributions to this volume. We are fortunate indeed to have assembled a distinguished group of clinicians and educators of recognized ability and accomplishment in their respective areas of expertise in diseases of the adrenal glands. The editor and authors are grateful for the untiring efforts of our secretaries and editorial assistants. I thank Mr. Jay Knipstein, medical illustrator, whose skillful modifications of classic adrenal surgical drawings illuminate and clarify this book. My special thanks also to Mrs. Leah Hayes, Managing Editor at Lippincott Williams & Wilkins, for infinite patience, continual encouragement, and invaluable assistance in bringing this work to publication.

I am particularly indebted to the Department of Urology and Henry Ford Hospital for the support and resources integral to the completion of this endeavor. Finally, the editor and authors are especially grateful for the understanding and forbearance of our often neglected families. As my wife Patti knows too well, in the schedule of a busy clinician, even a labor of love such as this adrenal text is undertaken only at the expense of countless weekend and evening hours. I am deeply appreciative of her unwavering support and devotion.

Medical and Surgical Management
of Adrenal Diseases

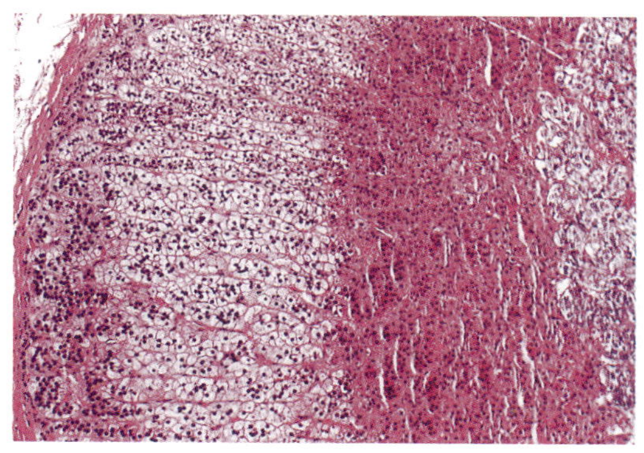

COLOR PLATE 1. Histologic section of a normal adrenal gland demonstrating the zona glomerulosa, zona fasciculata, and medulla.

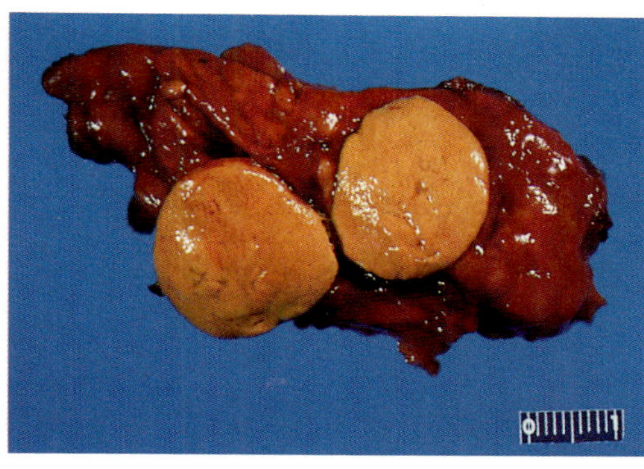

COLOR PLATE 2. An aldosterone-producing cortical adenoma (aldosteronoma) with its typical bright yellow color.

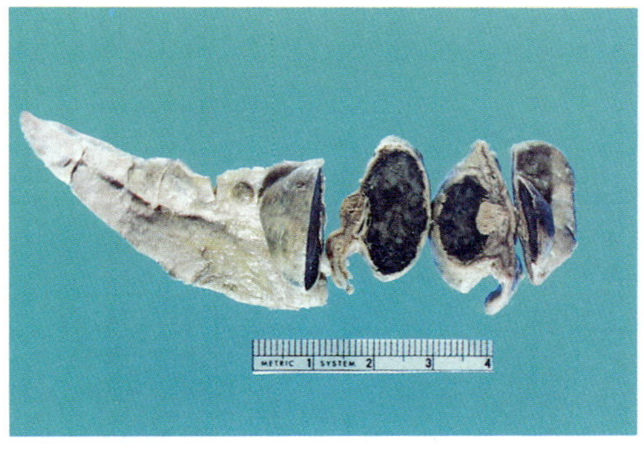

COLOR PLATE 3. A non-functional pigmented cortical adenoma.

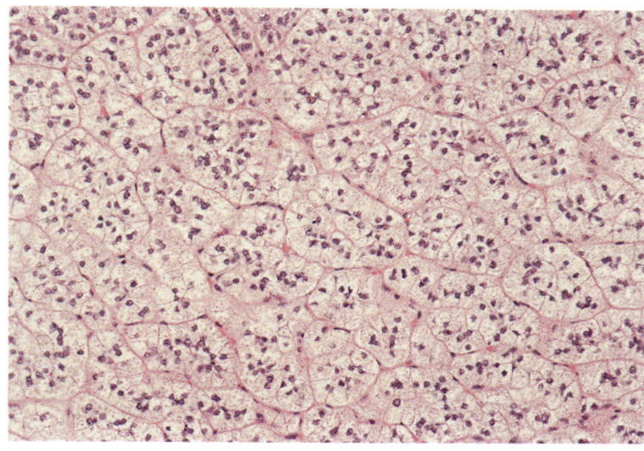

COLOR PLATE 4A. Histologic sections of cortical adenomas. Cortical adenoma (aldosteronoma) cells with clear cytoplasm.

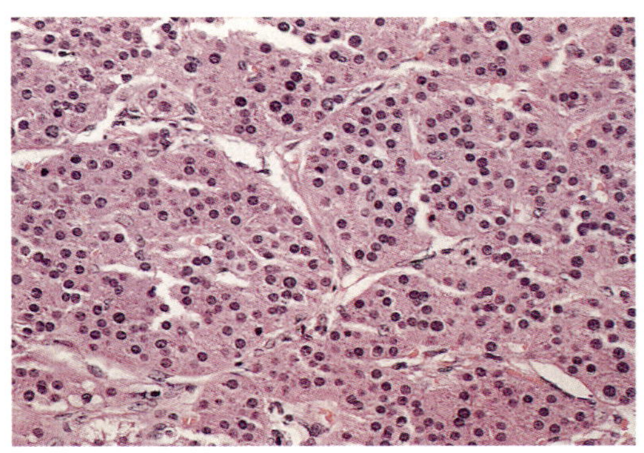

COLOR PLATE 4B. Histologic sections of cortical adenomas. Cortical adenoma cells with eosinophilic cytoplasm.

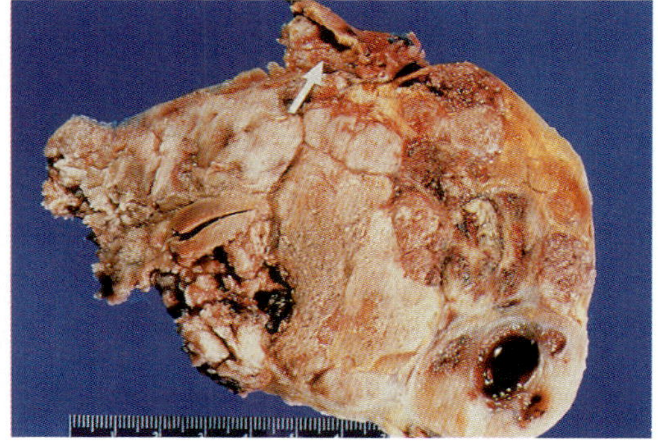

COLOR PLATE 5. A large adrenal cortical carcinoma has a nodular variegated appearance, with areas of hemorrhage and necrosis.

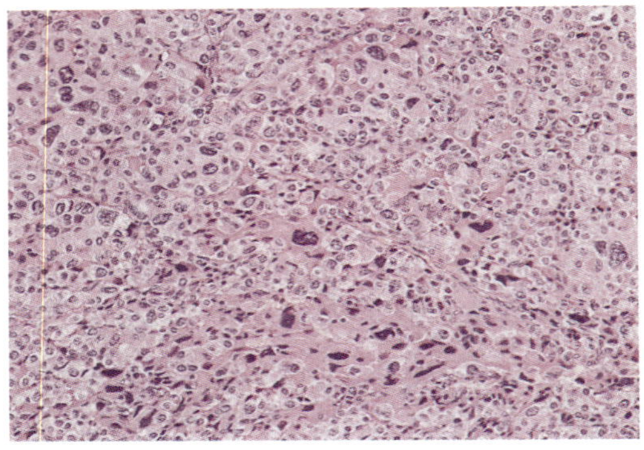

COLOR PLATE 6A,B,C. Three different adrenal cortical carcinomas demonstrating various degrees of cellular pleomorphism and nuclear atypia.

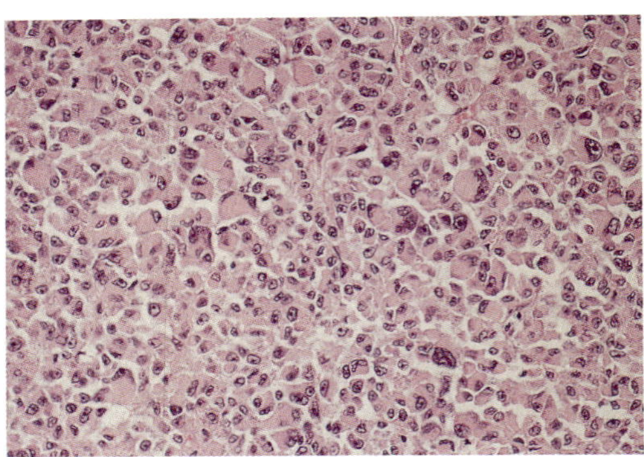

COLOR PLATE 6B.

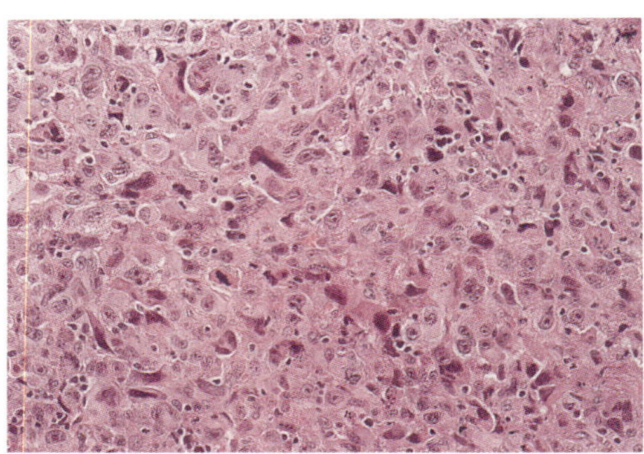

COLOR PLATE 6C.

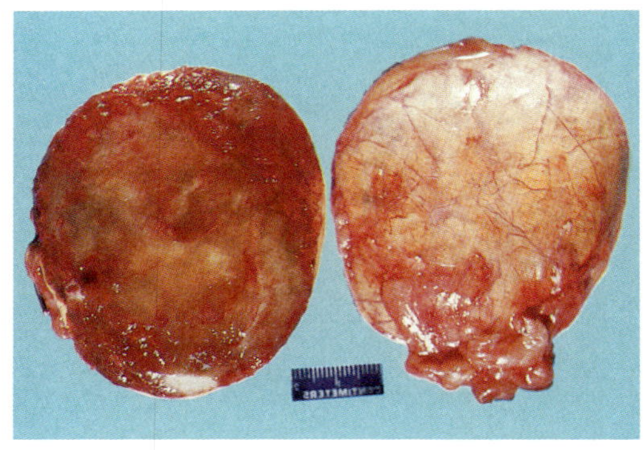

COLOR PLATE 7A. Adrenal myelolipoma. A circumscribed tumor with a yellow and red color.

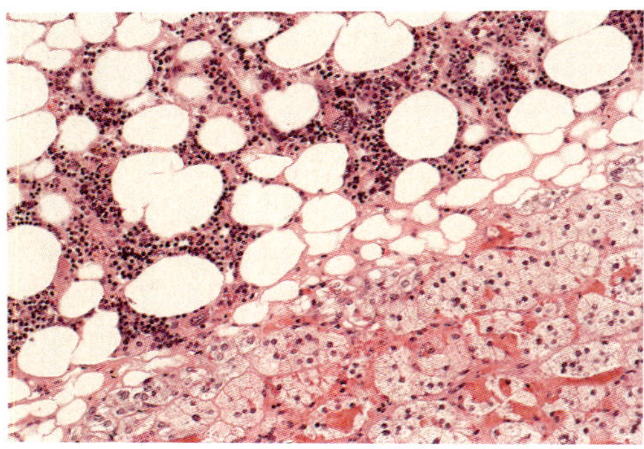

COLOR PLATE 7B. Adrenal myelolipoma. Hematopoietic and adipose tissue adjacent to the adrenal cortex.

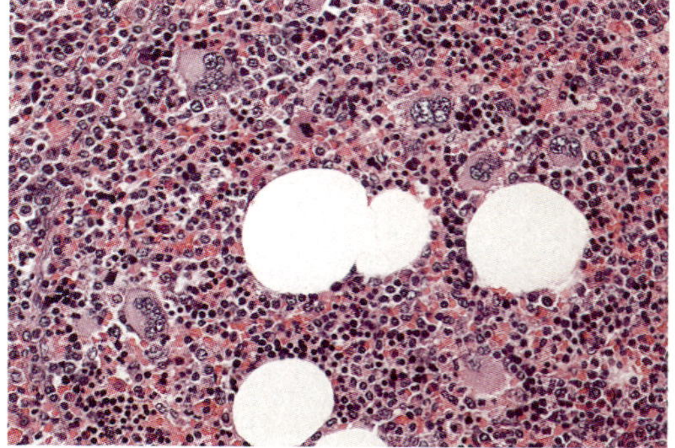

COLOR PLATE 7C. Adrenal myelolipoma. High-power view of hematopoietic elements with characteristic megakaryocytes.

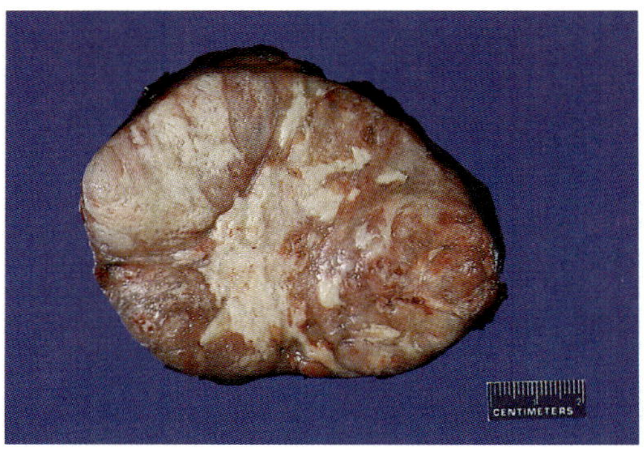

COLOR PLATE 8A. Metastatic renal cell carcinoma to the adrenal gland. The adrenal gland has been replaced by a large tan tumor with areas of necrosis.

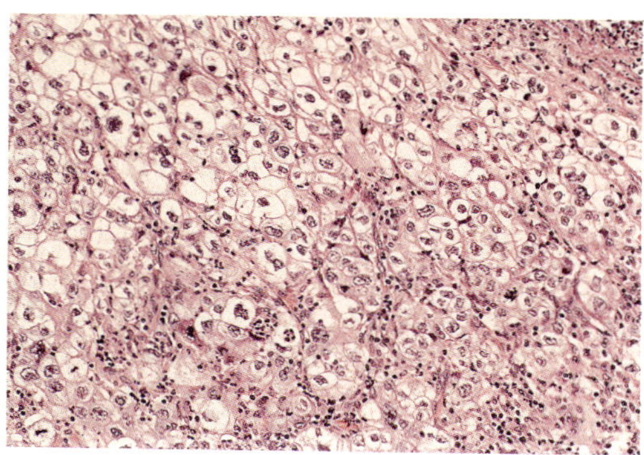

COLOR PLATE 8B. Metastatic renal cell carcinoma to the adrenal gland. Large malignant cells have abundant clear cytoplasm.

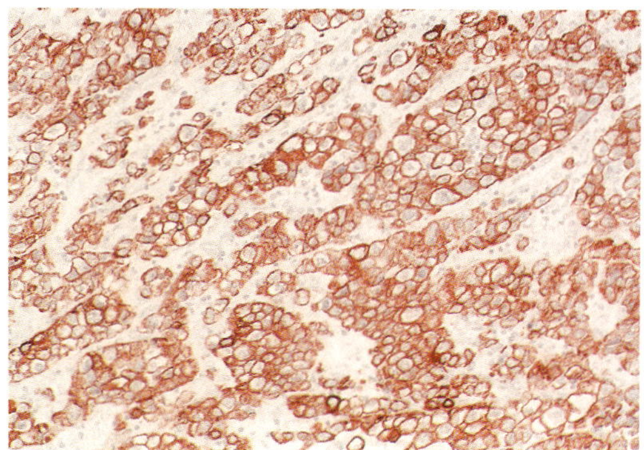

COLOR PLATE 8C. Metastatic renal cell carcinoma to the adrenal gland. Strong, diffuse immunoreactivity to cytokeratin supports the histologic impression of metastatic renal cell carcinoma.

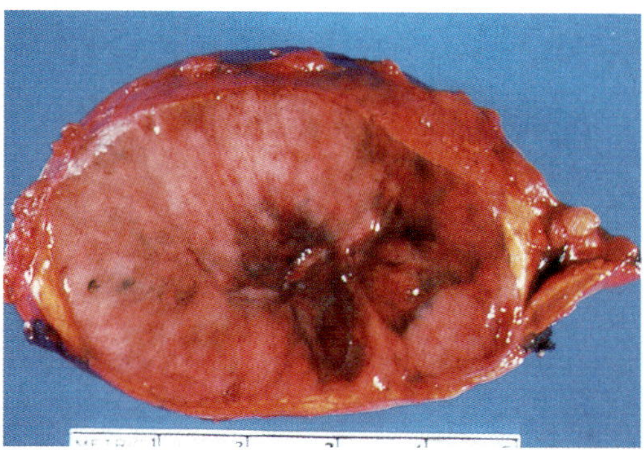

COLOR PLATE 9A. Two different adrenal pheochromocytomas. A small portion of adrenal cortex is present at the periphery of the tumor.

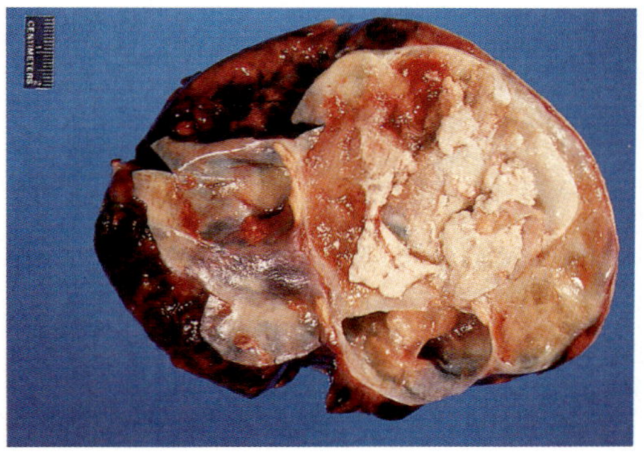

COLOR PLATE 9B. Extensive cystic change is present in this pheochromocytoma.

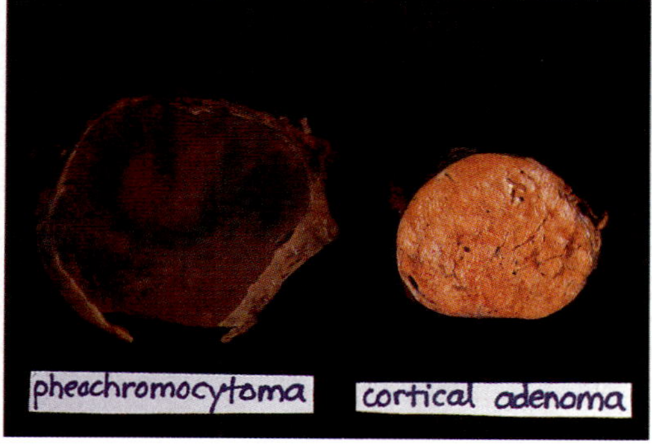

COLOR PLATE 10. A comparison of pheochromocytoma and adrenal cortical adenoma. The chromaffin reaction demonstrates dark brown staining of the pheochromocytoma.

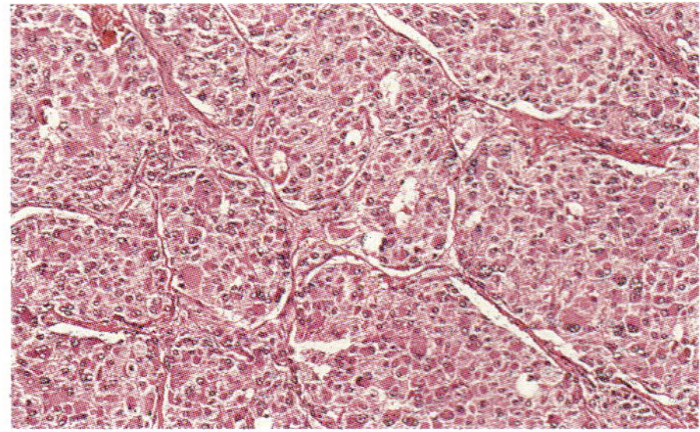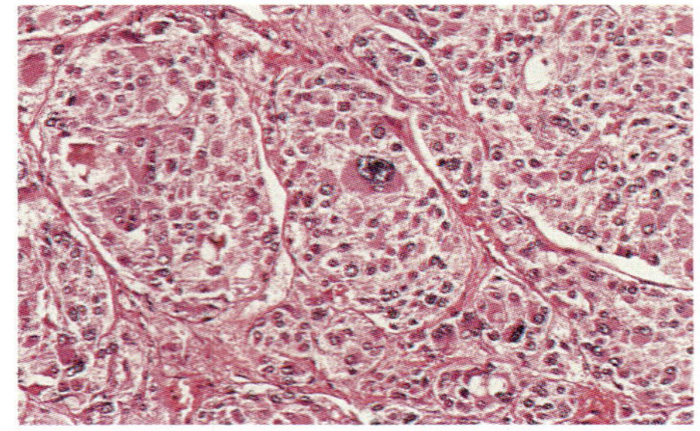

COLOR PLATE 11A. Histologic sections of pheochromocytomas demonstrate an alveolar (zellballen) pattern and cellular pleomorphism.

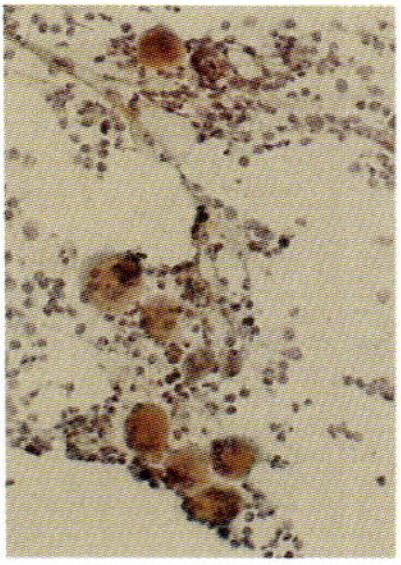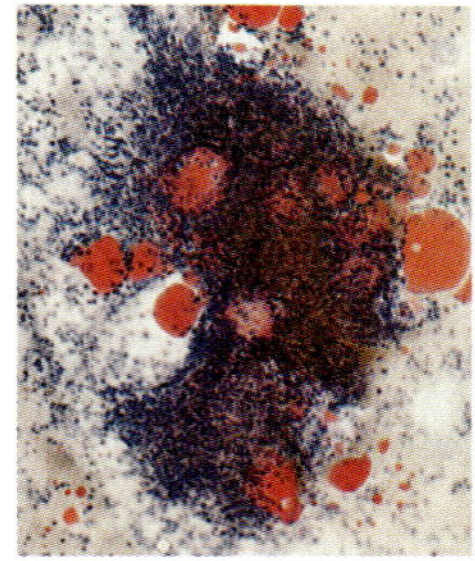

COLOR PLATE 12. Aspiration specimens of myelolipomas are characterized by a polymorphic cellular population including megakaryocytes (**left:** Papanicolaou stain) and lipid droplets (**right:** oil red O stain).

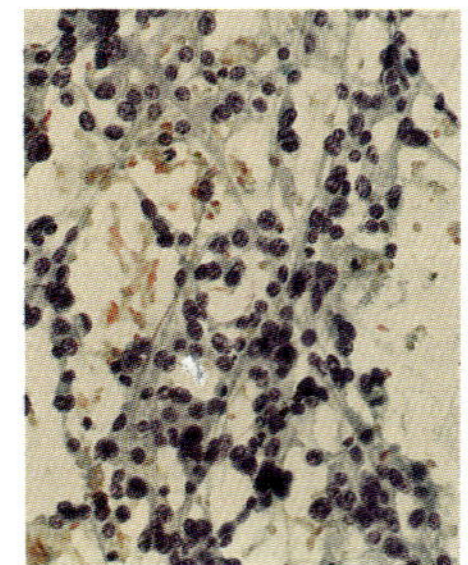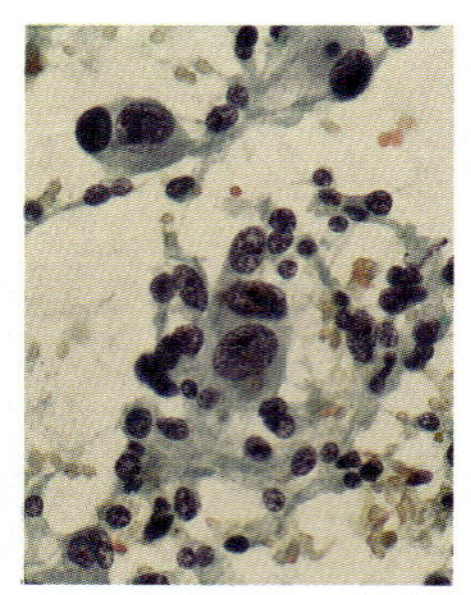

COLOR PLATE 14. This cytologic specimen of a pheochromocytoma demonstrates polygonal cells, spindled cells, and a few giant cells. The basophilic cytoplasm is coarsely granular (Papanicolaou stain).

COLOR PLATE 13. An adrenal aspirate from an 80-year-old woman with Cushing's syndrome and an 8-cm left adrenal mass. The cellular specimen contains loosely cohesive, large pleomorphic cells with macronucleoli. Histologically and clinically, the tumor is an adrenal cortical carcinoma (Papanicolaou stain).

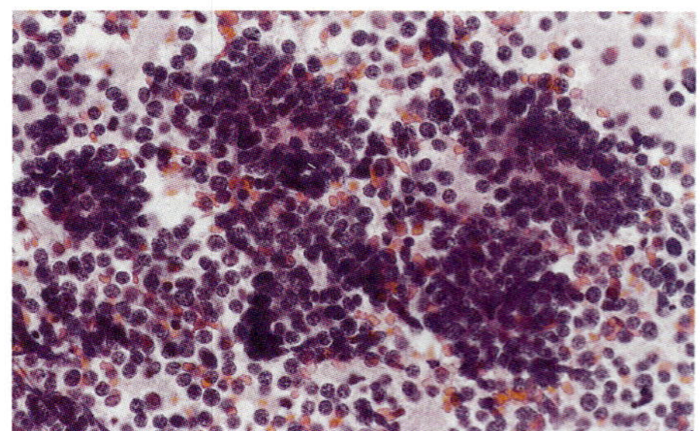

COLOR PLATE 15. Cytologic features of neuroblastoma include neoplastic cells with scant cytoplasm, high nuclear:cytoplasmic ratios, coarsely granular chromatin, and inconspicuous nucleoli. Rosette formations are quite characteristic (Papanicolaou stain).

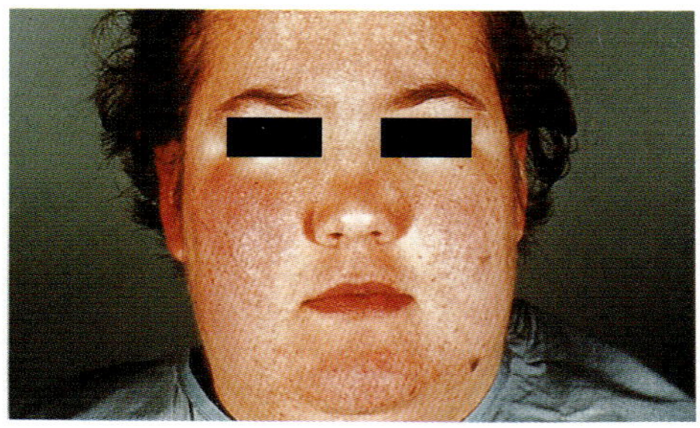

COLOR PLATE 16. Typical appearance of a patient with florid Cushing's syndrome.

*Medical and Surgical Management of
Adrenal Diseases,* edited by Joseph C. Cerny.
Lippincott Williams & Wilkins, Philadelphia © 1999.

1

Surgical Anatomy, Embryology, and Histology of Adrenal Glands

Sugandh D. Shetty and James O. Peabody

Department of Urology, Henry Ford Hospital, Detroit, Michigan 48202

SURGICAL ANATOMY

Adrenal glands are paired retroperitoneal structures situated in close proximity to the superior pole of the kidneys anterior to the crura of the diaphragm at the level of the eleventh thoracic vertebra. Each gland consists of a cortex and a medulla, which are structurally, functionally, and embryologically distinct from each other. These glands are bright golden yellow in color and can be easily distinguished from the surrounding adipose tissue by their tightly packed architecture. The right adrenal is an irregular tetrahedron, and the left adrenal is semilunar, slightly larger, and at a more superior level. Each gland weighs about 5 g and the medulla is about one-tenth of the total weight. The dimensions of the adult gland are approximately $50 \times 30 \times 10$ mm.

Anatomic Relations

The right adrenal is related to the upper pole of the right kidney, separated by a thin extension of perinephric fascia (Gerota's fascia). The adrenal is surrounded by adipose tissue and is enveloped by Gerota's fascia, to which it is anchored by fine strands, making it immobile during respiration. The anterior surface of the right adrenal is divided into a medial part, which lies behind the infrahepatic inferior vena cava (IVC), and the lateral part, which lies behind the liver and is in contact with its bare area (Fig. 1-1). A small portion of the anterior surface below the liver is covered by the peritoneal reflection from the inferior layer of the coronary ligament, which needs to be divided during hepatic mobilization to approach the right adrenal (1). Posteriorly, it is related to the right crus of the diaphragm and to the superior pole and adjacent anterior surface of the right kidney. The diaphragm separates the gland from the posterior pleural reflection and the lung (Fig. 1-2). The medial border is related to the right celiac ganglion and the right inferior phrenic artery coursing superolaterally on the right crus of the diaphragm.

The left adrenal gland is crescentic and occupies the anteromedial surface of the upper pole of the left kidney. The gland has a convex medial border, a concave lateral border, and a sharp upper border, and the inferior border is rounded. The anterior surface of the left adrenal has a superior portion that is covered by the peritoneum of the lesser sac, and the inferior portion is related to the posterior surface of the pancreas and the splenic artery (see Fig. 1-1). Because of its posterior location to the lesser sac, this adrenal can be approached via the lesser sac in bilateral adrenalectomy through a transperitoneal route. The hilum of the left adrenal faces ventrocaudally

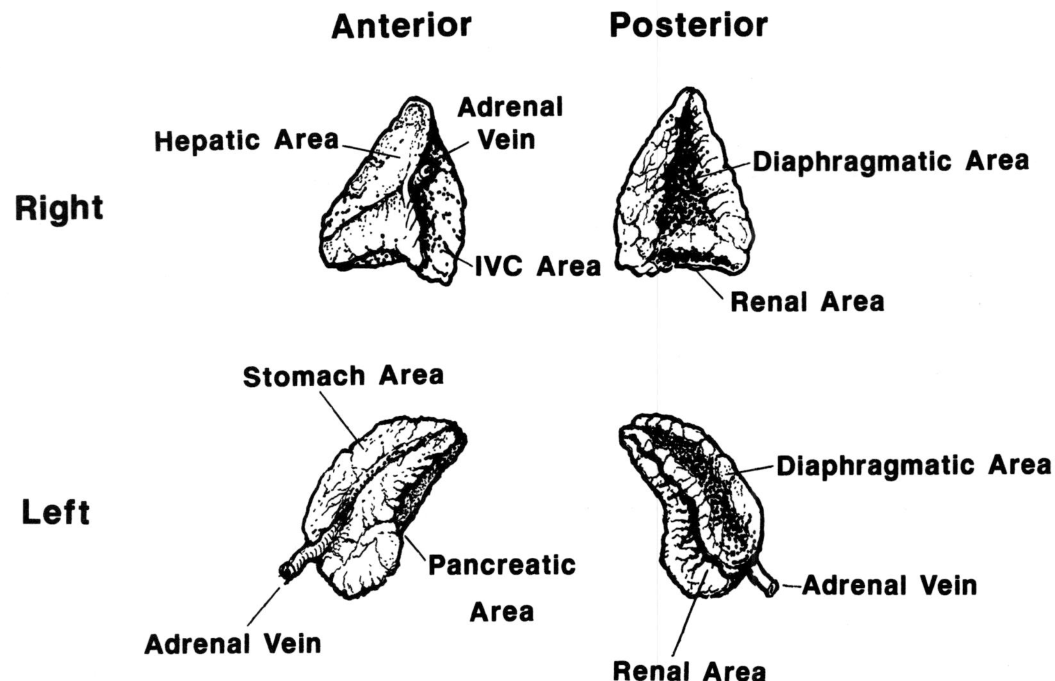

FIG. 1-1. Anterior and posterior relations of the adrenal gland. (Modified from ref. 3.)

on the lower anterior surface, and the left adrenal vein emerges to join the left renal vein. The posterior surface is related to the left crus of the diaphragm medially (which separates it from the pleural recess and the lung) and the superior pole of the kidney laterally. The medial border is related to the left celiac ganglion, and to the left inferior phrenic and left gastric arteries ascending on the left crus.

Cross-Sectional Anatomy

Because computed tomography (CT) has become the mainstay of adrenal imaging, it is essential to be familiar with the cross-sectional anatomy of the retroperitoneum. The adrenal gland on a CT cross-sectional image appears as a thin, folded structure with an anteromedial ridge and two posterolateral limbs (2). These wing-shaped limbs are close to-gether on the superior aspect of the gland and are far apart as the gland straddles the antero-medial aspect of the upper pole of the kidney. The angles between the limbs may exceed 120 degrees at the base. The more cephalad sec-tion shows the adrenal to have a linear ap-pearance with a directly anteroposterior ori-entation. Sections at the midportion of the gland usually produce an inverted Y-shaped structure (Fig. 1-3). The more inferior sec-tions show the inverted Y to have wider an-gles. The medial wing is shorter than the lat-eral wing. In some cases, the anteromedial ridge is not developed or is small, resulting in a cross-sectional image of an inverted V-shaped gland.

Arterial Supply

Each adrenal gland is supplied by a supe-rior adrenal artery from the inferior phrenic

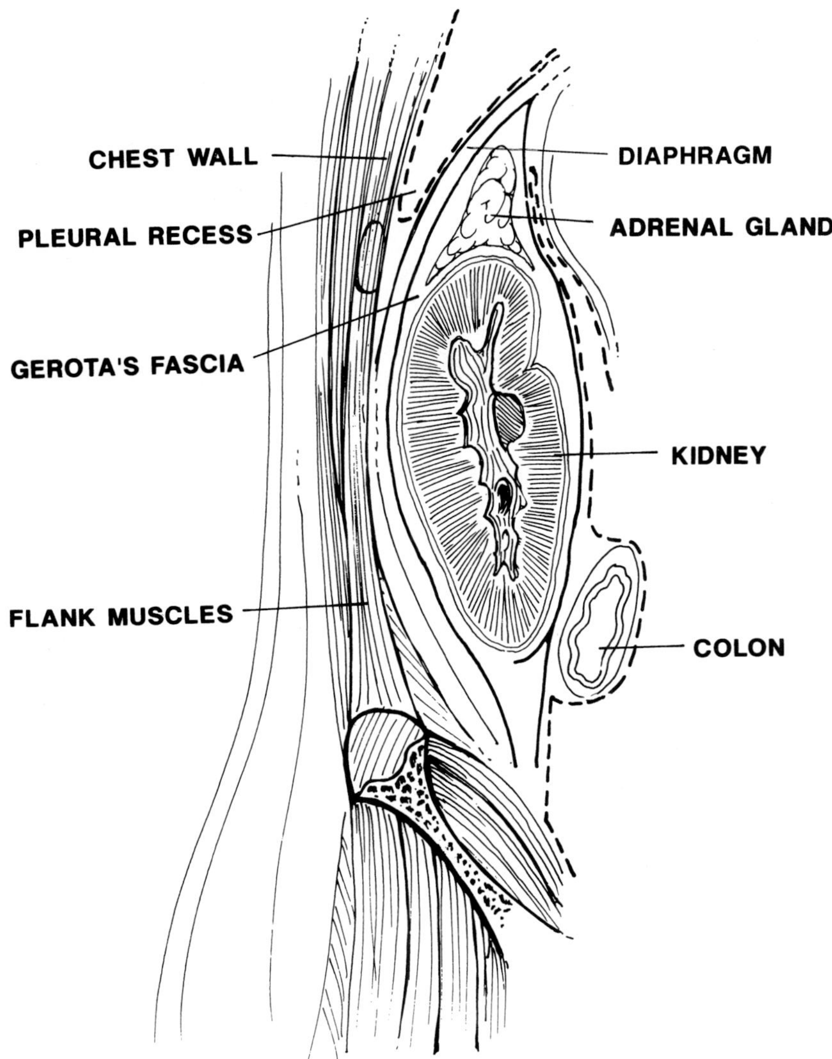

FIG. 1-2. Sagittal section through the right adrenal gland and kidney. (Modified from ref. 3.)

artery, a middle adrenal artery from the abdominal aorta, and an inferior adrenal artery from the renal artery (Fig. 1-4A) (3). The inferior phrenic artery is the major source of the arterial supply to the adrenal (4,5). The arterial branches form a plexus around the capsule, from which several penetrating vessels enter the zona glomerulosa, and between the columns in the zona fasciculata to a deeper plexus within the zona reticularis. The medulla also receives blood from arterial branches, which bypass the cortex.

Venous Drainage

The right adrenal vein emerges from the anterior surface and enters the IVC via a short trunk. It is vulnerable to injury during dissection of the IVC from the upper pole of the right kidney and the adrenal gland. This short,

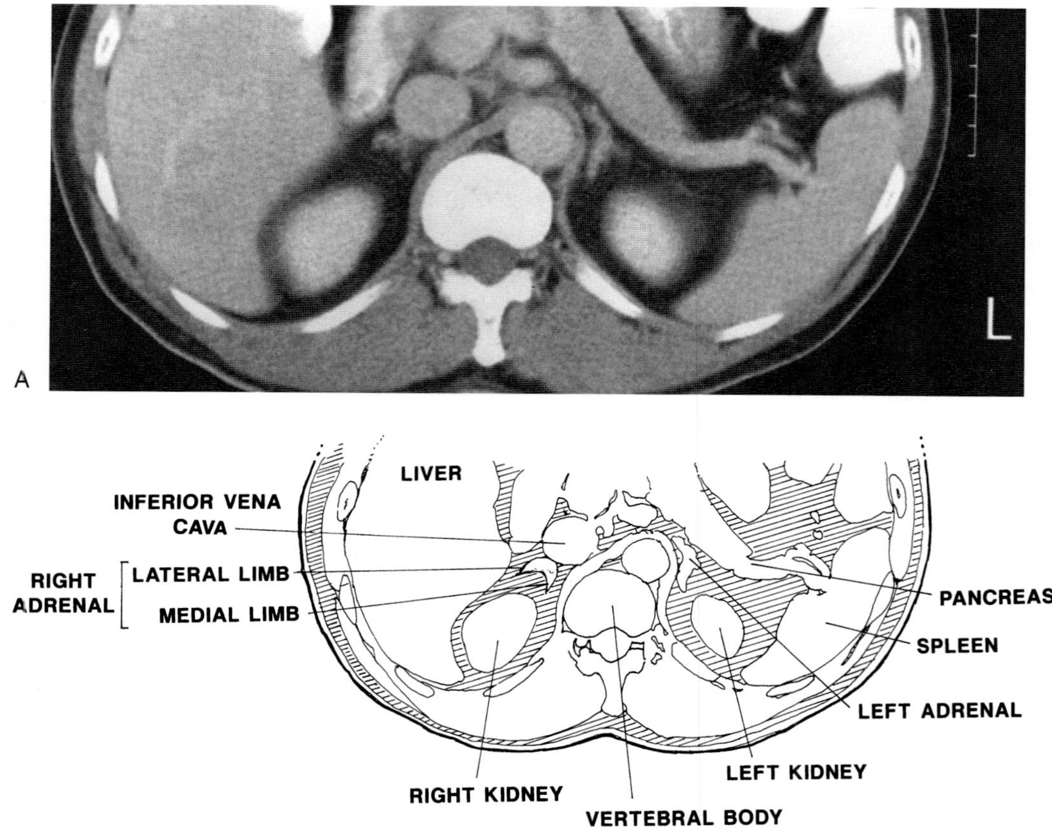

FIG. 1-3. A: Computed tomography section of a normal adrenal gland. **B:** Schematic representation of structures seen in **(A)**.

distinct vessel should be carefully ligated and divided. The left adrenal vein is larger and easily identifiable as it joins the left renal vein along its superior border (see Fig. 1-4B). The vein emerges from the anterior surface of the adrenal gland. The left adrenal vein also communicates with the inferior phrenic vein, which should be carefully ligated and divided during adrenalectomy.

Lymphatic Drainage

The lymphatics from both the adrenals drain into the paraaortic nodes.

Nerve Supply

The adrenal gland has a rich nerve supply, predominately of sympathetic origin, and innervates the medulla. There is no evidence of innervation of the cortex, which is under the control of adrenocorticotropic hormone and renin. The preganglionic sympathetic fibers originate at T10 to L1, pass through the sympathetic ganglia, and emerge as the splanchnic nerves. These synapse with the adrenal medullary chromaffin cells. The adrenal medulla functions as a sympathetic ganglion. The blood vessels of the adrenal also receive postganglionic innervation.

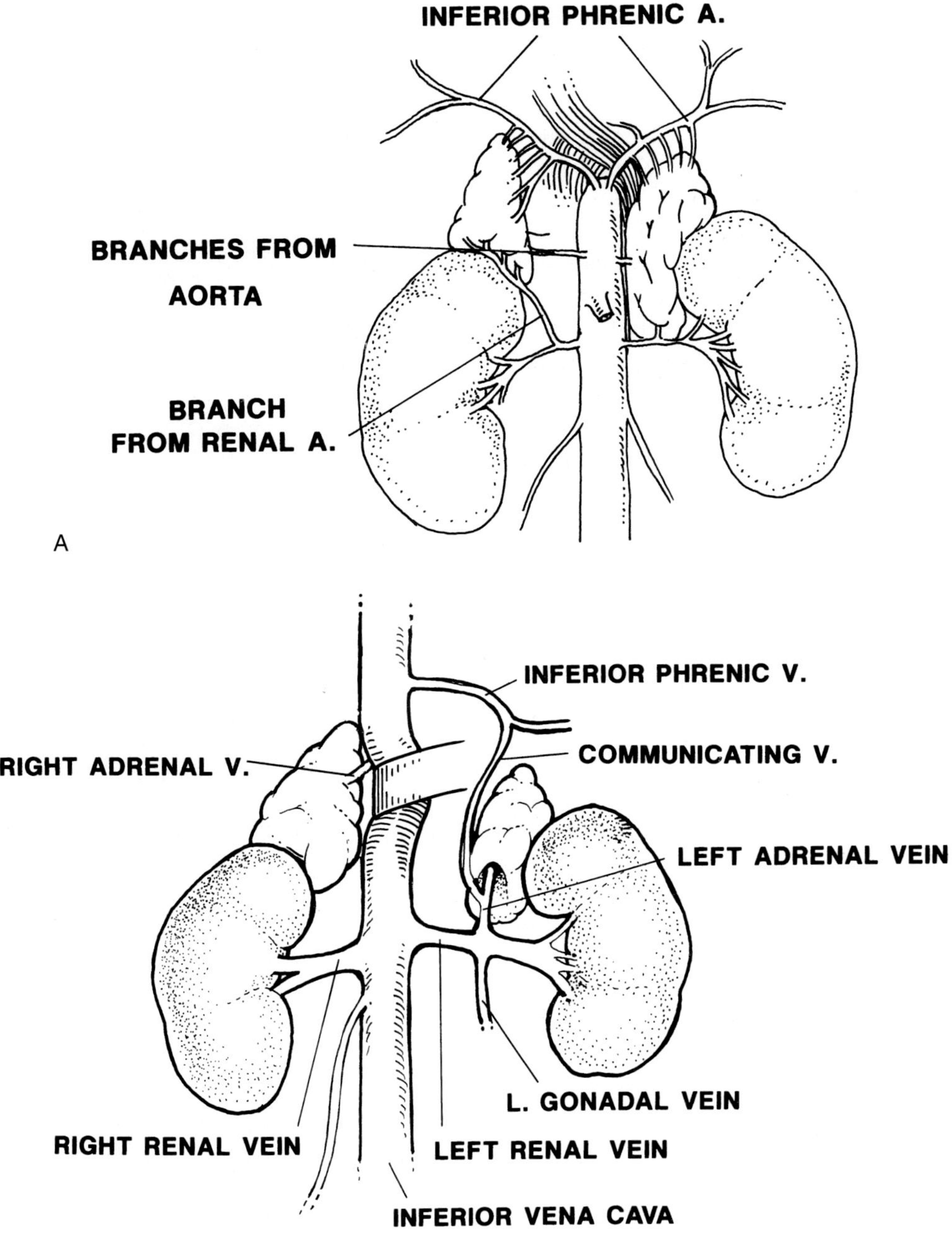

FIG. 1-4. A: Arterial branches to the adrenal gland. **B:** Venous drainage of the adrenal gland.

EMBRYOLOGY

Adrenal Cortex

The adrenal cortex evolves in two stages. The primitive cortex is derived from the celomic mesothelium at the cranial end of the mesonephric blastema, between the mesenteric root and the gonadal primordium, when the embryo is at the 6-mm stage. This fetal adrenocortical primordium proliferates rapidly; by the 10-mm stage, it separates from the celomic mesothelium and penetrates the mesenchyme of the retroperitoneum. A second wave of celomic epithelial cell proliferation begins and invades the mesenchyme at the 16-mm stage. By the 20-mm stage, it completely envelopes the fetal cortex and eventually forms the definitive adult cortex. An additional cell type arises from the mesonephron close to Bowman's capsule (6,7). The adrenal at this stage of the fourth fetal month attains maximum size and is larger than the developing kidney. The fetal cortex begins involuting slowly after the fourth fetal month, and shortly after birth there is a dramatic reduction in the adrenal mass as a result of rapid degeneration of the fetal cortex (8). The outer zone of the definitive cortex constitutes one-fourth of the adrenal gland. The cells of the fetal cortex are engulfed by those of the definitive cortex, and they remain grossly and histologically distinct from it. The adrenal cortex at birth, therefore, contains the involuting fetal cortex and the overlying definitive cortex; the latter, by this time, has differentiated in the zona glomerulosa and zona fasciculata. The adult reticular zone is absent at birth and is not recognizable until about the end of the third year of life (9). Because fetal adrenals are relatively large, they can be mistaken for kidneys on imaging in cases of unilateral renal agenesis. They may be traumatized during childbirth, causing severe adrenal hemorrhage. Spontaneous adrenal hemorrhage can also occur during rapid involution of the fetal cortex.

Adrenal Medulla

Cells from the neural crest migrate to the medial aspect of the fetal adrenal cortex by the tenth week of intrauterine life. By the eighteenth week, these cells are completely enveloped by the adrenal gland. The medulla remains relatively small compared to the chromaffin tissue in the paravertebral region. After birth, most of the extraadrenal chromaffin tissue involutes except for that found near the celiac axis, near the superior mesentric artery, and around the inferior mesenteric artery and aortic bifurcation (organ of Zuckerkandl) (Fig. 1-5). Because the kidneys essentially develop in the pelvic area and then ascend to their normal position, abnormalities of renal development such as agenesis or ectopia are not associated with adrenal malposition.

Aberrant Adrenal Tissue

The location of aberrant adrenal cortical tissue is variable but generally follows the path of migration of structures derived from the urogenital ridge. Heterotopical adrenal tissue is fairly constant in its relation to the kidney (10). Accessory adrenal tissue is most often present in broad ligament, spermatic, or ovarian vessels, spermatic cord, testis, ovary, and uterus (11,12). The aberrant adrenal tissue may undergo hyperplasia after adrenalectomy or may undergo neoplastic transformation.

Paraganglia

Paraganglia are extraadrenal aggregations of chromaffin tissue distributed near or in the autonomic nervous system. These contain small, intensely fluorescent cells, which are neuroectodermal in origin and synthesize and store catecholamines. The dispersed array of extraadrenal chromaffin tissue is the main source of fetal catecholamine while the adrenal medulla is still developing. Many

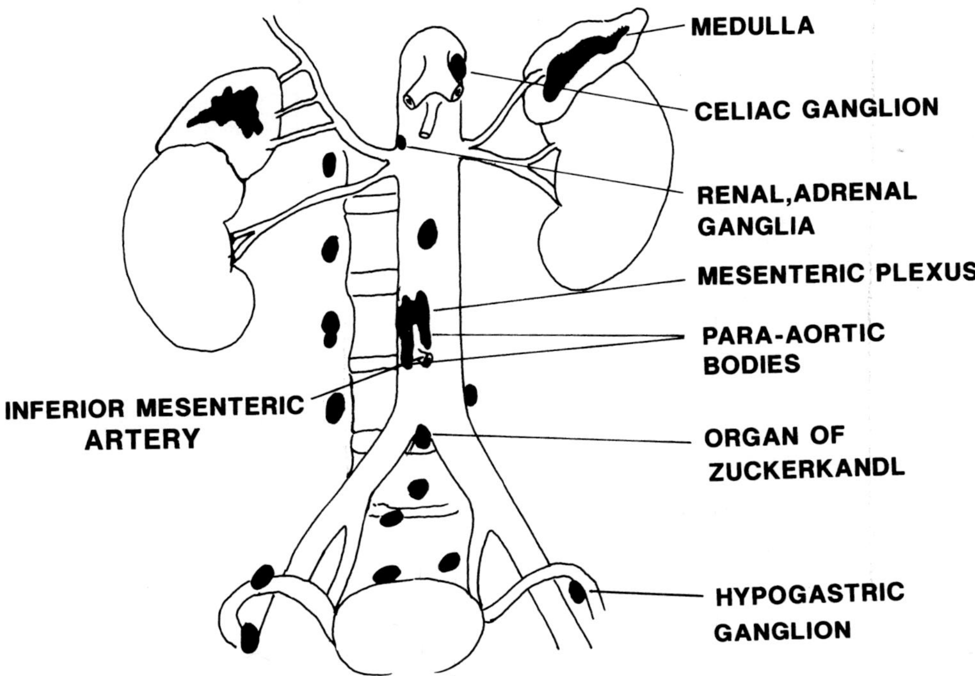

FIG. 1-5. Aberrant adrenal tissue and the paraganglion system. (Redrawn from Hinman F. *Atlas of Urosurgical Anatomy*. Philadelphia: WB Saunders, 1993.)

paraganglia degenerate after birth, but several remain in the mediastinum and retroperitoneum (see Fig. 1-5). Neuroblastoma, pheochromocytoma, schwannoma, and ganglioneuroma can all arise from these paraganglia.

HISTOLOGY

A cross section of the adrenal gland reveals the outer yellow cortex forming the main mass of the gland and a thin medulla, one-tenth the size of the cortex, which is dark red or pearl gray, depending on its blood content. The medulla is completely surrounded by the cortex except at its hilum. The gland has a thick, collagenous capsule, which sends deep trabeculae into the cortex along with its rich arterial plexus.

The adrenal cortex has three distinct zones: glomerulosa, fasciculata, and reticu-laris (Fig. 1-6A). The outer zone, the zona glomerulosa, consists of large polyhedral cells in rounded groups or curved columns with deeply staining nuclei, scanty basophilic cytoplasm, and a few lipid droplets. Ultrastructurally, the cytoplasm displays many microtubules, long mitochondria, and abundant smooth endoplasmic reticulum. Deep to this zone is the zona fasciculata, which consists of large polyhedral basophilic cells arranged in straight columns, two cells wide, with parallel fenestrated venous sinusoids between them. The cells are rich in lipid droplets, phospholipids, fats, fatty acids, and cholesterol embedded in complex smooth endoplasmic reticulum. The mitochondria are spherical, with tubular cristae, and the Golgi complex is extensive. The innermost part of the cortex, the zona reticularis, consists of branching, interconnected columns of round cells with abundant

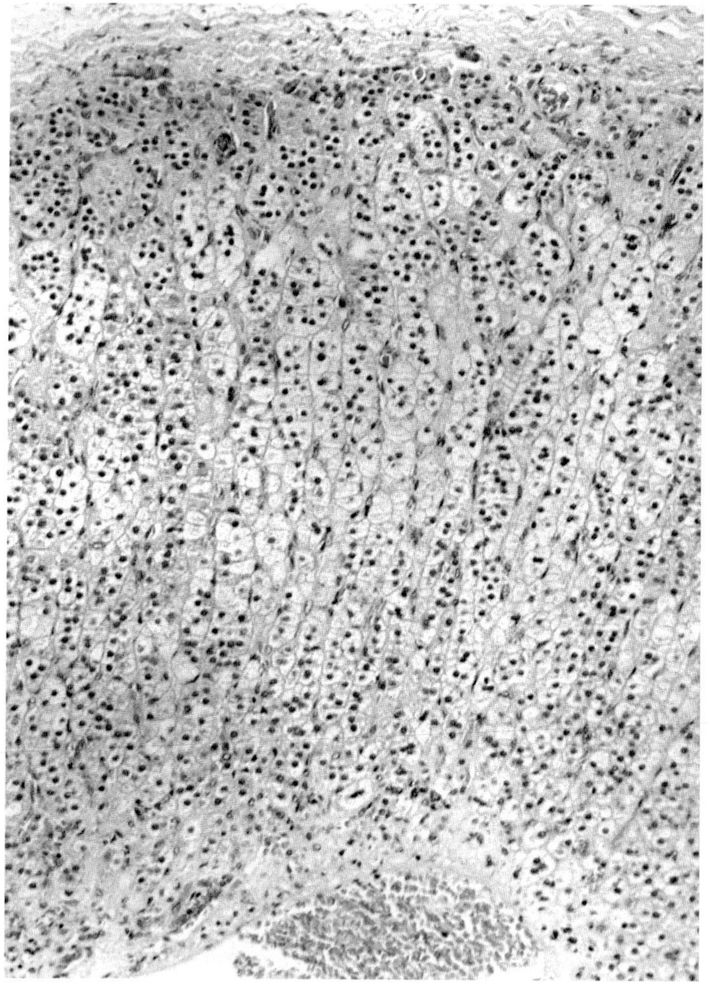

FIG. 1-6. A: Adrenal cortical histology showing the zonae glomerulosa, fasciculata, and reticularis from above downward; low-power view (H & E stain). **B:** Adrenal medulla with chromaffin cells; high-power view (H & E stain).

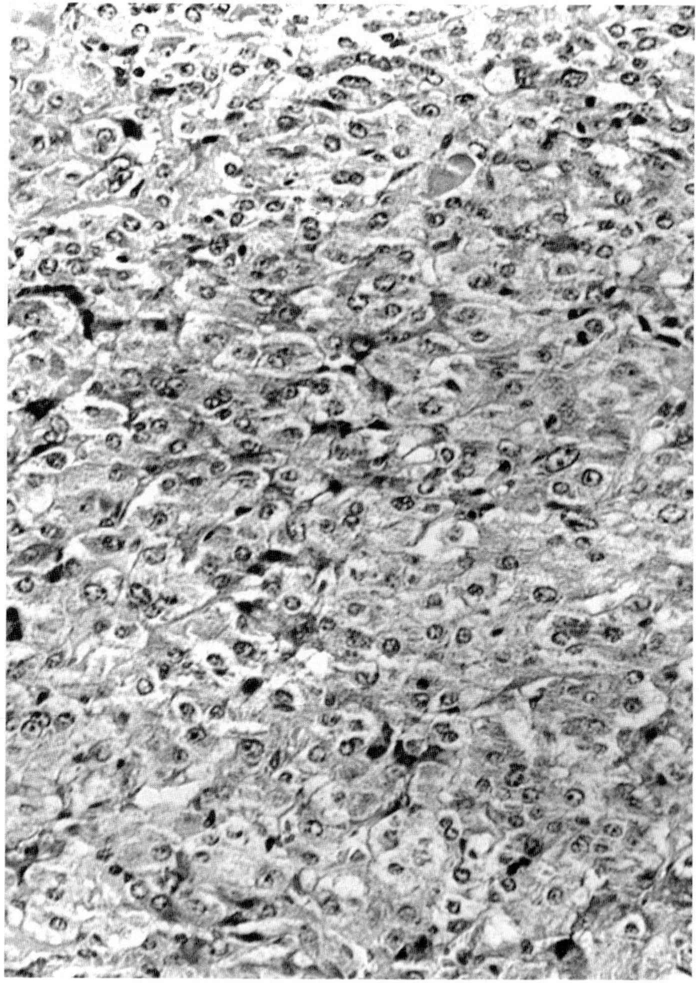

smooth endoplasmic reticulum containing lysosomes and pigment bodies. The cells of the adrenal cortex produce several hormones. The zona glomerulosa produces aldosterone, the zona fasciculata produces cortisol, and the zona reticularis produces sex hormones.

The adrenal medulla consists of columns of chromaffin cells (pheochromocytes) separated by venous sinusoids. Several neurons can be seen in the medulla (Fig. 1-6B). Chromaffin cells synthesize and store noradrenaline and adrenaline, the release of which is under sympathetic nervous system control. The cells are large and columnar, forming single rows along the venous sinusoids. The cell bases and nuclei synapse with the nerve endings. The cytoplasm is basophilic, with abundant rough endoplasmic reticulum, mitochondria, Golgi complexes, and many storage vesicles. The noradrenaline vesicles are typically rounded or ellipsoid, whereas the adrenaline vesicles are more pale, often with a clear zone between the granular contents and the membrane. In humans, adrenal chromaffin cells with both types of vesicles have been seen, suggesting the presence of adrenaline and noradrenaline in the same cell (13). The vesicle contents are released at the cell apices into the perivascular spaces and enter the circulation through the fenestrated endothelium of the sinusoids.

REFERENCES

1. Prinz R. Mobilization of the right lobe of liver for right adrenalectomy. *Am J Surg* 1990;159:336–338.
2. Mitty H. Adrenal embryology, anatomy, and imaging techniques. In: Pollock HM, ed. *Clinical urography.* Philadelphia: WB Saunders, 1990:2291–2295.
3. Williams PL, et al. Suprarenal glands. In: Williams PL, Warwick R, Dyson M, et al, eds. *Gray's anatomy.* Edinburgh: Churchill Livingstone, 1989:1468–1472.
4. Pick J, Anson BJ. The inferior phrenic artery: origin and suprarenal branches. *Anat Rec* 1940;78:413–427.
5. Dobbie J, Symington T. The human adrenal gland with special reference to the vasculature. *J Endocrinol* 1966;34:479–489.
6. Crowder R. The development of adrenal gland in man. *Carnegie Contrib Embryol* 1957;36:193–207.
7. Glen F, Peterson R, Mannix H. Embryology, anatomy, and histology of the adrenal gland. In: *Surgery of adrenal gland.* New York: MacMillan, 1968.
8. Benner M. Studies on the involution of fetal cortex of the adrenal gland. *Am J Pathol* 1940;16:787–798.
9. Sucheston ME, Cannon M. Development of zonular patterns in the human adrenal gland. *J Morphol* 1968;126:477–492.
10. Schechter D. Aberrant adrenal tissue. *Ann Surg* 1968;167:421–426.
11. Falls J. Accessory adrenal cortex in the broad ligament. *Cancer* 1955;8:143–148.
12. Culp O. Adrenal heteropia: a survey of the literature and report of a case. *J Urol* 1959;41:303–311.
13. Brown W, Barajas L, Latta H. The ultrastructure of the human adrenal medulla: with comparative studies of the white rat. *Anat Rec* 1970;169:173–183.

Medical and Surgical Management of
Adrenal Diseases, edited by Joseph C. Cerny.
Lippincott Williams & Wilkins, Philadelphia © 1999.

2

Pathology of the Adrenal Glands

Terri L. Johnson and *Mahul B. Amin

Department of Pathology, St. Joseph Mercy Hospital, Ann Arbor, Michigan 48106;
**Department of Pathology, Emory University Hospital, Atlanta, Georgia 30322*

ANATOMY AND PHYSIOLOGY

The adrenal glands are paired endocrine organs located superomedial to the kidneys within Gerota's fascia. The pyramid-shaped right adrenal lies medial to the right lobe of the liver, and the crescent-shaped left adrenal is posterior to the pancreas. A normal adult adrenal gland weights 4 to 5 g, with the cortex accounting for 80% to 90% of the total weight (1). The cortex and medulla are distinct functional units with separate embryologic origins. The steroid-producing cortex is derived from mesoderm and the catecholamine-producing medulla develops from the neural crest (2).

Histologically, the cortex is divided into the zona glomerulosa, zona fasciculata, and zona reticularis (Fig. 2-1; see color plate 1). The zona glomerulosa is a thin layer of small cells located just beneath the capsule and is the site of mineralocorticoid production. The middle layer, the zona fasciculata, is composed of columns of lipid-rich cells and accounts for about 75% of the cortical volume. Together with the inner zona reticularis layer, the zona fasciculata produces glucocorticoids and sex steroid hormones. Mineralocorticoid production is controlled by the renin-angiotensin system, and glucocorticoid production is regulated by pituitary release of adrenocorticotropic hormone (ACTH).

The medulla, composed of chromaffin cells and occasional ganglion cells, is the major source of the circulating catecholamines—epi-

nephrine, norepinephrine, and dopamine. Membrane-bound secretory granules are the characteristic ultrastructural feature of medullary cells. The adrenal medulla is one component of the autonomic paraganglion system, which also includes extraadrenal paraganglia distributed throughout the body, especially in the head and neck and the periaortic region.

HETEROTOPIC ADRENAL NODULES

Heterotopic adrenal nodules result from incomplete embryologic migration of cortical tissue. Nodules of the ectopic adrenal cortex most frequently occur in the retroperitoneum but may also occur within or near the gonads, celiac plexus, kidney, or liver (2). Hernia sacs and hydroceles occasionally contain ectopic nodules

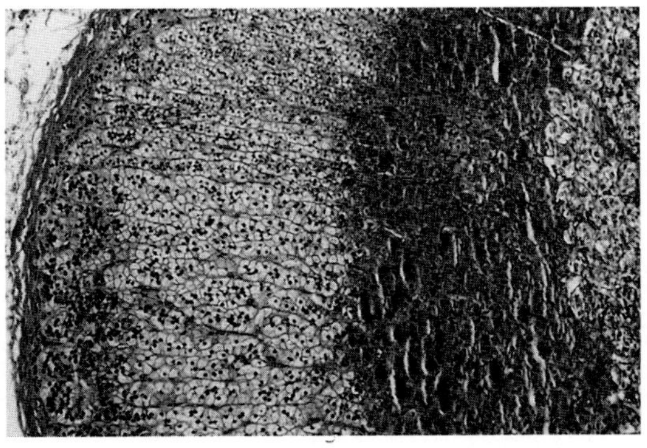

FIG. 2-1. Histologic section of a normal adrenal gland demonstrating the zona glomerulosa, zona fasciculata, and medulla.

TABLE 2–1. *Hyperfunctioning adrenal cortical lesions*

	Hyperplasia	Adenoma	Carcinoma
Cushing's syndrome (↑ cortisol)	70%–80% (adults)[a] 30%–40% (children)	10%–20% 50% (children)	10% (adults)
Conn's syndrome (↑ aldosterone)	30%	70%	Rare
Adrenogenital syndrome (↑ sex steroids)	Majority are congenital adrenal hyperplasia		Cancer more often than adenoma in children

[a]Pituitary adenomas account for most cases of adrenal cortical hyperplasia in adults; 10%–15% of cases are attributed to ectopic adrenocorticotropic hormone.

of adrenal cortical tissue. The heterotopic nodules occur as circumscribed yellow tumors ranging from 0.1 to 2 cm in diameter. Histologically, the nodules resemble normal adrenal cortex, with clear cells arranged in cords and nests.

ADRENAL CORTICAL HYPERPLASIA

Adrenal hyperplasia manifests as bilateral cortical expansion that is frequently associated with elevated serum ACTH levels (1,2). Cortical hyperplasia may occur as a congenital or acquired condition and may have a nodular or diffuse appearance. Nodular hyperplasia is characterized by multiple nodules up to 3 cm in size, but the distinction between nodular and diffuse hyperplasia is vague and combined patterns occur frequently.

Congenital adrenal hyperplasia (CAH) is an autosomal recessive disorder resulting from inborn errors of cortical steroid metabolism (1,2). The enlarged adrenal glands often have a tan or brown cerebriform appearance. From 85% to 95% of cases are due to a 21-hydroxylase deficiency resulting in decreased production of cortisol and aldosterone and overproduction of testosterone. The patients are virilized and may have electrolyte disturbances. Deficiency of 11-β-hydroxylase is the second most frequent cause of CAH and results in virilization and hypertension.

Acquired cortical hyperplasia most frequently presents as Cushing's syndrome, with enlarged yellow adrenal glands weighing 6 to 12 g (see also Cushing's Syndrome) (Table 2-1). Pituitary overproduction of ACTH is the most common cause of acquired adrenal hyperplasia and is referred to as Cushing's disease.

Paraneoplastic ectopic ACTH production is the second most frequent cause of adrenal cortical hyperplasia (ACH) and is characterized by massively enlarged adrenal glands that weigh up to 20 g. Small cell carcinomas of the lung and carcinoid tumors account for more than 90% of the neoplasms associated with ectopic ACTH; islet cell tumors, pheochromocytomas, and medullary thyroid carcinomas are associated less frequently (1,3).

Primary pigmented nodular adrenal cortical hyperplasia (PNACH) is a morphologically distinct, ACTH-independent lesion (2). Multiple small dark brown to black nodules occur unilaterally or bilaterally, without significant enlargement of the adrenal glands. The circumscribed nodules contain cortical cells with darkly pigmented cytoplasm. PNACH may occur as a component of a complex syndrome characterized by spotty cutaneous pigmentation, cutaneous and cardiac myxomas, myxoid fibroadenomas of the

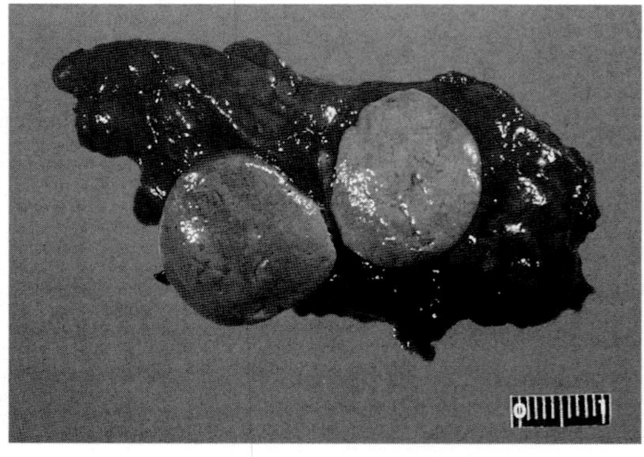

FIG. 2-2. An aldosterone-producing cortical adenoma (aldosteronoma).

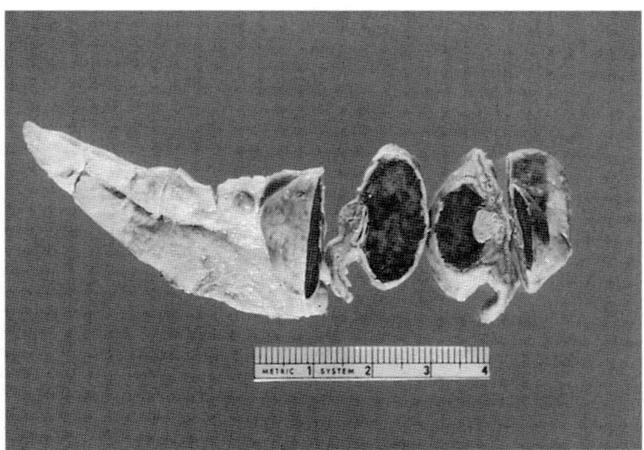

FIG. 2-3. A non-functional pigmented cortical adenoma.

breast, pituitary tumors, and Sertoli cell tumors of the testis (4).

ADRENAL CORTICAL ADENOMA

Adrenal cortical adenomas are benign neoplasms that may be associated with cortical steroid overproduction. Glucocorticoid-producing tumors (Cushing's syndrome) are the most frequent type of functional adenomas in adults, and aldosteronomas (Conn's syndrome) are the second most frequent type (3). Adrenogenital syndromes are rarely associated with cortical adenomas in adults, but virilization combined with Cushing's syndrome is the most common presentation of adenomas in children (see Table 2-1) (3).

Most cortical adenomas are solitary, circumscribed, solid, yellow-orange or tan tumors less than 5 cm in diameter (Fig. 2-2; see color plate 2) (2,3). Atrophy of nonneoplastic parenchyma resulting from feedback inhibition is characteristic of functional adenomas but is not a feature of nonfunctional tumors. Some adenomas are pigmented, with a dark brown or black appearance resulting from the intracellular accumulation of lipofuscin; most pigmented adenomas are nonfunctional (Fig. 2-3; see color plate 3) (2,3).

Cortical adenomas usually have a bland microscopic appearance resembling that of normal adrenal cortex (Fig. 2-4; see color plate 4), although some tumors are composed of pleomorphic cells. Histologic features do not reliably predict which hormone is being produced by a particular tumor, but ultrastructural features may be helpful (see color plate 4). Compared to aldosteronomas, glucocorticoid tumors are more likely to exhibit cellular pleomorphism and to be associated with lymphocytic aggregates or myelolipomas.

Oncocytic adrenal cortical adenomas have been described recently and are characterized by abundant granular eosinophilic cytoplasm, vesicular nuclei, and prominent nucleoli (5). The tumors are grossly similar to conventional adenomas but are characterized ultrastructurally by numerous intracytoplasmic mitochondria.

A 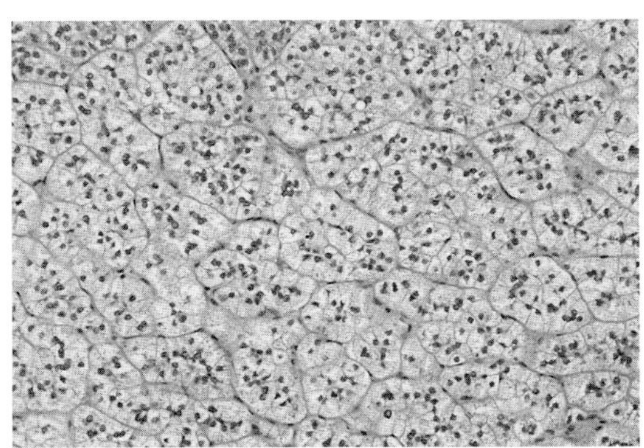 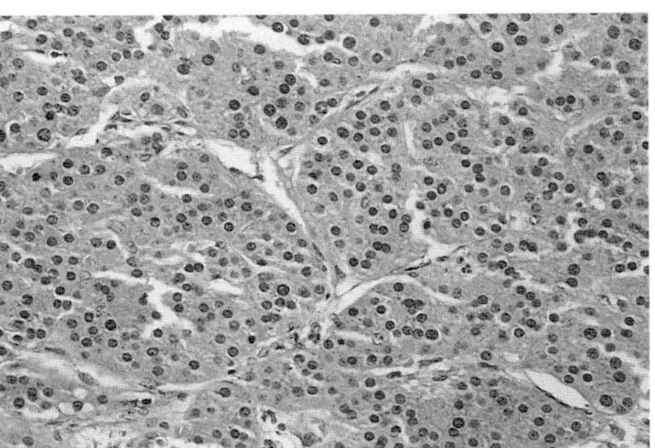 B

FIG. 2-4. Histologic sections of cortical adenomas. **A:** Cortical adenoma (aldosteronoma) cells with clear cytoplasm; **B:** cortical adenoma cells with eosinophilic cytoplasm.

ADRENAL CORTICAL CARCINOMA

Adrenal cortical carcinoma (ACC) is a rare and highly malignant neoplasm (2,6,7). It accounts for approximately 0.02% of all cancers, with an annual incidence of 0.5 to 2 cases per million people (3,8–10). Men and women are affected equally, and the average age at diagnosis is 45 to 50 years (2,7). Complete surgical excision is the treatment of choice, but the overall prognosis is poor. The mean length of survival is 6 to 30 months, and the 5-year survival rate is 20% to 30% (1,3,7–9,11). Common sites of metastasis include the lungs, lymph nodes, bones, and serosal surfaces (2,3).

About one-half of cortical carcinomas are clinically functional, with symptoms of cortical steroid overproduction (2). Functional carcinomas occur more frequently in younger women, whereas nonfunctional tumors are more common in men and in older patients (1,6,10). Pediatric cases of ACC are usually hormonally functional, with symptoms of Cushing's syndrome or virilization (3,10). There is an increased incidence of ACC in patients with Beckwith-Wiedemann syndrome and Li-Fraumeni syndrome (3).

Cortical carcinomas often are quite large (>5 cm, >100 g), with a variegated nodular appearance and soft, friable areas of hemorrhage and necrosis (Fig. 2-5; see color plate 5) (1,3,7). The tumors may invade into the adrenal vein or inferior vena cava. Most tumor cells are polygonal, with eosinophilic or reticulated cytoplasm and a variable degree of cytologic atypia (Fig. 2-6; see color plate 6). Some carcinomas are composed of minimally atypical cells that resemble benign cortical cells, whereas other tumors contain large, bizarre cells or spindle-shaped cells (3). The malignant cells typically lack cytoplasmic mucin and glycogen but may contain eosinophilic hyaline globules (3). Ultrastructural features of ACC include abundant smooth and rough endoplasmic reticulum and mitochondria with lamellar or tubulovesicular cristae.

The histologic features of ACC overlap with those of cortical adenoma; there is no single pathologic parameter that reliably distinguishes benign from malignant adrenal cortical neoplasms (2,3). Three diagnostic systems have been proposed to separate ACC from cortical adenoma (Table 2-2). The Weiss system is probably the most widely used and is based on nine histologic parameters (11):

- Nuclear grade
- Mitotic rate
- Atypical mitotic figures
- Eosinophilic cytoplasm
- Diffuse architecture
- Necrosis
- Venous invasion
- Sinusoidal invasion
- Capsular invasion

Originally, four of the nine features were required for a diagnosis of malignancy, but the requirement was subsequently changed to three of nine features. Three parameters [mitotic rate >5 per 50 high-power fields (HPF), atypical mitotic figures, and venous invasion] were present only in malignant tumors. The Van Slooten system assigns numeric values, ranging from 1.6 to 9.0, to seven histologic parameters and determined that a histologic index >8 correlated with malignant clinical behavior (12). The seven parameters are

- Regressive changes
- Loss of structure
- Nuclear atypia
- Nuclear hyperchromasia

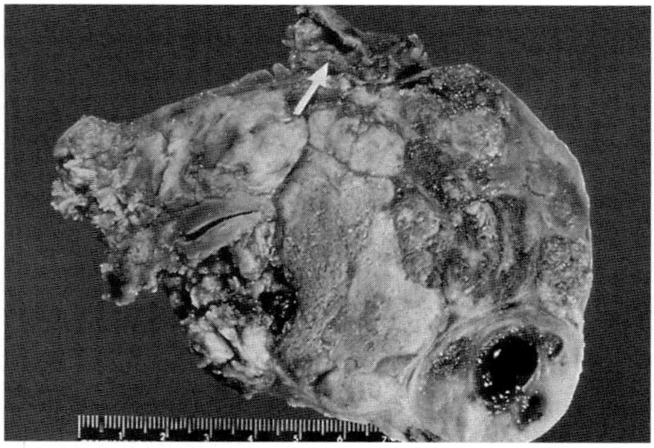

FIG. 2-5. A large adrenal cortical carcinoma has a nodular variegated appearance, with areas of hemorrhage and necrosis.

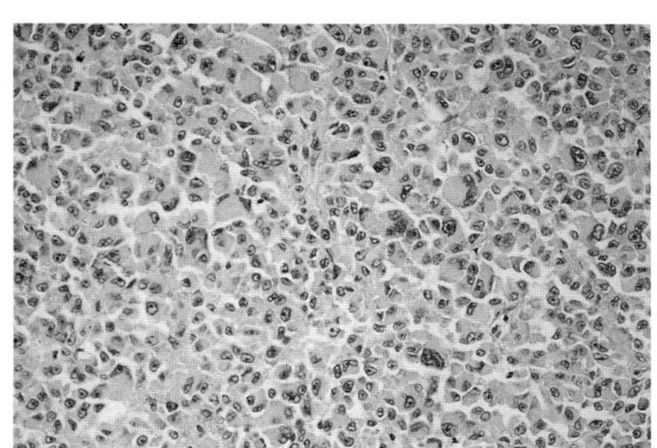

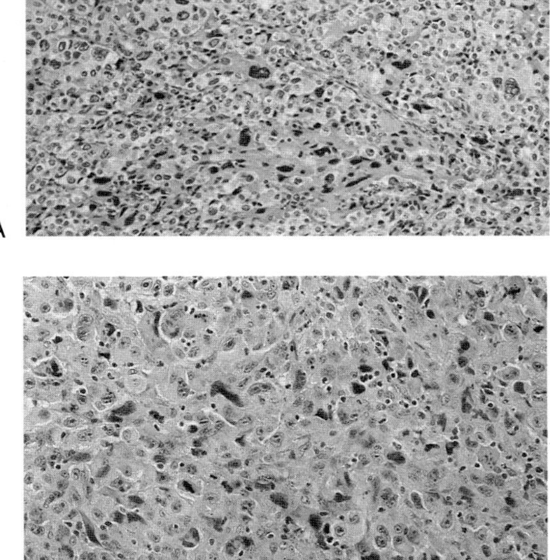

FIG. 2-6. Three different adrenal cortical carcinomas demonstrating various degrees of cellular pleomorphism and nuclear atypia.

- Abnormal nucleoli
- Mitotic activity
- Vascular or capsular invasion

In the Hough system, numeric values are assigned to five nonhistologic criteria and seven histologic parameters:

- Diffuse growth pattern
- Vascular invasion
- Necrosis
- Fibrous bands
- Capsular invasion
- Mitotic rate
- Pleomorphism

TABLE 2–2. *Histologic criteria of malignancy in adrenal cortical neoplasms*

Hough system (1979)	Weiss system (1984)	Van Slooten system (1985)
Diffuse growth (0.92)	High nuclear grade	Regressive changes (5.7)
Vascular invasion (0.92)	>5 mitoses/50 HPF[a]	Loss of structure (1.6)
Tumor necrosis (0.69)	Atypical mitoses[a]	Nuclear atypia (2.1)
Fibrous bands (1.00)	≥75% eosinophilic cells	Hyperchromasia (2.6)
Capsular invasion (0.37)	≥33% diffuse architecture	Abnormal nucleoli (4.1)
>1 mitosis/10 HPF (0.60)	Necrosis	>2 mitoses/10 HPF (9.0)
Pleomorphism (0.39)	Venous invasion[a]	Vascular or capsular invasion (3.3)
Also includes five nonhistologic criteria	Sinusoidal invasion	
	Capsular invasion	
Mean Histologic Indexes		
Malignant 2.91	Presence of three or more	Histologic index >8 indicates
Indeterminate 1.00	features indicates	malignancy
Benign 0.17	malignancy	

[a]Only in malignant tumors.
HPF, high-power fields.

TABLE 2–3. *Staging system for adrenal cortical carcinoma*

Stage I:	localized tumor ≤5 cm
Stage II:	localized tumor >5 cm
Stage III:	locally invasive tumor not involving adjacent organs, or localized tumor with regional lymph node metastasis
Stage IV:	tumor invading adjacent organs, locally invasive tumor (stage III) with regional lymph node metastasis, or any tumor with distant metastasis

These values range from 0.37 to 1.00 for the histologic features and from 0.42 to 2.00 for the nonhistologic features. The mean histologic index for malignant tumors is 2.91, for indeterminate tumors is 1.00, and for benign tumors is 0.17.

The pathologic evaluation of adrenocortical neoplasms involves two major issues. The first issue is to distinguish benign from malignant tumors. In general, malignant tumors are more likely to exhibit marked nuclear pleomorphism, abnormal mitotic figures, a diffuse growth pattern, necrosis, vascular and capsular invasion. The second issue is related to the prognosis of malignant tumors. Although tumor size may have prognostic significance, tumor stage and mitotic rate are probably the most important prognostic factors (Table 2-3). Tumor size is important in predicting the clinical behavior of malignant adrenal cortical tumors, but it should not be used to distinguish benign adenomas from cortical carcinomas (8). Several small (<100 g) but clinically malignant ACCs have been reported (13). Histologic examination of the excised tumor is required to assess the malignant potential of an adrenal cortical neoplasm. Weiss and colleagues (14) found that mitotic rate was the most important pathologic determinant of survival and proposed that a rate of 20 mitoses per 50 HPF be used to separate low-grade from high-grade cancers. There is a correlation between aneuploidy and malignant behavior, but DNA content is not a useful prognostic feature for individual tumors (3,8). Cellular proliferation markers, Ki-67 (MIB-1), and proliferating cell nuclear antigen have been noted to correlate with mitotic rate.

The differential diagnosis of ACC includes renal cell carcinoma (RCC), metastatic carcinoma (especially large cell lung cancer), hepatocellular carcinoma (HCC), melanoma, and pheochromocytoma. RCC and HCC present special diagnostic challenges because of morphologic similarities to ACC and proximity to the adrenal glands. Histologic features that may be diagnostically helpful include gland formation and periodic acid-Schiff (PAS)-positive glycogen granules in RCC, eosinophilic cytoplasmic hyaline globules in ACC, and the bile pigment in HCC (2). Immunohistochemistry may be useful in confirming the diagnosis of ACC (Table 2-4).

TABLE 2–4. *Differential diagnosis by immunohistochemistry*

	ACC	RCC	HCC	Melanoma	Pheochromocytoma	Metastatic adenocarcinoma
CK	0[a]	+	AE1/3 negative CAM 5.2 positive	0	0	+
Vim	+	Most positive	+/−	+/−	0	0
EMA	0	Most positive	+/−	0	0	+
AFP	0	0	Often positive	0	0	0
CEA	0	0	Canalicular (polyclonal CEA)	0	0	+
HMB-45	0	0	0	+	0	0
CHR	0	0	0	0	+	0
S-100	0	0	0	+	0	0

[a]Frozen tissue from adrenal cortical adenoma (ACC) may express cytokeratin.

RCC, renal cell carcinoma; HCC, hepatocellular carcinoma; CK, cytokeratin; Vim, vimentin; EMA, epithelial membrane antigen; AFP, alphafetoprotein; CEA, carcinoembryonic antigen; CHR, chromogranin.

ACC is characteristically positive for vimentin and negative for epithelial membrane antigen (EMA), carcinoembryonic antigen (CEA), α-fetoprotein (AFP), and S-100 protein. Although frozen ACC tissue may express cytokeratin, formalin-fixed tissue is usually cytokeratin negative unless pretreated with proteases (8,15). RCC typically coexpresses cytokeratin and vimentin, and many tumors are positive for EMA. Metastatic carcinomas are usually positive for cytokeratin, EMA, and CEA, but negative for vimentin. HCC stains positively for cytokeratin CAM 5.2 but is negative for cytokeratins AE1 and AE3. A canalicular staining pattern with polyclonal CEA is characteristic of HCC, and many cases are AFP positive. Immunohistologic markers of melanoma and pheochromocytoma are HMB-45 and chromogranin, respectively.

CUSHING'S SYNDROME

In considering the syndromes of cortical steroid overproduction, it is important to consider both etiology and adrenal morphology. Cushing's syndrome is caused by excessive levels of glucocorticoids and is manifested by truncal obesity, moon facies, weakness and fatigability, hypertension, and glucose intolerance (2). The syndrome may have exogenous (i.e., therapeutic administration of corticosteroids) or endogenous causes. Endogenous causes of Cushing's syndrome include (a) pituitary hypersecretion of ACTH, (b) ectopic ACTH-producing tumors, and (c) ACTH-independent adrenal cortical neoplasms. Cushing's syndrome may be associated morphologically with cortical hyperplasia, adenoma, or carcinoma.

Prolonged therapeutic administration of corticosteroids is the most common cause of Cushing's syndrome. Exogenous Cushing's syndrome is characterized by decreased pituitary secretion of ACTH and bilateral adrenal gland atrophy. Steroid therapy must be tapered gradually to prevent adrenal insufficiency.

Pituitary hypersecretion of ACTH accounts for 65% to 70% of cases of endogenous Cush-

ing's syndrome. Pituitary-induced glucocorticoid overproduction, also known as Cushing's disease, occurs most often in young adult women and is usually associated with bilateral diffuse cortical hyperplasia (2).

Ectopic ACTH-producing tumors account for 10% to 15% of endogenous Cushing's syndrome and most frequently affect men in the fifth or sixth decade of life. As previously noted (see Adrenal Cortical Hyperplasia), neoplasms that may be associated with ectopic ACTH production include small cell anaplastic lung cancers, carcinoid tumors, islet cell tumors, medullary thyroid carcinomas, and pheochromocytomas (2).

Adrenal cortical neoplasms account for 20% to 25% of endogenous Cushing's syndrome. In adults, the incidence of adenomas and ACC is approximately equal, but in children, malignant neoplasms occur significantly more often than benign tumors. ACC accounts for about 50% of the pediatric cases of Cushing's syndrome. The clinical symptoms of Cushing's syndrome are usually more prominent in malignant neoplasms than in benign tumors.

CONN'S SYNDROME

Conn's syndrome refers to primary hyperaldosteronism and is characterized by hypertension, hypokalemia, sodium retention, and decreased levels of renin (2). The biochemical abnormalities may be accompanied by neuromuscular disorders including weakness, paresthesias, and tetany.

Adrenal cortical adenomas account for 65% to 70% of cases, and adrenal hyperplasia is associated with most of the remaining cases; Conn's syndrome is rarely associated with ACC (2).

Aldosteronomas are usually solitary yellow tumors that tend to be smaller than glucocorticoid-producing tumors (1–3). They affect women more often than men and occur most frequently in the fourth and fifth decades of life. Mast cells are often associated with aldosteronomas and may provide a histologic clue to mineralocorticoid production (3). Distinctive eosinophilic cytoplasmic inclusions may occur in tumor cells and adjacent zona glomerulosa in patients undergoing treatment with spironolactone (1,2). Spironolactone bodies range from 2 to 15 μm in diameter and are composed of lamellar whorls of smooth endoplasmic reticulum (3).

ADRENOGENITAL SYNDROME

Adrenogenital syndromes are associated with overproduction of cortical sex steroids, and about half of the cases occur in children (2). Precocious puberty in boys and virilization in girls and women are the most common clinical presentations; symptoms of virilization are difficult to detect in men. Feminization that results from adrenal lesions is rare and almost always indicates a malignant tumor. Malignancy is also likely in cases of mixed virilization and Cushing's syndrome.

Congenital adrenal hyperplasia (CAH) is the most common cause of adrenogenital syndromes in children, but a significant proportion of pediatric cases are related to ACC (2,3). As previously noted (see Adrenal Cortical Hyperplasia), CAH is an autosomal recessive disorder with inborn errors in cortical steroid biosynthesis resulting in the overproduction of testosterone.

ADRENAL CYSTS

Cystic lesions of the adrenal include pseudocysts, infectious cysts, and true cysts. In addition, any primary or metastatic adrenal neoplasm may undergo cystic degeneration. Pseudocysts and cystic neoplasms are the most common adrenal cysts; true cysts are rare (3). Percutaneous needle aspiration can be a useful diagnostic and therapeutic procedure for adrenal cysts.

The etiology of pseudocysts is uncertain, but some lesions appear to arise from vascular or lymphatic channels (1,3). Pseudocysts may be large (>10 cm) and often contain brown or bloody fluid. The lesions lack an epithelial lining; they are composed of necrotic material and clusters of cortical cells surrounded by a fibrous wall. Calcifications, foamy histiocytes, and hemosiderin may occur within the wall.

Infectious adrenal cysts are most commonly related to echinococcal, mycobacterial, or fungal infections. Both adrenal glands are often involved, and adrenal insufficiency may result. Identification of the microorganisms is required to distinguish infectious cysts from pseudocysts.

True cysts are characterized by an epithelial or mesothelial lining. These rare lesions are usually small and asymptomatic.

MYELOLIPOMA

Myelolipomas are rare benign adrenal tumors that usually occur as incidental radiographic or autopsy findings (1–3). The lesions are thought to arise from metaplasia of adrenocortical cells or from multipotential mesenchymal cells (7). Large tumors may cause pain, a mass, or intraabdominal hemorrhage caused by rupture.

Myelolipomas are circumscribed yellowish-red masses surrounded by residual adrenal parenchyma or occasionally found in association with cortical neoplasms (Fig. 2-7A; see color plate 7A). Although most tumors are small, the size range is broad, with some tumors exceeding 1,000 g.

Myelolipomas are composed of varying proportions of mature adipose tissue and hematopoietic elements, including megakaryocytes, myeloid precursors, and erythroid precursors (Figs. 2-7B,C; see color plates 7B,C); bony trabeculae are present in some tumors.

ADRENAL INCIDENTALOMA

Adrenal incidentalomas are unexpected, radiologically detected adrenal lesions (1,16). They are reported in about 1% to 2% of abdominal computed tomography (CT) scans (3,16), but as technical improvements allow detection of smaller lesions, their incidence will probably increase.

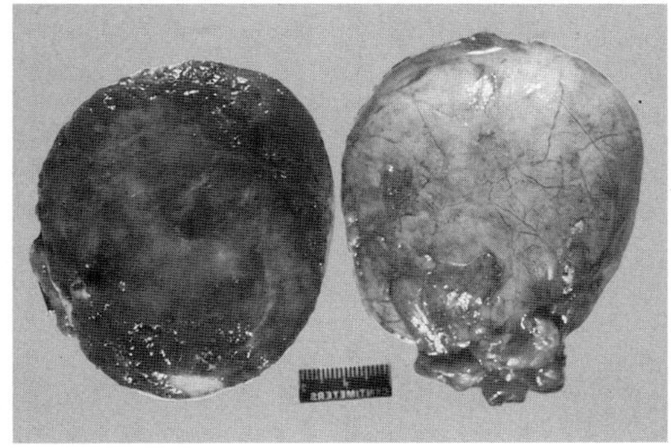

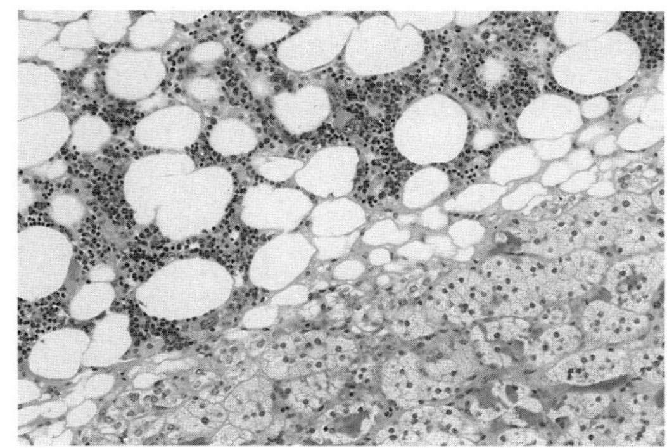

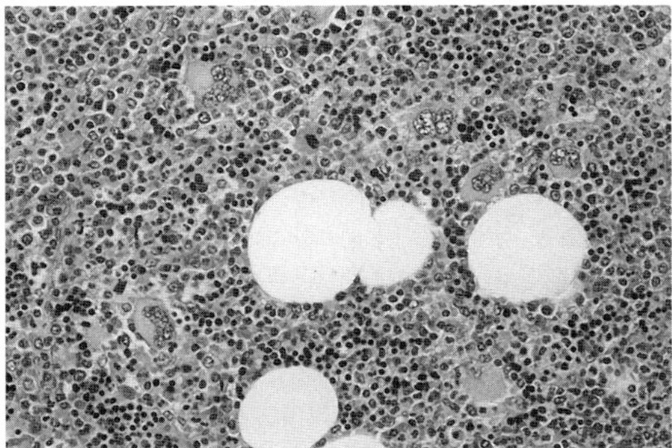

FIG. 2-7. Adrenal myelolipoma. **A:** A circumscribed tumor which had a yellow and red color; **B:** hematopoietic and adipose tissue adjacent to the adrenal cortex; **C:** high-power view of hematopoietic elements with characteristic megakaryocytes.

Patient management is guided by tumor size, radiologic features, and medical history. The general approach includes laboratory evaluation for cortical steroid or catecholamine overproduction and surgical excision of all functional tumors. Fine needle aspiration of nonfunctional adrenal lesions is indicated in patients with a previous diagnosis of malignancy to exclude the possibility of an adrenal metastasis. Nonfunctional solid masses can be stratified by size into high- and low-risk groups; surgical excision is recommended for larger tumors, whereas smaller lesions may be followed up conservatively with serial CT scans.

The differential diagnosis of adrenal incidentalomas includes adrenal cortical neoplasms, metastatic tumors, pheochromocytomas, myelolipomas, and adrenal cysts. After the possibility of metastasis has been excluded, approximately 80% to 90% of incidental adrenal masses are nonfunctional cortical adenomas, 5% to 10% are functional adenomas, 5% are pheochromocytomas, and less than 0.1% are cortical carcinomas (16).

METASTATIC TUMORS

The adrenal gland is a common site for metastatic tumors. Metastases are often bilateral, and massive involvement may cause adrenal insufficiency (2). Radiographic findings suggestive of malignancy in adrenal nodules include irregular borders, evidence of invasion, enlargement on serial CT examinations, and tumor size >3 cm. Knowledge of the patient's medical history and attention to histologic patterns are important clues in the accurate diagnosis of metastatic tumors. Lung and breast cancers account for about 60% of metastatic adrenal tumors (1). Solitary adrenal metastasis is relatively common in lung cancer, but breast cancer usually involves other sites (i.e., lungs, liver, bones) by the time adrenal metastases occur. Other malignancies that may metastasize to the adrenal gland include gastrointestinal malignancies, RCC, thyroid carcinoma, and melanoma (Fig. 2-8; see color plate 8) (2,3). Lymphomas may secondarily involve the

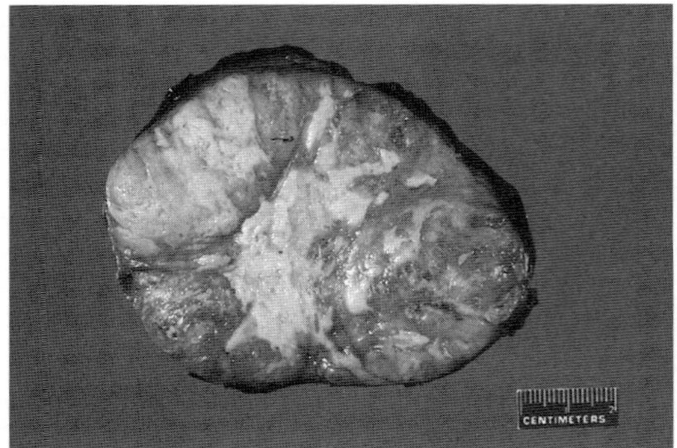

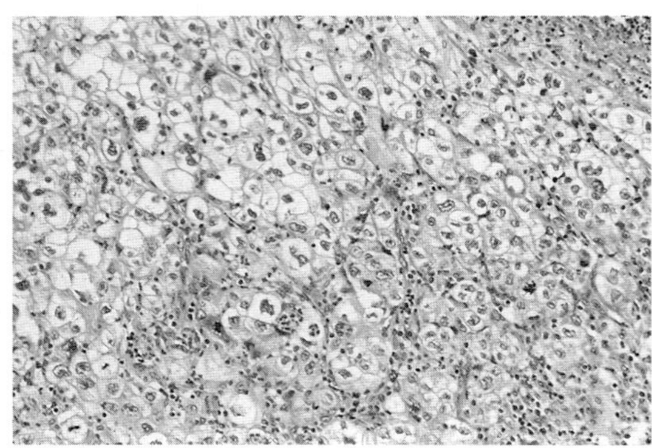

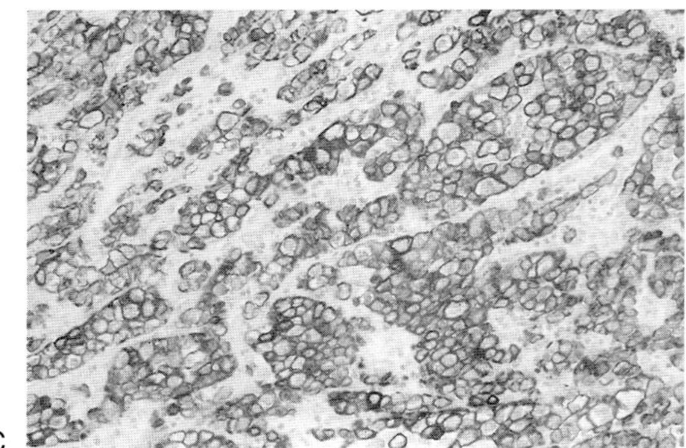

FIG. 2-8. Metastatic renal cell carcinoma to the adrenal gland. **A:** The adrenal gland has been replaced by a large tumor with areas of necrosis; **B:** large malignant cells have abundant clear cytoplasm; **C:** strong, diffuse immunoreactivity to cytokeratin supports the histologic impression of metastatic renal cell carcinoma.

adrenal and rarely may arise in this site. Immunohistochemistry is often helpful in distinguishing cortical carcinomas from metastatic cancers (see Table 2-4).

PHEOCHROMOCYTOMA

Pheochromocytomas are uncommon catecholamine-producing neoplasms of the adrenal medulla, with an annual incidence of approximately 8 cases per million people (1). Most tumors occur sporadically, but 10% are familial and may be associated with the multiple endocrine neoplasia syndromes (MEN IIA, MEN IIB), von Hippel-Lindau syndrome, or neurofibromatosis (Table 2-5) (1–3). Sporadic pheochromocytomas affect men and women equally, with a peak incidence between the ages of 35 and 50 years, and 10% to 15% are bilateral. Nonsporadic or familial pheochromocytomas tend to occur in younger patients, including children, and about 70% are bilateral (1,2).

Overproduction of norepinephrine, epinephrine, or dopamine by pheochromocytomas causes hypertension, headache, tachycardia, and sweating (7,17). Pheochromocytomas may follow a benign or malignant clinical course, but the prognosis cannot always be predicted based on histologic features. Although large tumor size, high mitotic rate, and extensive necrosis often correlate with aggressive behavior, documenting distant metastasis is the only reliable feature in identifying clinically malignant tumors (1,17). The most common metastatic sites are the liver, lung, lymph nodes, and bone (17).

TABLE 2–5. *Clinical features of pheochromocytoma*

	Solitary	Bilateral	Extraadrenal
Sporadic (90%)	80%–90%	10%	10%
Familial (10%)	20%–30%	70%	<10%
Children (10%)	50%	20%–30%	10%–20%

Pheochromocytomas are usually well-circumscribed tumors surrounded by a rim of compressed adrenal tissue. The tumors range in size from 1 to 4,000 g (average, 100 g) and are usually yellow-white, gray, or brown, with areas of hemorrhage, necrosis, or cystic degeneration (Fig. 2-9; see color plate 9) (1). Sporadic neoplasms usually occur as solitary tumors surrounded by normal-appearing medulla, whereas familial tumors are often multicentric and associated with medullary hyperplasia (3).

The chromaffin reaction is positive in up to 90% of pheochromocytomas under optimal conditions (2,3). When fresh tumor tissue is placed in potassium dichromate at pH 5 to 6, a dark brown color results from the oxidation and polymerization of catecholamine granules (Fig. 2-10; see color plate 10). Similarly, a purple or magenta color results when tumor tissue is placed in potassium iodate. Zenker's fixative may be used for the chromaffin reaction, but the results are suboptimal because of the presence of acetic acid. Formaldehyde-induced fluorescence is an alternative method of demonstrating catecholamines in which unstained sections of tumor emit a yellow-green fluorescence when exposed to formaldehyde vapors. The Grimelius histochemical stain is used to demonstrate cytoplasmic argyrophilia, which is indicative of neuroendocrine origin.

Pheochromocytomas are highly vascular tumors composed of large polygonal cells with abundant granular cytoplasm arranged in alveolar (zellballen), trabecular, or diffuse sheetlike patterns (Fig. 2-11; see color plate 11). Some tumors are composed of spindle-shaped cells or extremely bizarre cells with large, hyperchromatic nuclei, but these histologic variations do not have prognostic significance (1,2). The nuclei are round to oval with prominent nucleoli and a variable degree of pleomorphism. Intranuclear cytoplasmic pseudoinclusions are present in 30% to 50% of pheochromocytomas.

From 30% to 50% of pheochromocytomas contain acid-fast, PAS-positive hyaline cytoplasmic globules, and about 10% to 20% of tumors have scattered ganglion cells (1,3). Other features that occasionally occur in pheochromocytomas include oncocytic metaplasia, cytoplasmic pigment, and amyloid deposits. Rarely, pheochromocytomas may coexist with ganglioneuroblastomas (GNBs) or ganglioneuromas (GNs).

Pheochromocytomas and normal adrenal medullary tissue are immunoreactive to chromogranin (CHR), synaptophysin, and neuron-specific enolase (NSE). CHR staining is usually stronger in normal than in neoplastic tissues. Pheochromocytomas may also express neurofilaments, enkephalins, ACTH, calcitonin, vasoactive intestinal peptide, or somatostatin (1,3).

Sustentacular cells are spindle-shaped cells distributed at the periphery of neoplastic cell

A 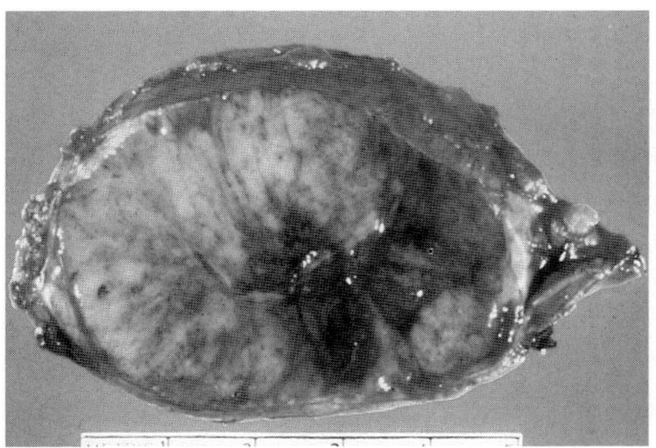 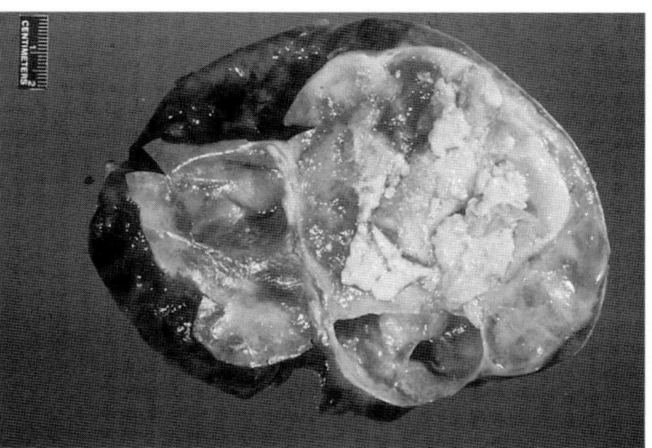 B

FIG. 2-9. Two different adrenal pheochromocytomas. **A:** A small portion of adrenal cortex is present at the periphery of the tumor; **B:** extensive cystic change is present in this pheochromocytoma.

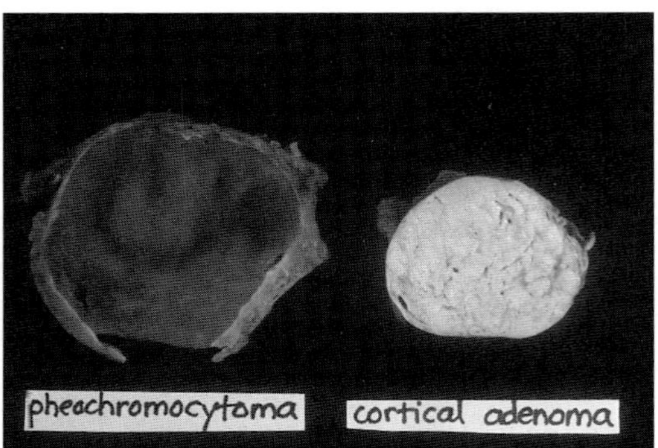

FIG. 2-10. A comparison of pheochromocytoma and adrenal cortical adenoma. The chromaffin reaction demonstrates staining of the pheochromocytoma.

clusters. They have small, hyperchromatic nuclei and are immunoreactive to S-100 protein. Compared to sporadic tumors, MEN-associated pheochromocytomas have more numerous sustentacular cells.

The differential diagnosis of pheochromocytoma includes medullary hyperplasia, neuroblastoma, adrenal cortical neoplasms, and metastatic carcinomas (3). Nodular medullary hyperplasia and pheochromocytomas are arbitrarily separated by size; lesions smaller than 1 cm are classified as hyperplasia. Neuroblastic tumors and pheochromocytomas are both derived form the neural crest and may have some overlapping histologic features. Neuroblastomas occur in young children and are composed of undifferentiated cells, often associated with neurofibrillary stroma or Homer-Wright rosettes. Both neuroblastomas and pheochromocytomas are NSE positive, but CHR staining is usually weak or negative in neuroblastic tumors. The chromaffin reaction and Grimelius stain can be useful in distinguishing pheochromocytomas from adrenal cortical neoplasms. Cytoplasmic lipid is characteristic of cortical tumors but is rarely identified in pheochromocytomas.

NEUROBLASTOMA

Neuroblastoma is the most common solid tumor in infants younger than 1 year old and the third most common malignancy—after leukemia/lymphoma and central nervous system tumors—in children of all ages (1,3). The annual incidence is approximately one case of neuroblastoma per 7,000 children younger than 15 years of age. Most tumors occur in children younger than 6 years old, with a peak incidence at 2 years (2). Boys are affected more often than girls, and European-Americans are affected more often than African-Americans. Occasional cases have a familial incidence pattern or an association with Beckwith-Wiedemann syndrome or neurofibromatosis (1,2). Nearly all patients have elevated urinary levels of homovanillic acid and vanillylmandelic acid. Neuroblastomas have a 5-year survival rate of about 50% to 60%.

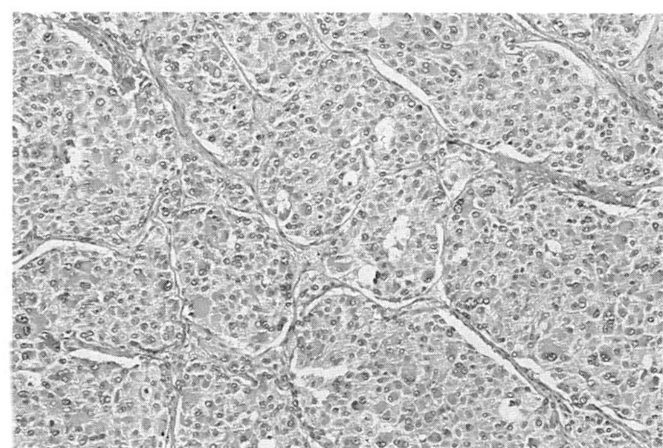

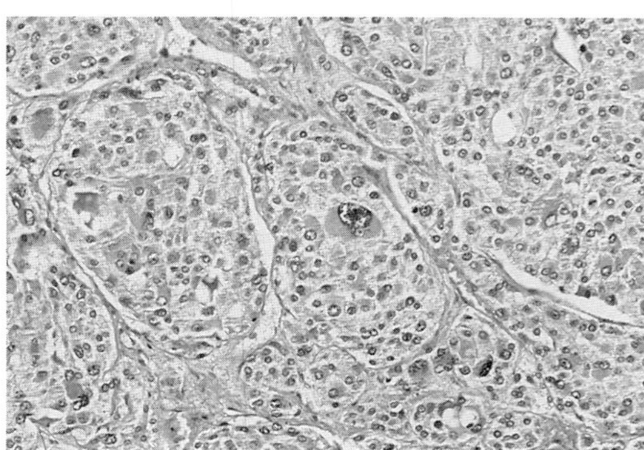

A   B

FIG. 2-11. Histologic sections of **(A, B)** pheochromocytomas demonstrate an alveolar (zellballen) pattern and cellular pleomorphism.

The adrenal glands and retroperitoneum are the most common tumor sites, but neuroblastomas may also arise in the thorax, mediastinum, neck, or pelvis (1). Approximately 30% of patients have metastases at the time of diagnosis, usually involving the liver, bones, or lymph nodes (1). Important prognostic features include age at diagnosis, tumor stage, and amplification of the N-*myc* oncogene (3) (Table 2-6). Infants younger than 1 year of age have the best prognosis, with a 90% long-term survival rate. Infants and patients with stage IV-S disease have the highest incidence of spontaneous tumor maturation or regression. Stage I, II, and IV-S tumors have a significantly better prognosis than stage III or IV tumors (Table 2-7). Amplification of the N-*myc* oncogene is a poor prognostic indicator associated with rapid clinical progression. In contrast to most other neoplasms, aneuploidy is associated with a favorable prognosis in neuroblastoma.

TABLE 2–6. *Prognostic factors for neuroblastoma*

Age at diagnosis: younger patients have better prognosis; infants <1 year old have 90% long-term survival[a]
Tumor stage[a]
N-*myc* oncogene: amplification associated with worse prognosis[a]
Tumor location: extraadrenal tumors have a better prognosis
Histologic differentiation: more abundant cytoplasm, larger nuclei, vesicular chromatin, prominent nucleoli
    Undifferentiated: 0% differentiated cells
    Poorly differentiated: <5% differentiated cells
    Differentiating: >5% differentiated cells
Lymphocytic infiltration: may be associated with a better prognosis
DNA index: aneuploidy associated with a better prognosis
MKI (Shimada)
    MKI <100: favorable prognosis
    MKI >200: unfavorable prognosis
Calcification and mitotic rate (Joshi et al.[19])
    Grade 1: calcification present and MR ≤10/10 HPF
    Grade 2: calcification present or MR ≤10/10 HPF
    Grade 3: no calcification and MR ≥10/10 HPF

[a]Most important factors.
MKI, mitosis karyorrhexis index; HPF, high-power fields; MR, mitotic rate.

TABLE 2–7. *Staging system for neuroblastoma*

Stage I:	tumor confined to organ or structure of origin
Stage II:	unilateral tumor extension beyond organ or structure of origin
Stage III:	tumor extension beyond organ or structure of origin across the midline
Stage IV:	distant disease
Stage IV-S:	stage I or II tumors with distant disease involving liver, skin, and/or bone marrow, but without radiographic bone involvement

[a]Reprinted with permission from Evans classification (*Cancer* 1971;27:374).

Neuroblastomas are usually large, tan or gray, circumscribed tumors with a bulging, lobulated cut surface and foci of hemorrhage, necrosis, and calcification (2,3). The tumors are composed predominantly of undifferentiated cells with scant, indistinct cytoplasm and round, hyperchromatic nuclei with coarsely granular chromatin. The nuclei are slightly larger than lymphocytes. From 25% to 40% of neuroblastomas contain Homer-Wright rosettes, characterized by a ring of nuclei around a fibrillary tangle of neurites (1–3). Features that may occasionally be present in neuroblastomas include spindle-shaped cells, intranuclear cytoplasmic pseudoinclusions, pseudorhabdoid change, and dark cytoplasmic pigmentation (3). Tumor cells usually have a nesting arrangement surrounded by thin fibrovascular septa. Less common architectural patterns include sclerosing, pseudoalveolar, papillary, angiomatoid, and starry-sky patterns (3).

Neuroblastomas are immunologically positive for NSE, neurofilaments, and other neural-related antigens (2). Ultrastructurally, the tumors contain 50- to 200-nm neurosecretory granules, primitive cell processes, abundant basal lamina, and occasional neurofilaments (3). Secretory granules tend to concentrate in the periphery of the cells.

Neuroblastomas are derived from neuroectodermal cells of the neural crest and are distinguished from other neuroblastic tumors (GNBs and GNs) by a lack of cellular maturation (18). GNBs and GNs usually occur out-

TABLE 2–8. *Classification systems of neuroblastic tumors[a]*

Conventional	Shimada	Modified (POG)
Classic NB (<5% differentiated cells)	NB, stroma poor, and undifferentiated	Undifferentiated NB Poorly differentiated NB
GNB (>5% ganglion cells)	NB, stroma poor, and differentiated	Differentiating NB
Composite GNB (nodules of NB in GN)	NB stroma rich	GNB
	Nodular	Nodular
	Intermixed	Intermixed
	Well differentiated	Borderline
GN	GN	GN

NB, neuroblastoma; GNB, ganglioneuroblastoma; GN, ganglioneuroma; POG, Pediatric Oncology Group.
[a]From ref. 18 with permission.

side the adrenal glands in the retroperitoneum of mediastinum. GNs are benign neoplasms with a favorable prognosis, and GNBs have a prognosis intermediate between those of neuroblastoma and GN.

Several classification systems have been used for neuroblastic tumors (Table 2-8) (18). The modified conventional classification system, recommended by the Pediatric Oncology Group, is probably the most widely accepted and easiest to apply (Table 2-9) (18,19).

Neuroblastomas are subclassified based on the percentage of differentiated cells in the tumor. Tumor cell differentiation is characterized by the presence of abundant cytoplasm, cell processes, large nuclei, and prominent nucleoli. Undifferentiated neuroblastomas completely lack cellular differentiation, whereas poorly differentiated tumors have greater than 5% differentiated cells and differentiating tumors have greater than 5% differentiated cells.

The Shimada prognostic scheme for neuroblastic tumors (Table 2-10) is based on the relative proportion of stroma, the patient's age, and the mitosis-karyorrhexis index (MKI). The MKI is defined as the number of mitotic figures and karyorrhectic nuclei per 5,000 cells. The classification and prognostic systems for neuroblastomas are applicable only to adequately sampled (one section per maximal dimension in centimeters) and untreated tumors.

The differential diagnosis of neuroblastoma includes other small cell neoplasms of childhood, such as leukemia/lymphoma, rhabdomyosarcoma, medulloblastoma, retinoblastoma, and Ewing's sarcoma (1–3). In many cases, immunohistochemistry or ultrastructural studies are required for a definite diagnosis. Neuroblastomas are immunoreactive to NSE and neurofilaments but are nonreactive to cytokeratin, leukocyte common antigen, vimentin, and muscle markers (desmin, actin, myoglobin). Neurosecretory granules are a helpful ultrastructural finding in neuroblastomas. Cytogenetic studies may be useful in

TABLE 2–9. *Modified conventional classification of neuroblastic tumors recommended by the pediatric oncology group[a]*

Tumor type	Definition	Subtypes
NB	>50% neuroblasts and neurophil May have a minor GN component	Undifferentiated Poorly differentiated Differentiating
GNB	>50% GN <50% NB	Nodular Intermixed Borderline
GN	100% mature ganglion cells, neurites, Schwann cells, and fibrous tissue	

GN, ganglioneuroma; NB, neuroblastoma; GNB, ganglioneuroblastoma.
[a]From ref. 18 with permission.

TABLE 2–10. *Shimada prognostic classification of neuroblastic tumors*

Favorable histology
  SR, well differentiated
  SR, intermixed
  SP, <18 mo; MKI <200
  SP, 18–60 mo differentiated; MKI <100
Unfavorable histology
  SR, nodular
  SP, <18 mo; MKI >200
  SP, >60 mo
  SP, 18–60 mo undifferentiated
  SP, 18–60 mo differentiated; MKI >100

SR, stroma rich; SP, stroma poor; mo, months of age; MKI, mitosis karyorrhexis index.

making the differential diagnosis because deletions of chromosome 1p are characteristic of neuroblastoma, whereas translocations t(11;22)(q24;q12) are typical of Ewing's sarcoma.

FINE-NEEDLE ASPIRATION BIOPSY OF ADRENAL GLANDS

Fine-needle aspiration biopsy (FNAB) of the adrenal gland is a relatively safe and effective method of evaluating solid and cystic mass lesions (20,21). Sensitivity rates vary from 80% to 95% and specificity rates from 95% to 100% (22). Complications rarely occur with adrenal FNAB and consist primarily of pneumothorax and hemorrhage (7,20). Because of the proximity of the left adrenal gland to the pancreas, aspiration of this gland may cause pancreatitis. Clinical symptoms of catecholamine excess are a contraindication to adrenal biopsy in that aspiration of pheochromocytomas can precipitate a hypertensive crisis (7).

Because benign and malignant primary adrenal cortical tumors have overlapping features and often cannot be distinguished cytologically, the primary function of FNAB is to exclude metastatic malignancy. FNAB of the adrenal is a useful technique in the diagnosis of metastatic adrenal tumors. Cytologic evaluation of adrenal masses is especially helpful in patients with a history of lung cancer in that solitary adrenal metastases are relatively common in this clinical setting. FNAB may also be useful to confirm a characteristic radiographic abnormality such as myelolipoma (Fig. 2-12; see color plate 12).

Aspirates of adrenal cortical nodules and adenomas yield benign cortical cells with fragile vacuolated cytoplasm. Nuclei are often stripped of cytoplasm, and in some aspirates bare nuclei may aggregate in a pattern mimicking that of small cell carcinoma (7,22). Cytologic features are not always reliable in distinguishing benign from malignant cortical neoplasms, but nuclear uniformity and a clean background (i.e., lack of tumor necrosis) occur more frequently in benign lesions. ACC may have cytologic features indistinguishable from those of RCC and immunocytochemistry is often required (Fig. 2-13; see color plate 13).

Although a clinical suspicion of pheochromocytoma is a contraindication for adrenal FNAB, unexpected tumors are occasionally as-

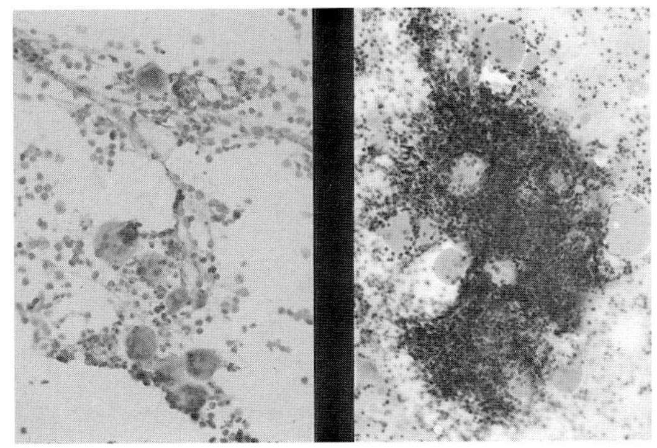

A   B

FIG. 2-12. Aspiration specimens of myelolipomas are characterized by a polymorphic cellular population including megakaryocytes (**A**, Papanicolaou stain) and lipid droplets (**B**, oil red O stain).

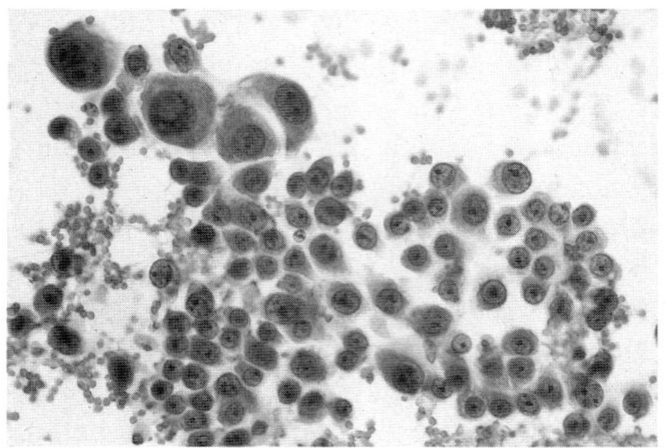

FIG. 2-13. This is an adrenal aspirate from an 80-year-old woman with Cushing's syndrome and an 8-cm left adrenal mass. The cellular specimen contains loosely cohesive, large pleomorphic cells with macronucleoli. Histologically and clinically, the tumor is an adrenal cortical carcinoma (Papanicolaou stain).

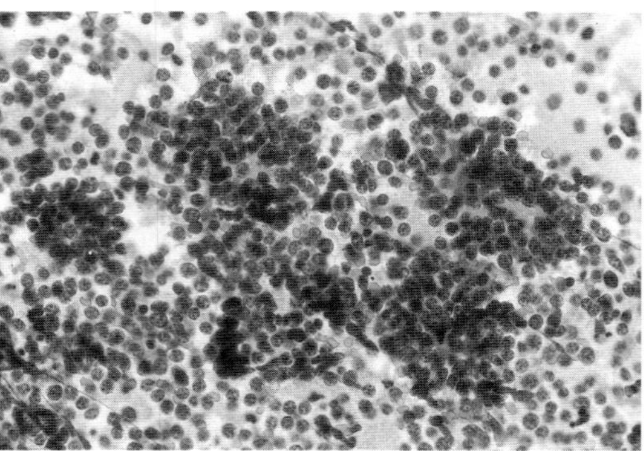

FIG. 2-15. Cytologic features of neuroblastoma include neoplastic cells with scant cytoplasm, high nuclear:cytoplasmic ratios, coarsely granular chromatin, and inconspicuous nucleoli. Rosette formations are quite characteristic (Papanicolaou stain).

pirated (7,22). Aspirates of pheochromocytomas tend to be highly cellular and composed of a polymorphic population of polygonal cells, giant cells, and occasional spindle-shaped cells. The cytoplasm is usually granular and eosinophilic, but it may be amphophilic or basophilic (Fig. 2-14; see color plate 14). Hyperchromatic nuclei have coarsely granular chromatin and prominent nucleoli. The cytologic differential diagnosis of pheochromocytoma includes adrenal cortical tumors, neuroblastoma, RCC, HCC, melanoma, and sarcomas. Im-

munocytochemical and ultrastructural studies may be indicated in some cases.

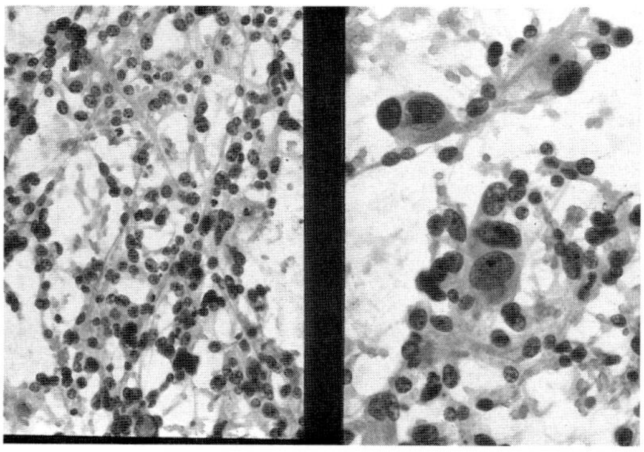

Aspirates of neuroblastomas are generally highly cellular and contain small, undifferentiated cells occurring as single cells, in small clusters, and occasionally in pseudorosettes (7,22). The cells have scant cytoplasm and high nucleocytoplasmic ratios (Fig. 2-15; see color plate 15). A fibrillar matrix and cytoplasmic processes extending from the neoplastic cells are characteristic features. The nuclei have finely granular chromatin and often demonstrate a molding arrangement. In addition to undifferentiated cells, differentiating neuroblastomas contain a population of larger cells with eosinophilic cytoplasm or ganglion cells.

FIG. 2-14. This cytologic specimen of a pheochromocytoma demonstrates polygonal cells, spindled cells, and a few giant cells. The cytoplasm is coarsely granular (Papanicolaou stain).

REFERENCES

1. DeLellis RA. The adrenal glands. In: Sternberg SS, ed. *Diagnostic surgical pathology*, Vol. 1. New York: 1989: 445–446.
2. Rosai J. Adrenal gland and other paraganglia. In *Ackerman's surgical pathology*, 7th ed. St. Louis: Mosby, 1989:789–818.
3. Medeiros LJ, Weiss LM. The difficult diagnosis in surgical pathology. In: Noel Weidner, ed. *Adrenal gland: tumors and tumor-like lesions*. Philadelphia: WB Saunders, 1996.
4. Carney JA, Hruska LS, Beauchamp GD, et al. Dominant inheritance of the complex syndrome of myxomas, spotty pigmentation, and endocrine overactivity. *Mayo Clin Proc* 1986;61:165–172.

5. Sasano H, Suzuki T, Sano T, et al. Adrenocortical onco-cytoma: a true nonfunctioning adrenocortical tumor. *Am J Surg Pathol* 1991;15:949–956.

6. Brennen MF. Adrenocortical carcinoma. *CA* 1987;37 (6):348–365.

7. Katz RL. Kidney, adrenal and retroperitoneum. In: Bibbo M, ed. *Comprehensive cytopathology*. Philadelphia: WB Saunders, 1991:789–796.

8. Medeiros LJ, Weiss LM. New developments in the pathologic diagnosis of adrenal cortical neoplasms: a review. *Am J Clin Pathol* 1992;97:73–83.

9. Venkatesh S, Hickey RC, Sellin RV, et al. Adrenal cortical carcinoma. *Cancer* 1989;64:765–769.

10. Wooten MD, King DK. Adrenal cortical carcinoma—epidemiology and treatment with mitotane and a review of the literature. *Cancer* 1993;72:3145.

11. Weiss LM. Comparative histologic study of 43 metastasizing and nonmetastasizing adrenocortical tumors. *Am J Surg Pathol* 1984;8:163–169.

12. Van Slooten H, Schaberg A, Smeenk D, et al. Morphological characteristics of benign and malignant adrenal cortical tumors. *Cancer* 1985;55:766–773.

13. Gandour MJ, Grizzle WE. A small adrenocortical carcinoma with aggressive behavior: an evaluation of criteria for malignancy. *Arch Pathol Lab Med* 1986;110:1076–1079.

14. Weiss LM, Medeiros J, Vickery AL. Pathologic features of prognostic significance in adrenocortical carcinoma. *Am J Surg Pathol* 1989;13:202–206.

15. Wick MR, Cherwitz DI, McGlennen RC, et al. Adrenocortical carcinoma: an immunohistochemical comparison with renal cell carcinoma. *Am J Pathol* 1986;122:343–352.

16. Gajraj H, Young AE. Adrenal incidentaloma. *Br J Surg* 1993;80:422–426.

17. Medeiros LJ, Wolf BC, Balogh K, et al. Adrenal pheochromocytoma: a clinicopathologic review of 60 cases. *Hum Pathol* 1985;15:580–589.

18. Joshi VV, Silverman JF. Pathology of neuroblastic tumors. *Semin Diagn Pathol* 1994;11:107–117.

19. Joshi VV, Cantor AB, Altshuler G, et al. Recommendations for modification of terminology of neuroblastic tumors and prognostic significance of Shimada classification. *Cancer* 1992;69:2183–2196.

20. Katz RL, Patel S, Mackay B, et al. Fine needle aspiration cytology of the adrenal gland. *Acta Cytol* 1984;28:269–282.

21. Wadih GE, Nance KV, Silverman JF. Fine needle aspiration cytology of the adrenal gland: fifty biopsies in 48 patients. *Arch Pathol Lab Med* 1992;116:841–846.

22. Suen KC, Chan NH. Fine needle aspiration biopsy of the adrenal gland: cytologic features and clinical applications. *Endocrinol Pathol* 1992;3:173–181.

*Medical and Surgical Management of
Adrenal Diseases,* edited by Joseph C. Cerny.
Lippincott Williams & Wilkins, Philadelphia © 1999.

3

Imaging of the Adrenal Glands

Milan V. Pantelic

*Department of Diagnostic Radiology and Medical Imaging, Henry Ford Hospital,
Detroit, Michigan 48202*

The adrenal glands are subject to a wide spectrum of pathologic conditions, including a variety of benign and malignant primary tumors, functional abnormalities, involvement by metastasis, inflammatory and infectious diseases, and hemorrhage. Imaging of the adrenals has always been difficult because of their small size, relatively inaccessible location, and proximity to other structures. However, the maturation of cross-sectional imaging by ultrasound (US) and computed tomography (CT) since the 1970s, the rapid, ongoing evolution of magnetic resonance imaging (MRI), the availability of specific radiopharmaceuticals, and the development of widespread expertise in guided percutaneous biopsy techniques have greatly increased morphologic, physiologic, and histologic information available to the clinician for accurate diagnosis.

INDICATIONS FOR IMAGING

Adrenal gland imaging is necessitated in a variety of clinical situations: when there is a biochemical abnormality or clinical signs and symptoms of a functional adrenal lesion, its nature (e.g., cortical adenoma, hyperplasia, pheochromocytoma) and location (unilateral, bilateral, extraadrenal) must be demonstrated; when there are symptoms or signs of abdominal or retroperitoneal mass; in the staging of malignancy with a predisposition for metastasis to the adrenal (e.g., bronchogenic or breast carcinoma), or in the search for an unknown primary tumor. Finally, imaging is used for further characterization of the incidentally discovered adrenal mass (Table 3-1).

IMAGING MODALITIES

Radiographic and Angiographic Techniques

Radiographic methods no longer have a primary role in the detection and diagnosis of primary adrenal disease. Abdominal radiographs can show large adrenal masses, and excretory urography with tomography can detect up to 80% of adrenocortical tumors and pheochromocytomas; however, the detection of most adrenal lesions in this fashion is serendipitous.

Radiographs can detect calcification associated with adrenal disease, such as prior hemorrhage, granulomatous disease, cysts, and some tumors. Review of radiographs may also reveal urolithiasis and changes in bone mineralization associated with adrenal disease or show evidence of osseous metastases in the setting of a primary or metastatic adrenal tumor. Retroperitoneal pneumography, once a mainstay of adrenal imaging, has been relegated to a historical footnote by the advent of cross-sectional imaging.

Although a sensitive, if nonspecific, test for the detection of adrenal masses, arteriography and venography are no longer indicated for their primary assessment. Arteriography is

TABLE 3–1. *Suggested imaging strategies*

Clinical scenario	Primary imaging modality			Problem-solving modality	Second-tier problem solving	Notes
Child/neonate: question of adrenal hemorrhage	US			MRI CT		Indeterminate lesions should be followed to exclude underlying neoplasm
Child: suspected adrenal mass or palpable mass	US	Hormonally inactive		MRI CT		
		Active: steroidal excess		MRI Radiocholesterol scintigraphy	Biopsy Adrenal venous sampling	
		Active: catecholamine excess		MRI MIBG	Biopsy Bone scintigraphy	
Adult: suspected adrenal mass	CT	Hormonally inactive or incidental	Large (>5 cm) or malignant features	Biopsy		
			Indeterminate (<5 cm)	MRI Radiocholesterol scintigraphy	Octreotide scan	Malignant: biopsy Benign features and 3–5 cm: follow with CT or MRI
		Active: catecholamine excess		MIBG MRI		Adrenal venous sampling is rarely needed
		Active: steroidal excess	Large (>5 cm) or malignant features	Biopsy		
				Radiocholesterol scintigraphy MRI	Adrenal venous sampling	
Adult: acute adrenal insufficiency	CT					Noncontrast CT
Large mass: uncertain origin by CT	MRI			Biopsy	Angiography	
Adrenal mass: question of vascular invasion	MRI			Angiography Inferior vena cavography		

CT, computed tomography; MRI, magnetic resonance imaging; MIBG, guanethidine, iodine-131-metaiodobenzylguanidine.

generally reserved for the clarification of equivocal findings on cross-sectional imaging, for preoperative road mapping, or as a prelude to embolization. When there is a large retroperitoneal mass or hemorrhage, the organ of origin may be difficult or impossible to determine by noninvasive imaging, and angiographic demonstration of an adrenal arterial supply can add specificity to the diagnosis (1). Adrenal venography is generally used to provide support for selective adrenal venous sampling. In patients with primary hyperaldosteronism, adrenal venous sampling has a reported accuracy of nearly 100% both in distinguishing bilateral from unilateral disease and in determining the side of a unilateral lesion (1).

Cross-Sectional Techniques

Ultrasound

Sonographic evaluation of the adrenal remains a challenge despite the routine availability of high-resolution, real-time equipment. Because the adrenal glands are central within the upper abdomen, acoustic windows may be limited, depending on the patient habitus. Even though a skilled sonographer is still required, the adrenal glands in the adult can be visualized in up to 90% of patients. Although US has been reported to detect up to 90% of known adrenal masses, a prospective study found an overall accuracy of only 70% for sonography in patients with suspected adrenal disease (2). Sonography remains the study of choice for the initial evaluation of the adrenal gland in the pediatric population. It can be useful for the characterization of adrenal lesions, particularly in discriminating solid from cystic masses, and it can provide a simple means of following up lesions under conservative management.

Computed Tomography

CT remains the technique of choice for imaging the adult adrenal glands, with a reported sensitivity of 84%, a specificity of 98%, and an accuracy of 90% in suspected adrenal disease (2). The adrenal glands are visualized by CT in nearly 100% of patients (1,3). Adrenal abnormalities are generally evident as mass lesions that obliterate or distort the normal gland configuration or present as localized or diffuse enlargement.

The newest generation of spiral (helical) and electron-beam CT scanners has the ability to image the entire abdomen in a breath-hold and may further enhance adrenal imaging with improved resolution, reduced respiratory artifacts, better reformations or three-dimensional reconstructions, and the ability to perform dynamic contrast-enhanced studies and CT angiography. Their impact on the imaging of subtle adrenal disease or mass characterization remains to be demonstrated.

Magnetic Resonance Imaging

MRI is the newest modality available for adrenal imaging; although it has become widely available, it is still undergoing rapid technologic evolution. Among the greatest strengths of MRI are its superb soft-tissue contrast, the ability to obtain images in arbitrary planes, the natural enhancement of many pathologic lesions resulting from their greater water content, the lack of ionizing radiation, and the ability to depict and quantitate blood flow noninvasively. MRI has the potential to differentiate benign from malignant lesions by the use of chemical-shift imaging, to evaluate for vessel invasion or tumor thrombus, and to provide dynamic evaluation of enhancement patterns with breath-hold sequences following bolus intravenous injection of gadolinium chelate contrast material. Tissue characterization and the interrogation of physiologic processes with in vivo MR spectroscopy continue to be areas of active research. Chang and colleagues (4) have shown that MRI can demonstrate the normal adrenal glands on T1-weighted images in more than 90% of patients and can detect lesions more than 1 cm in diameter with sensitivity comparable to that of CT. Even so, MRI remains primarily a problem-solving imaging modality in the assessment of adrenal lesions initially imaged by CT.

Nuclear Medicine Techniques

Scintigraphic methods maintain an important role in the diagnosis of adrenal cortical and medullary disease. Although unable to achieve the level of anatomic detail possible with the cross-sectional techniques, nuclear imaging provides physiologic information about adrenal gland function or an adrenal mass, which cannot be obtained by any other noninvasive method, and is well suited to whole body imaging. Scintigraphy can determine whether a morphologic adrenal abnormality corresponds to abnormal function or whether disease is bilateral or unilateral. This can be critical in the selection of the most appropriate therapy and in the assessment of its results. These methods are complementary to those of cross-sectional imaging and biochemical assay; no adrenal scintigraphic study should be undertaken without knowledge of the clinical and biochemical findings, the results of prior imaging, and the specific clinical question to be answered.

Adrenal Cortical Scintigraphy

Steroid production by the adrenal cortex uses cholesterol from the circulating pool as its primary raw material; thus, radiolabeled cholesterol analogues have been used for adrenal cortical scintigraphy. Several related agents have been developed; the two in greatest use are iodine-131-6β-iodomethylnorcholesterol (NP-59) and selenium-75-6β-selenomethylnorcholesterol (Scintidren). Of these, only NP-59 is available in the United States under Investigational New Drug guidelines. These agents have comparable imaging efficacy (5).

Adrenocortical scintigraphy should be undertaken only after all pertinent clinical, biochemical, and imaging data have been reviewed because it can be a moderately expensive and prolonged examination and can

result in significant patient radiation exposure. Nevertheless, it can be useful in differentiating between bilateral hyperfunctional disease (e.g., hyperplasia) and unilateral disease resulting from adenoma, and can in some situations demonstrate the side of abnormal function when sectional imaging does not confirm the presence of a mass. Additionally, it may be used to determine the function of a clinically or biochemically silent adrenal mass (6). Adrenocortical scintigraphy can also be used to localize functional adrenal cortical remnants or heterotopias following surgery when other imaging methods are inconclusive.

The sensitivity and specificity of adrenocortical scanning are essentially 100% in the setting of adrenocorticotropic hormone (ACTH)-independent Cushing's syndrome and hyperandrogenism; in the differentiation of aldosteronism caused by adenoma from hyperplasia, sensitivity is 90% and specificity is 90%, whereas sensitivity is 76% and specificity is 100% for assessment of the incidentally discovered adrenal mass. The safety of NP-59 has been established over many years. In a review of 729 doses of NP-59, adverse reactions were reported in only eight cases. Of these, seven were minor, self-limited reactions requiring no treatment. No severe, life-threatening reactions have been reported (6,7).

Adrenal Medullary Scintigraphy

Specific imaging of the adrenal medulla and related sympathetic tissues began with the development of a radiolabeled derivative of guanethidine, iodine-131-metaiodobenzylguanidine (MIBG) in 1980. Since then, MIBG has been used to detect many forms of pheochromocytoma and neuroblastoma and has shown affinity for other neuroendocrine tumors such as paragangliomas, carcinoid, and medullary thyroid carcinoma. It has also been used for radiation therapy in a limited way.

MIBG scintigraphy is clinically useful in a number of situations. While a patient with clinical and biochemical findings of pheochromocytoma and a definitive adrenal mass on CT or MRI rarely needs an MIBG scan, one can be obtained for confirmation of an equivocal lesion or for assessment of multiple lesions or potential sites of metastasis. Similarly, if cross-sectional imaging is negative and clinical and biochemical findings are present, an MIBG scan is indicated. MIBG is also useful in postsurgical pheochromocytoma patients with recurrent symptoms. Whereas general screening is inappropriate, patients at higher risk for sympathoadrenal lesions as indicated by a family history or by virtue of known predisposing disease such as neurofibromatosis, von Hippel-Lindau syndrome, or multiple endocrine neoplasias (MEN) type IIA or IIB may benefit. MIBG scintigraphy has a sensitivity of 80% to 100% and a specificity of 90% to 100% in the detection of pheochromocytomas (7). MIBG is similarly sensitive (75%–100%) and specific (nearly 100%) in the detection and localization of neuroblastoma. In the United States, only iodine-131 MIBG is commercially available; the iodine-123 form is available only at some centers, such as the University of Michigan. If possible, iodine-123 MIBG should be used because of its more optimal imaging and more favorable radiation dosimetry.

The only other commercially available radiopharmaceutical alternative to MIBG for assessment of some lesions, primarily paragangliomas and neuroendocrine (amine precursor uptake and decarboxylatin) tumors, is radiolabeled octreotide (indium-111 DTPA-D-Phe-1-octreotide), a synthetic octapeptide analogue of somatostatin (8). A number of other radiopharmaceuticals for adrenomedullary or sympathetic imaging have been investigated, including several positron emission tomography (PET) agents; none of these is generally available, aside from fluorine-18-2-fluorodeoxyglucose, a glucose metabolic agent that is not specific for sympathoadrenal tumors but may show dedifferentiated lesions of neuroblastoma and malignant pheochromocytoma that have lost their avidity for MIBG (9).

IMAGING OF ADRENAL PATHOLOGY

Pathologic conditions involving the adrenal gland can be divided along anatomic or physiologic lines. Anatomically, lesions may arise from the adrenal cortex or medulla or involve the entire gland; adrenal cortical disease may also be categorized by whether there is associated elevation or reduction of steroid hormone production or no effect on function (euadrenal lesions).

Diseases of Adrenal Cortical Origin

Hormonal Syndromes

Hypercortisolism

Cushing's Syndrome. Aside from iatrogenic causes, the most common cause of hypercortisolism in the adult is bilateral adrenal hyperplasia secondary to overstimulation by excess ACTH, termed Cushing's disease. Most pediatric cases are due to a primary adrenal neoplasm. In a small subgroup of adult patients, the source of ACTH is ectopic, most commonly from a bronchogenic small cell carcinoma or carcinoid tumor. The primary adrenal causes of adult hypercortisolism are almost evenly divided between benign and malignant neoplasms (adenoma or carcinoma); there is an even higher incidence of malignancy in the pediatric population.

Hyperplasia. When ACTH-dependent disease is present, the adrenal glands appear either normal or hyperplastic; when the glands are normal by CT, a diagnosis of hyperplasia is presumed. Marked bilateral enlargement is suggestive of an ectopic source of ACTH. Hyperplasia is present in up to 70% of patients with ACTH-independent disease and tends to be greater than that seen with hyperaldosteronism (10). Adrenal enlargement is most commonly smooth but may also be nodular. On MRI, hyperplasia is seen as homogenous, bilateral adrenal enlargement with preservation of the normal morphology, enhancement pattern, and signal characteristics on T1- and T2-weighted images. Adrenocortical scintigraphy shows bilateral adrenal uptake of radiocholesterol (6).

In 12% to 15% of cases of ACTH-dependent hypercortisolism, there can be bilateral masses related to macronodular hyperplasia, with contour distortion or discrete (<2 cm) nodularity on CT and MRI (11). As many as one-half of these patients can have asymmetric macronodular changes. If there is a significant size discrepancy, ACTH elevation may have to be confirmed by petrosal sinus sampling to prevent misclassification as unilateral disease (12).

Massive macronodular hyperplasia and primary pigmented nodular disease are uncommon causes of autonomous adrenal hypercortisolism. Macronodular hyperplasia results in complete replacement of the adrenal glands by nodules ranging from imperceptible up to 3 to 4 cm in diameter, with loss of the normal adrenal contours (13). Primary pigmented nodular disease is a cause of hypercortisolism in adolescents and young adults. In one published series, thin-section CT and MRI demonstrated nonenlarged glands with small (4- to 8-mm) nodules and atrophy of intervening parenchyma, giving a string-of-beads appearance. These nodules have a benign, low-signal appearance on T2-weighted MR images (14).

Hyperfunctioning Adenoma. In Cushing's syndrome, because of autonomous adrenal disease, there is most often a unilateral mass that may be an adenoma or a carcinoma, with a contralateral normal or atrophic adrenal gland on CT. An adrenal adenoma in this setting is most often 2 cm or larger in size and is readily detected by CT or MRI (15); adenomas are most often homogenous, round, or contour-deforming masses that are frequently hypodense relative to normal parenchyma by CT, occasionally resembling a cyst. On MRI, signal characteristics are homogenous, usually similar to those of the normal adrenal and liver, although many hyperfunctioning adenomas may show some increase in signal on T2-weighted images. Adrenal adenomas show mild, homogenous enhancement on CT and postgadolinium MRI, with relatively rapid washout of contrast on MRI (16). Chemical-shift MRI may show significant signal loss on out-of-phase images (17). Adrenocortical scintigraphy shows ipsilateral uptake corresponding to the adenoma, with suppression of uptake by the normal gland (6).

Adrenal Cortical Carcinoma. Adrenal cortical carcinoma is an uncommon malignancy that can occur at any age, usually presenting in the fifth decade of life. Approximately 50% of these carcinomas cause symptoms related to hormone excess. Whereas adrenal carcinoma is rare in the pediatric population, it is almost always functional. Most adult patients with functional adrenal cortical carcinoma are first seen with Cushing's syndrome, accounting for 10% to 20% of cases. These are aggressive malignant lesions that are most often large at the time of presentation, generally larger than 4 cm and not uncommonly in excess of 10 cm, and easily detected by CT and MRI (18).

Adrenal carcinomas often contain regions of necrosis and may also show calcification. By imaging, the diagnosis of malignancy is often suggested by the large size of the lesion. Sonography of smaller (3- to 6-cm) carcinomas shows well-delineated, round to lobular masses with homogenous echogenicity similar to that of renal cortex. Larger masses demonstrate heterogeneity from underlying necrosis, hemorrhage, and calcification. US is unable to distinguish benign from malignant lesions (19). CT demonstrates a soft-tissue mass that may have hypodense regions resulting from necrosis and heterogenous enhancement and can show calcifications (18). On MRI, these masses can be isointense or hypointense to liver on T1-weighted images and are almost always hyperintense on T2-weighted images (Fig. 3-1); carcinomas are often heterogenous on all sequences (4,20). Demonstration of internal hemorrhage is probably more common on MRI than on CT (20). Calcifications are often difficult to depict on MRI. Following intravenous contrast administration, enhancement is often rapid, with prolonged retention on delayed images, peripheral nodularity, and better demarcation

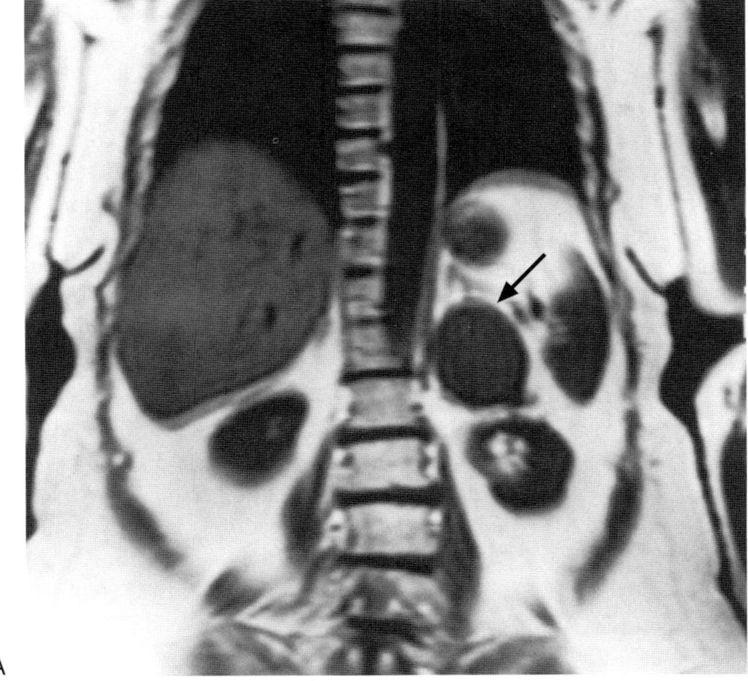

A

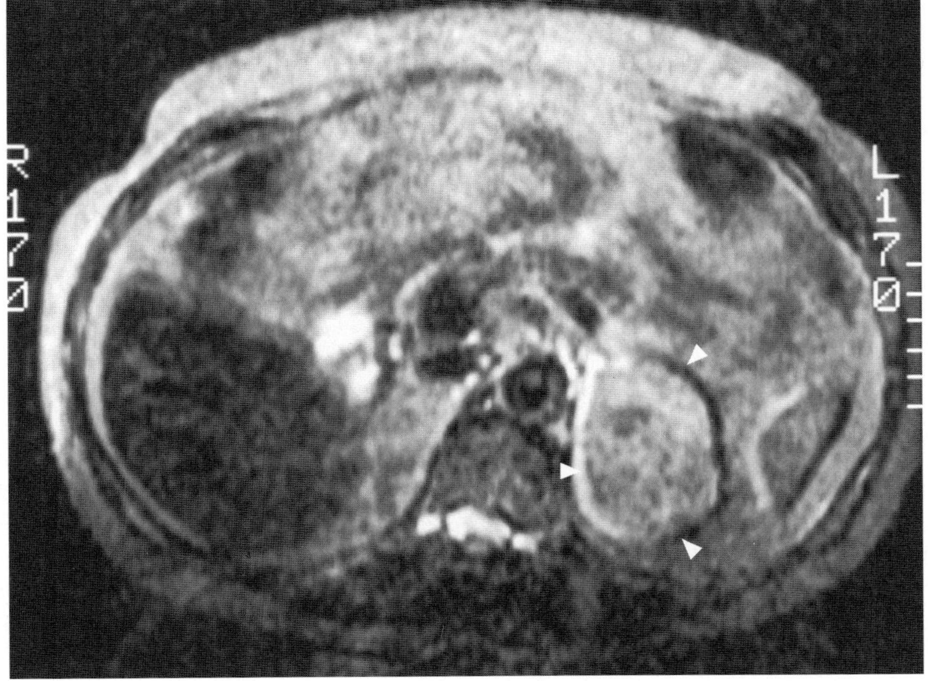

B

FIG. 3-1. A 70-year-old woman with new-onset Cushing's syndrome. **A:** Coronal T1-weighted MRI showed a round 5- to 6-cm adrenal mass (*arrow*) isointense to liver. **B:** An axial T2-weighted image showed heterogenous signal in this mass (*arrowheads*) greater than that of the liver or adjacent splenic tip. These findings were not that of adenoma. Biopsy revealed a functioning adrenal cortical carcinoma.

of areas of necrosis (16,20). Adrenocortical scintigraphy most frequently shows nonvisualization of either adrenal gland because of the relatively poor radiocholesterol concentration and relative inefficiency of glucocorticoid synthesis by the carcinoma (6).

Extraadrenal tumor spread is well imaged by CT; however, MRI can complement or surpass CT by allowing better assessment of regional organ invasion with sagittal or coronal imaging. Flow-sensitive MR sequences can also depict vascular invasion or thrombosis (20) (Fig. 3-2); in one series, MRI detected all cases of inferior vena cava tumor thrombi (21).

Hyperaldosteronism

Primary aldosteronism, termed *Conn's syndrome,* is due to unilateral adenoma in most (80%) cases. The remainder of cases (20%) result from bilateral adrenal hyperplasia. Even though patients with adrenal cortical carcinoma may have clinical features of mineralocorticoid excess, this is found most often in conjunction with excess cortisol or another steroid and almost never as pure, primary aldosteronism. Generally, patients with hyperaldosteronism are initially imaged with high-resolution CT, although adrenocortical scintigraphy and venous sampling are sometimes needed for final diagnosis. The ability of adrenocortical scintigraphy to determine the nature of hyperaldosteronism is at least equal to that of CT and has sensitivity and specificity reported at 90% (6).

Hyperfunctioning Adenoma (Conn's Syndrome). Most cases of aldosteronism result from a hypersecreting adenoma, usually unilateral. These adenomas tend to be small, in contrast to those causing hypercortisolism; they can be less than 1 cm in size and are rarely larger than 3 cm (22). Although CT should still be the initial examination of choice, the relatively smaller size of the aldosteronoma makes definitive detection by CT and MRI more difficult; in one series, CT was shown to detect only 70% of aldosteronomas (22). Unlike in Cushing's syndrome, negative or equivocal CT findings should not suggest hyperplasia; rather, indeterminate re-

sults of sectional imaging should be followed up by adrenocortical scintigraphy or adrenal venous sampling. The aldosterone-secreting adenoma is not otherwise differentiated from other adenomas by CT or MRI; unlike radiocholesterol scintigraphy, the functional status of an adrenal adenoma cannot be determined by sectional imaging (4,23). Unilateral, early visualization of the adrenal gland on adrenocortical scintigraphy performed under dexamethasone suppression is diagnostic of aldosteronoma (Fig. 3-3) (6).

Hyperplasia. Morphologically, adrenal gland hyperplasia associated with primary hyperaldosteronism is generally bilateral and may be micronodular or macronodular; unilateral macronodular hyperplasia causing aldosteronism has also been reported in the pediatric population. On CT scan, the glands may appear normal, may be homogenously enlarged, or may show nodular enlargement. Hyperplasia has been reported by US, but sonography generally has little to offer in this clinical setting. Adrenocortical scintigraphy typically shows bilateral, early adrenal gland visualization (Fig. 3-4) (6).

When there is evidence on sectional imaging of bilateral masses or a unilateral mass with enlargement of the contralateral gland, a diagnosis of hyperplasia is often assumed; however, in one series of 28 patients with hyperaldosteronism, eight of ten patients diagnosed by CT as having hyperplasia were ultimately shown by adrenal venous sampling and adrenalectomy to have adenoma (12). Because of the increased prevalence of nonhyperfunctioning adrenal nodules in older patients and in those with hypertension and hyperaldosteronism, closer evaluation with functional studies such as adrenocortical scintigraphy and venous sampling may be indicated before hyperplasia is assumed and the patient is denied a surgical cure.

Virilization and Feminization

This group of clinical syndromes arises from overproduction of sex steroid hormones. The symptoms and clinical features depend on the severity of the hormonal abnormality,

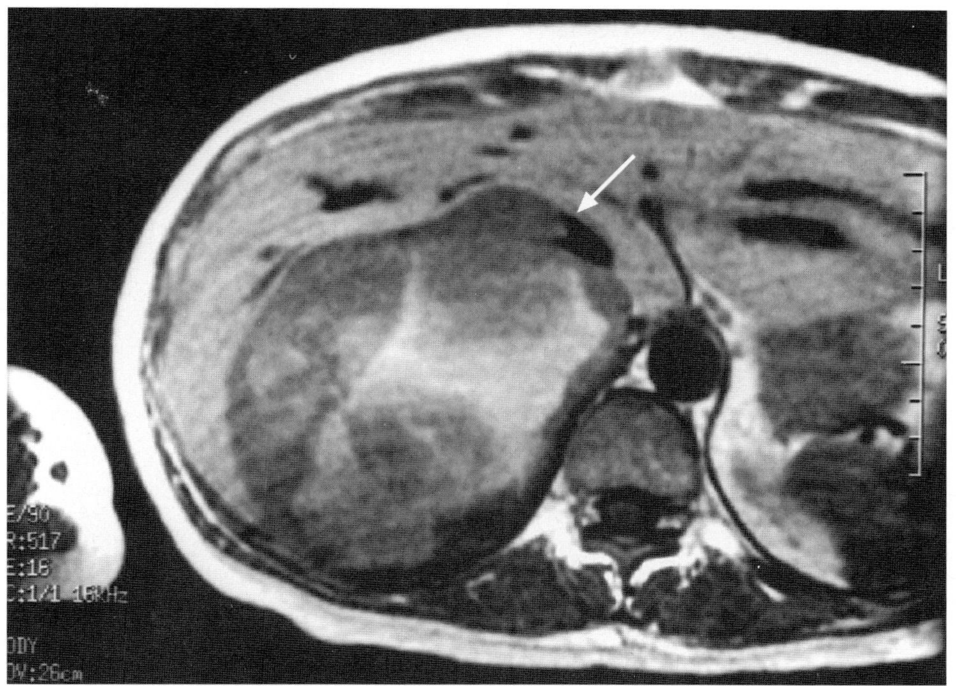

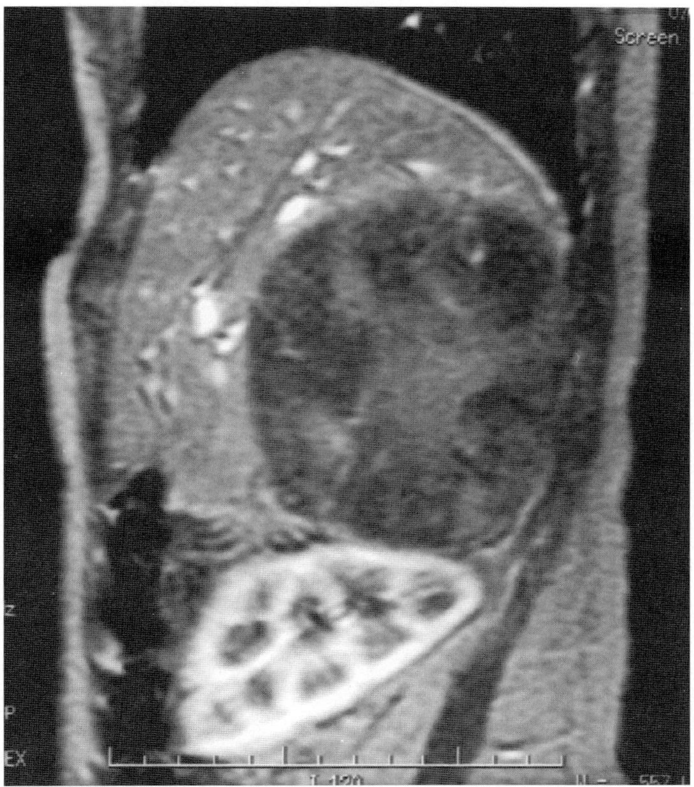

FIG. 3-2. A 37-year-old woman with a large adrenal cortical carcinoma was sent for magnetic resonance imaging study because there was concern about vascular invasion and tumor thrombus. **A:** An axial T1-weighted image showed a very large right adrenal mass, with central high signal resulting from hemorrhage and necrosis; there was tumor extending into the displaced inferior vena cava (*arrow*). **B:** A dynamic, breath-hold, sagittal gradient-echo image with bolus intravenous gadolinium contrast demonstrated the adrenal carcinoma to be hypovascular to the displaced right kidney and liver, with no sign of invasion of these organs.

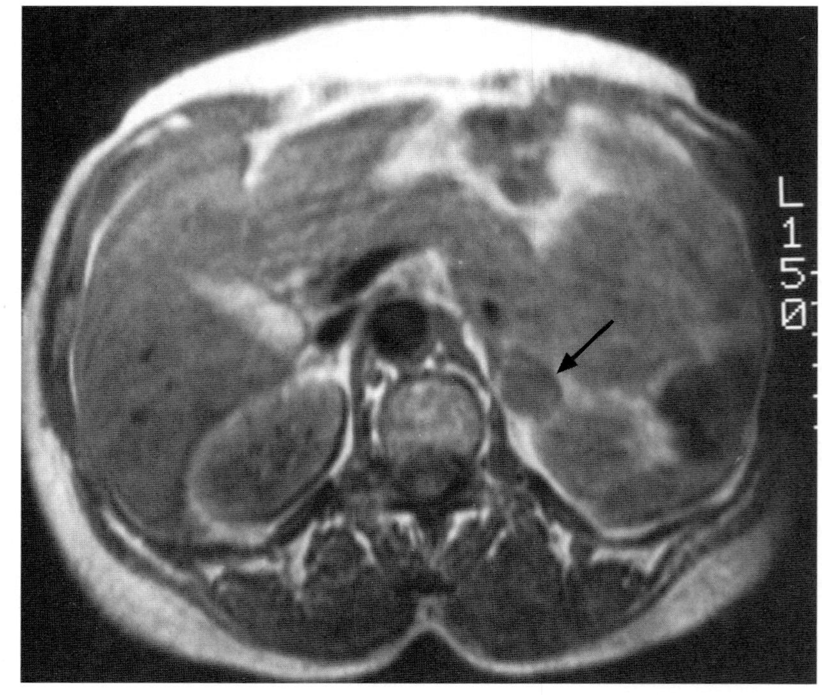
A
L 150

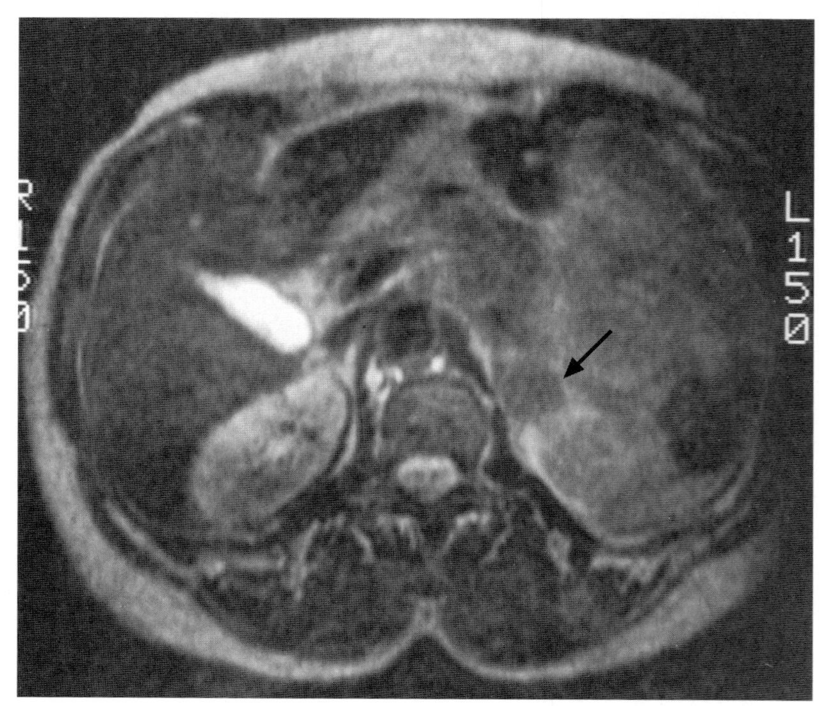
R
L 150
B

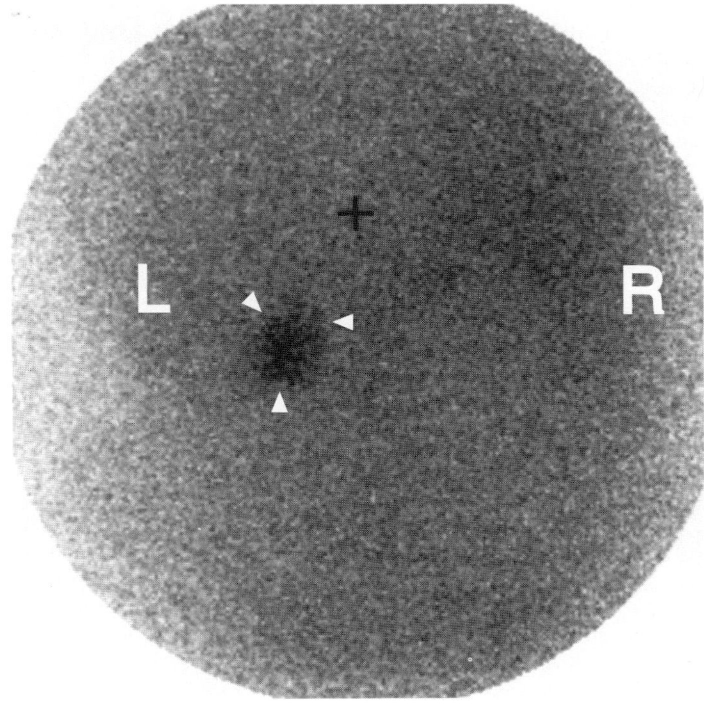

C

FIG. 3-3. A 47-year-old woman with signs and symptoms of hyperaldosteronism. **A:** Axial T1-weighted magnetic resonance imaging scan showed a 2-cm left adrenal mass (*arrow*), which was hypointense to the liver. This mass demonstrated low signal on T2-weighted **(B)** images. A posterior iodine-131 iodocholesterol (NP-59) scan **(C)** showed unilateral, early uptake in the left adrenal (*arrowheads*) concordant to the mass. These findings are all typical of adrenal adenoma.

the age of onset, and the sex of the patient. Clinical features may include virilization in women, precocious puberty, or pseudohermaphroditism. In male patients, feminizing lesions can result in gynecomastia, testicular atrophy, and decreased libido or impotence. The most frequent cause of virilization is due to congenital adrenal hyperplasia (CAH). Less common adrenal causes are adenoma or functioning carcinoma.

Hyperplasia. CAH is a group of autosomal recessive disorders arising from a congenital enzymatic defect in the steroid synthesis pathway, most often (90%) a 21-hydroxylase deficiency. Most of these patients have virilism from androgen excess. Most cases are diagnosed in childhood and, if severe, may be detected in the perinatal period. Sonography is useful to assess the adrenal glands and to determine whether a uterus is present (24).

On US, the adrenal glands in infants with CAH usually appear enlarged or at the upper limits of normal in size (24). There is preservation of corticomedullary differentiation. Adrenal hyperplasia may appear smooth or nodular on CT or MRI, as previously described. Adrenocortical scintigraphy performed under dexamethasone suppression typically shows bilateral, early adrenal visualization (6).

Hyperfunctioning Adenoma and Adrenal Cortical Carcinoma. These lesions are infrequently seen and have imaging characteristics indistinguishable from those of adrenal adenomas or adrenocortical carcinomas, as previously described. Adenomas are smaller masses, although generally not as small as those causing aldosteronism, frequently hypodense by CT, and have signal characteristics similar to those of liver or normal adrenal by

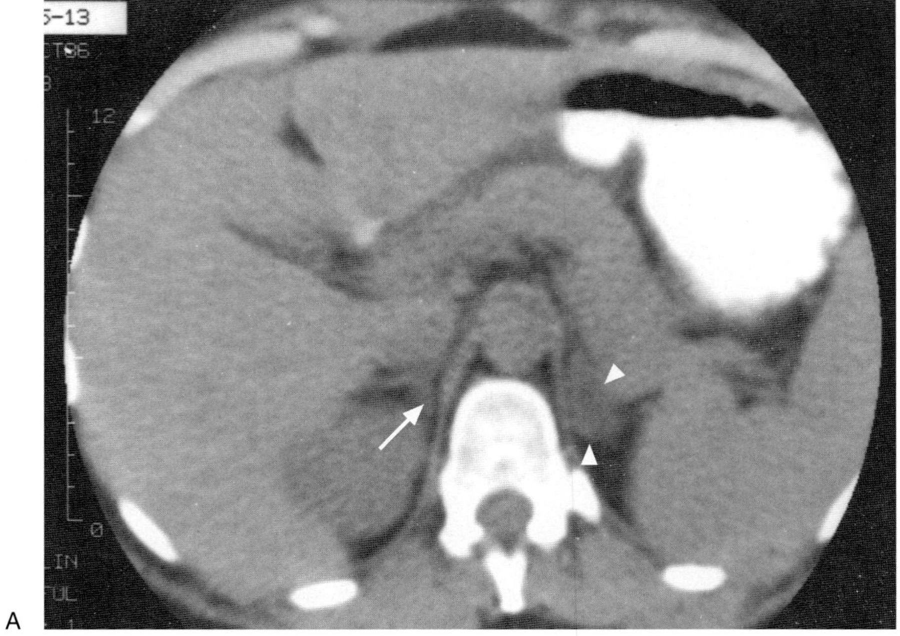
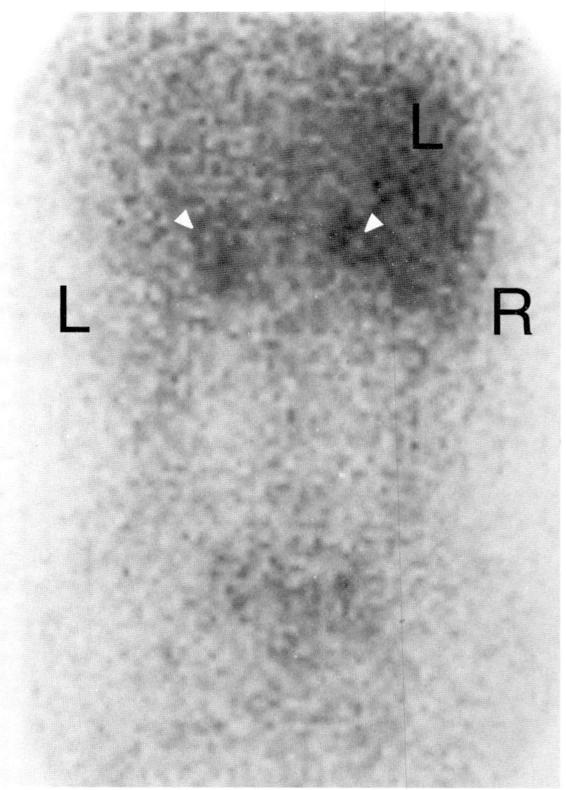

FIG. 3-4. A 38-year-old hypertensive man with clinical findings of hyperaldosteronism. **A:** Computed tomography showed rounded enlargement of the left adrenal (*arrowheads*), with thickening of the medial limb of the right adrenal (*arrow*). **B:** Iodine-131 iodocholesterol scan (NP-59) of the posterior abdomen on the fourth postinjection day showed prominent bilateral adrenal uptake (*arrowheads*) consistent with hyperplasia. Physiologic liver activity (*L*) is seen.

MRI. Carcinomas are usually considerably larger and can demonstrate necrosis or calcification by CT; MRI features include heterogeneity, low signal on T1-weighted images, and high signal on T2-weighted images. Primary carcinomas are often indistinguishable from other malignant adrenal masses by imaging features. On adrenocortical scintigraphy, unilateral, early adrenal visualization generally suggests an adenoma (6), although carcinoma has less commonly been demonstrated. Complete nonvisualization can be seen with extraadrenal causes, usually ovarian lesions or peripheral processes.

Adrenal Cortical Hypofunction (Addison's Disease)

Primary adrenocortical insufficiency requires loss of more than 90% of functional cortical tissue. The condition may be chronic, subacute, or acute. Even though cross-sectional imaging and imaging-guided biopsy are often useful in the diagnosis and management of subacute adrenal failure, imaging in acute adrenal insufficiency may be critical to patient management. In the United States, the most common cause of chronic adrenal cortical failure is idiopathic autoimmune atrophy. In this setting, the adrenal glands can appear normal or slightly decreased in size and imaging is rarely indicated (10). In other parts of the world, tuberculous adrenalitis is more common. Other causes of adrenal insufficiency include gland destruction by metastases, other granulomatous or fungal infections, bilateral hemorrhage, amyloid, hemochromatosis, congenital defects such as acid lipase deficiency or adrenoleukodystrophy, and surgical resection or ablation.

With longstanding adrenal failure from granulomatous infection, the glands can appear atrophic and may have dense calcifications. Although metastases are the most common cause of bilateral adrenal masses, they are a recognized cause of adrenal failure in less than 20% of these patients; particularly when calcification is not present or not appreciated, metastases may be indistinguishable from granulomatous disease on CT or MRI (25). Bilateral adrenal hemorrhage (apoplexy) is the most common cause of an acute addisonian crisis (Fig. 3-5).

Clinically Silent Adrenal Cortical Lesions

Nonhyperfunctioning Adenoma

Nonhyperfunctioning adenomas are common adrenal cortical lesions, which are most often seen by imaging as small, homogenous, round, contour-deforming masses (26); they are frequently hypodense relative to normal parenchyma by CT, reflecting their increased cellular lipid content, and occasionally even resembling a cyst. Radiographs and sonography do not show findings specific for adenoma, although US can be useful in excluding adrenal cyst. On MRI, signal characteristics are homogenous, usually resembling those of normal adrenal parenchyma, slightly hypointense relative to liver with T1-weighting, and isointense to mildly hyperintense with T2-weighting (27,28). Adrenal adenomas show early, mild, homogenous enhancement on contrast CT and postgadolinium MRI, with rapid washout of contrast on dynamic MRI (16,29). They most often lose signal on opposed-phase chemical-shift MRI images. Even though there is no endocrine excess, they are most often visible on adrenocortical scintigraphy and can appear symmetric to or more intense than the contralateral, normal gland (6,30).

Myelolipoma

Myelolipomas are rare, nonfunctioning, benign masses of the adrenal cortex, composed of varying proportions of mature fat and hematopoietic, myeloid elements. They are endocrinologically inactive and are typically discovered incidentally. Rarely, myelolipomas may be symptomatic on the basis of large size, necrosis, or hemorrhage, or may coexist with a functional lesion. The diagnosis is best established by the demonstration of fat in the lesion, usually by CT or MRI, although in

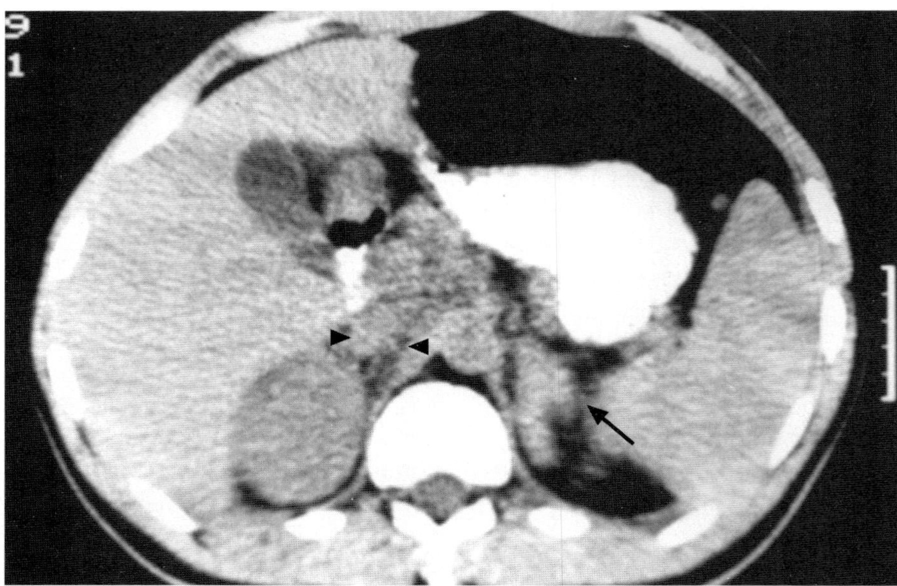

FIG. 3-5. A 36-year-old man with antiphospholipid antibodies. Noncontrast computed tomography scan showed diffuse enlargement and hyperdensity of the left adrenal (*arrow*) with enlargement of the partially seen right gland (*arrowheads*) consistent with adrenal hemorrhage.

cases in which there is little lipomatous tissue, biopsy may be required. Generally, the presence of macroscopic fat in a lesion on sectional imaging suggests a diagnosis of myelolipoma unless other malignant morphologic characteristics are present (Fig. 3-6). Differentiation from adrenocortical carcinoma or other malignant lesions can be difficult in cases in which there is a preponderance of myeloid elements or complications resulting from hemorrhage or infarction (31).

On radiographs or intravenous pyelography, a radiolucent mass displacing the kidney may be visible. The mass is frequently avascular at angiography. Ultrasonography typically shows a hyperechoic mass when abundant fat is present, which can be homogenous or heterogenous. Similarly, CT demonstration of a well-defined, mixed, fat and soft tissue or primarily fatty attenuation mass strongly suggests this diagnosis. CT may also show calcifications in these masses, and contrast enhancement may be visible in lesions with a significant myeloid component.

Lesions of the Adrenal Medulla

Pheochromocytoma

Pheochromocytoma is the most common tumor of the adrenal medulla. Most of these lesions arise sporadically, but they may occur with a familial predisposition or with hereditary diseases such as MEN IIA and IIB and neurocutaneous syndromes such as neurofibromatosis and von Hippel-Lindau syndrome. Approximately 10% of sporadic pheochromocytomas and 50% of familial pheochromocytomas are bilateral or multiple. Extraadrenal sites are present in 10% of sporadic cases. Malignant forms occur in more than 10% of cases. Because malignancy is more a corollary of the behavior of an individual lesion than a histologic determination, imaging has a significant role to play in diagnosis.

Most adrenal pheochromocytomas are 3 cm or larger at the time of presentation, are readily detected by CT (32), and can often be seen with US. The sonographic findings are not specific. A smaller mass may be rounded and have homogenous echogenicity. With a

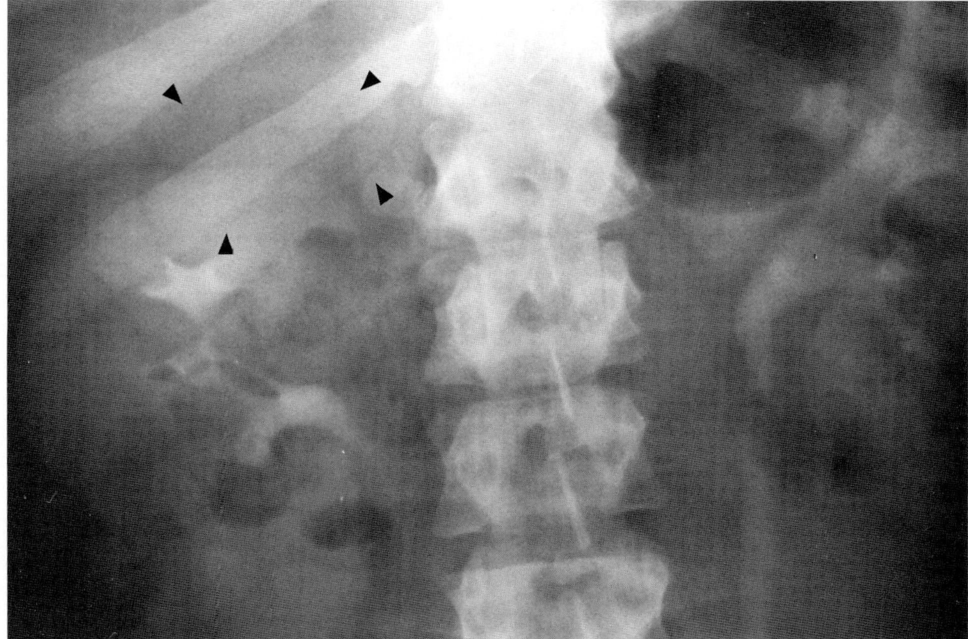

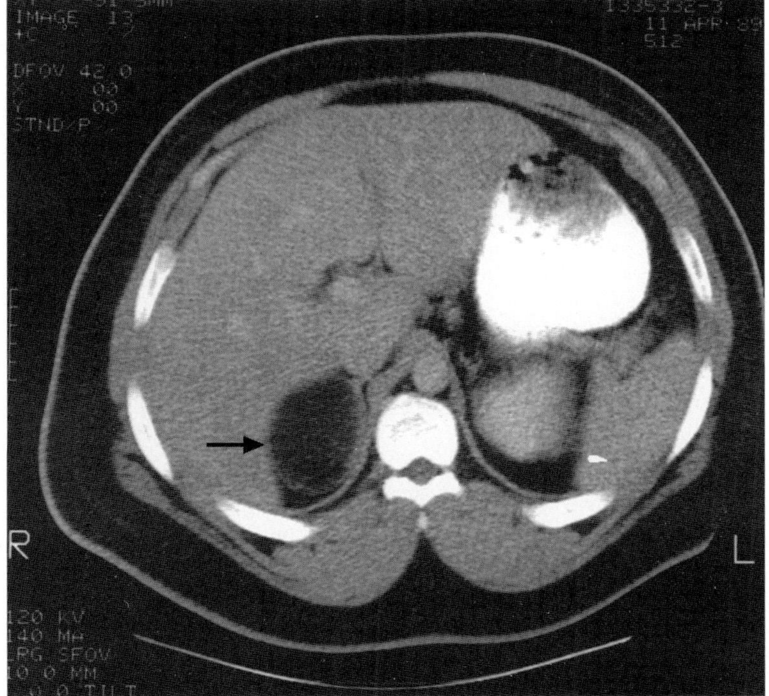

FIG. 3-6. A 20-year-old woman underwent excretory urography for suspected urolithiasis. **A:** A post-contrast radiograph showed displacement of the right upper renal pole by a mass (*arrowheads*). **B:** Computed tomography of the upper abdomen demonstrated a fat-attenuation mass splaying the limbs of the right adrenal (*arrow*) consistent with myelolipoma.

larger or necrotic mass, the echo pattern is heterogenous, with regions of hypoechoic change; echogenic calcification may be present, and if necrosis is massive, a complex cystic appearance may occur (33). On CT, pheochromocytomas are typically round, homogenous, soft-tissue attenuation masses that may also show central hypodense regions of necrosis and calcification (Fig. 3-7). Most adrenal lesions can be located by CT without the use of contrast; however, these tumors readily enhance with contrast administration, increasing the visibility of extraadrenal lesions. CT assessment of recurrent disease is less successful than for the initial diagnosis, possibly because of the smaller size of lesions or postoperative artifacts (32); MIBG scintigraphy and MRI play a greater role in evaluating these patients.

Adrenal and extraadrenal pheochromocytomas can be successfully localized by MRI (15,27). The typical MRI features include hypointensity on T1-weighted images and intense hyperintensity on T2-weighted images (27,28,34). The signal characteristics are frequently homogenous, particularly if a lesion is small (Fig. 3-8). If a tumor contains sufficient necrosis, hemorrhage, or calcification, heterogeneity may be present (Fig. 3-9) (15). Pheochromocytomas usually show intense, prolonged enhancement with intravenous contrast (16,29).

Nuclear medicine techniques in the evaluation of pheochromocytoma are well established and are more accessible since iodine-131 MIBG has become commercially available. Although still investigational, iodine-123 MIBG is the preferred agent for adrenal medullary scintigraphy. A recent review shows a combined sensitivity of 86% and a specificity of 99% in a pooled group of more than 1,900 reported patients (7). CT and MRI are more sensitive than MIBG scintigraphy for adrenal pheochromocytoma but are

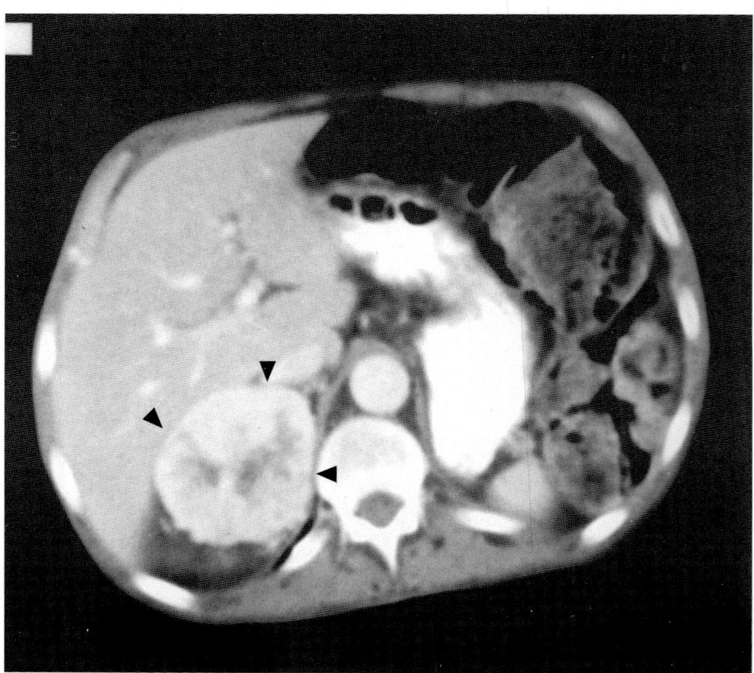

FIG. 3-7. A 56-year-old man with hypertension and elevated catecholamine levels. Contrast-enhanced computed tomography scan demonstrated a 7-cm enhancing, mixed-attenuation right renal mass (*arrowheads*). Pheochromocytoma was confirmed by metaiodobenzylguanidine scan, with subsequent resection.

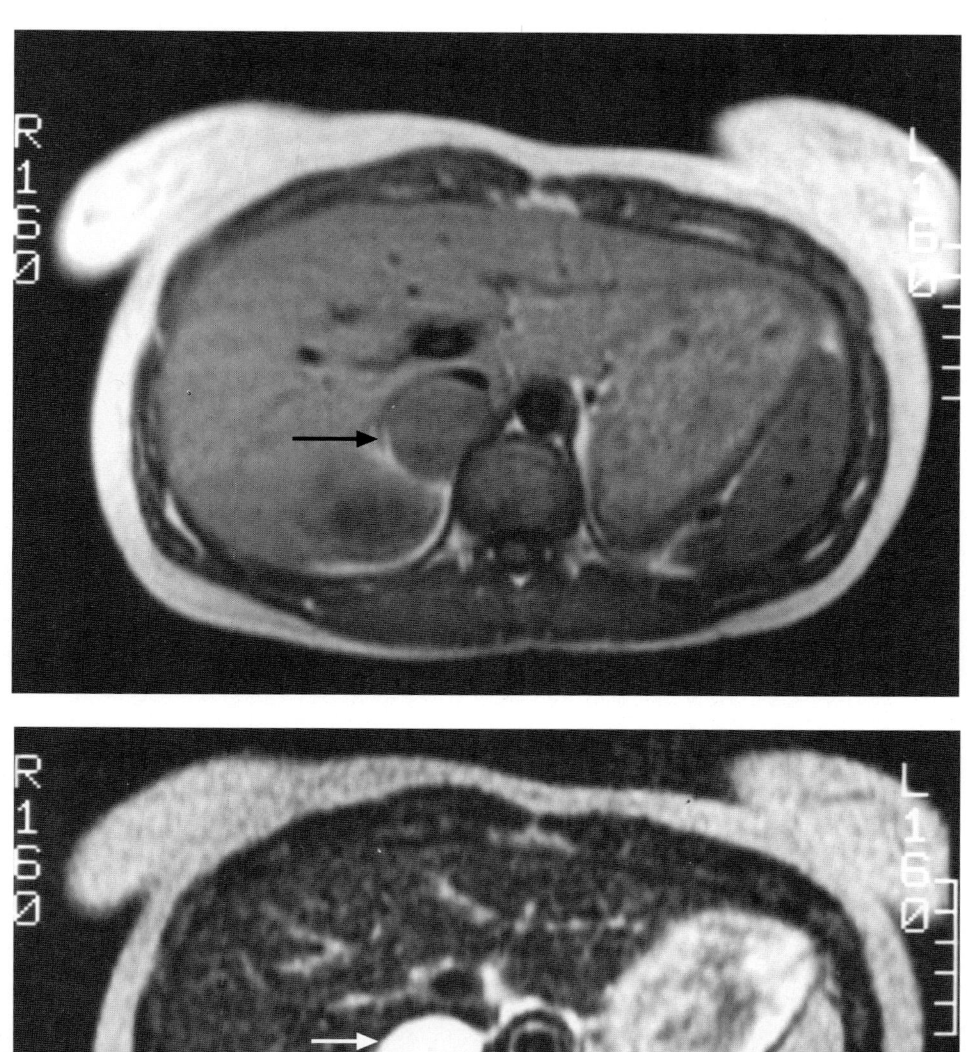

FIG. 3-8. A 22-year-old woman with labile hypertension and elevated catecholamine levels. **A:** T1-weighted axial magnetic resonance imaging scan demonstrated a 3- to 4-cm, well-demarcated, low-signal right adrenal mass (*arrow*), which was markedly hyperintense on T2-weighted images **(B)**, consistent with pheochromocytoma.

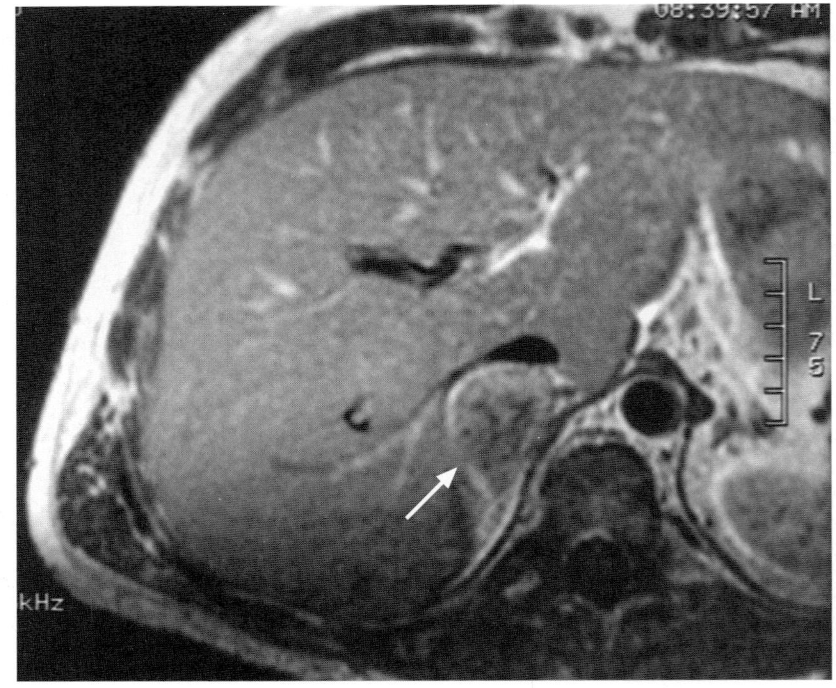

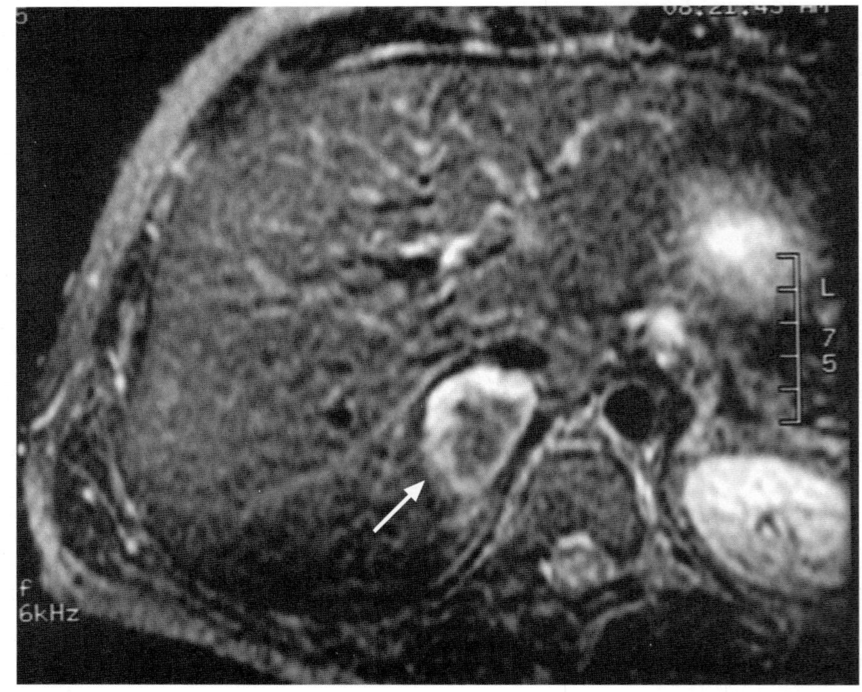

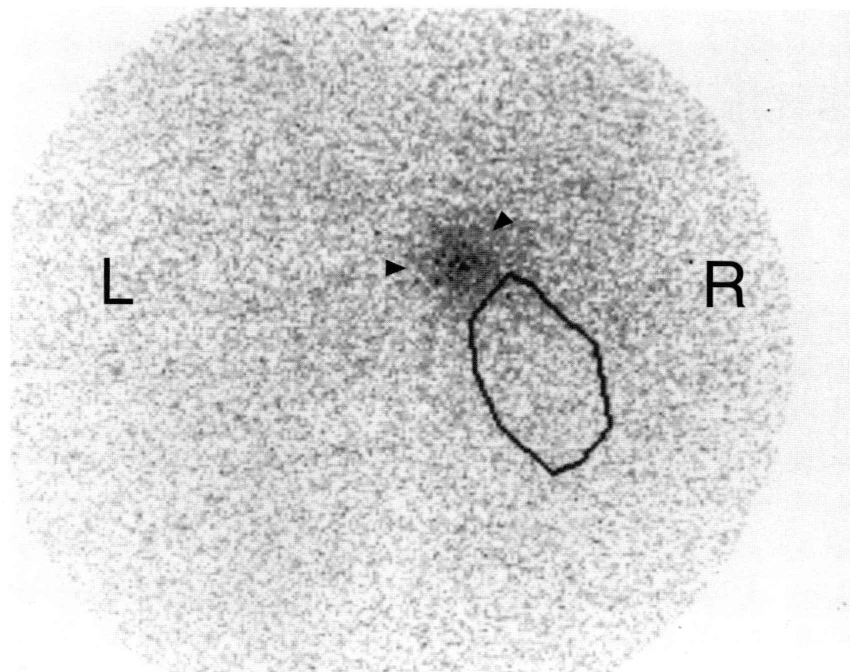

FIG. 3-9. A 41-year-old man with neurofibromatosis was referred for magnetic resonance imaging scan for suspected chest wall mass. **A:** An axial T1-weighted image showed an unsuspected heterogenous, primarily low-signal mass in the right adrenal gland (*arrow*), which was only peripherally hyperintense with T2 weighting **(B)** and contained central low signal resulting from hemorrhage or calcification. **C:** A posterior abdominal image from a subsequent iodine-131-metaiodobenzylguanidine scan confirmed the presence of a right suprarenal pheochromocytoma (*arrowheads*). The renal outline was traced from a concurrent diethylenetriaminepentaacetic acid (DTPA) renal scan used to confirm the anatomic location.

less specific (34); scintigraphy is better than CT for the assessment of extraadrenal disease and may be slightly better than MRI. Thallium-201 scintigraphy can image metastases from malignant pheochromocytoma, and indium-111-octreotide scintigraphy may also be useful in this setting (7,35).

The optimal imaging strategy in patients with pheochromocytoma has not been established. Initial evaluation may involve CT, MRI, or whole-body MIBG scanning, depending on the experience with and availability of these modalities at a given institution. CT has the advantages of speed and access, whereas MRI and MIBG scintigraphy are more sensitive but slightly more time-consuming and less available. MIBG scanning allows the entire body to be surveyed and is par-

ticularly useful if the iodine-123 labeled form can be used. Ultimately, a combination of these modalities may be the optimal strategy. Some authors have recommended MIBG screening of asymptomatic patients with MEN II, with further assessment of suspicious lesions by cross-sectional imaging, preferably MRI.

Neuroblastoma

Neuroblastoma is the most common extracranial solid tumor in children younger than age 5 years, and the adrenal medulla is the most common site of origin. Metastasis is frequent, with common sites of involvement including the lymph nodes, liver, skeleton, bone marrow, and skin. The initial imaging is most often done by radiography and US. Abdominal radiographs can demonstrate a mass or the presence of calcification; in this case, CT or preferably MRI should be performed. Otherwise, US is obtained to assess further for the presence of a mass. Neuroblastoma is usually a poorly marginated, predominantly solid suprarenal mass on sonography. It can be either hyperechoic or hypoechoic relative to the liver and is often heterogenous as a result of internal necrosis, hemorrhage, and calcification (36). Cystic change in the neonate has also been reported.

CT and MRI can both stage the extent of disease and assess visceral involvement and vascular encasement by this tumor; the multiplanar capabilities of MRI are particularly useful in demonstrating the organ of origin and assessing for vascular and spinal invasion. CT shows a variety enhancing solid mass and commonly identifies calcifications (Fig. 3-10). MRI visualizes calcifications poorly but shows neuroblastoma to be hyperintense to muscle, isointense to mildly hyperintense to liver on T1-weighted images, and hyperintense to both on T2-weighted images. Significant heterogeneity may be present. Unlike MIBG scanning, MRI is generally unaffected by ongoing therapy.

MIBG has high sensitivity (75%–100%) and a specificity of nearly 100% for the detection and localization of neuroblastoma (37); it is useful in the staging and follow-up of these patients (38). Iodine-123 MIBG is

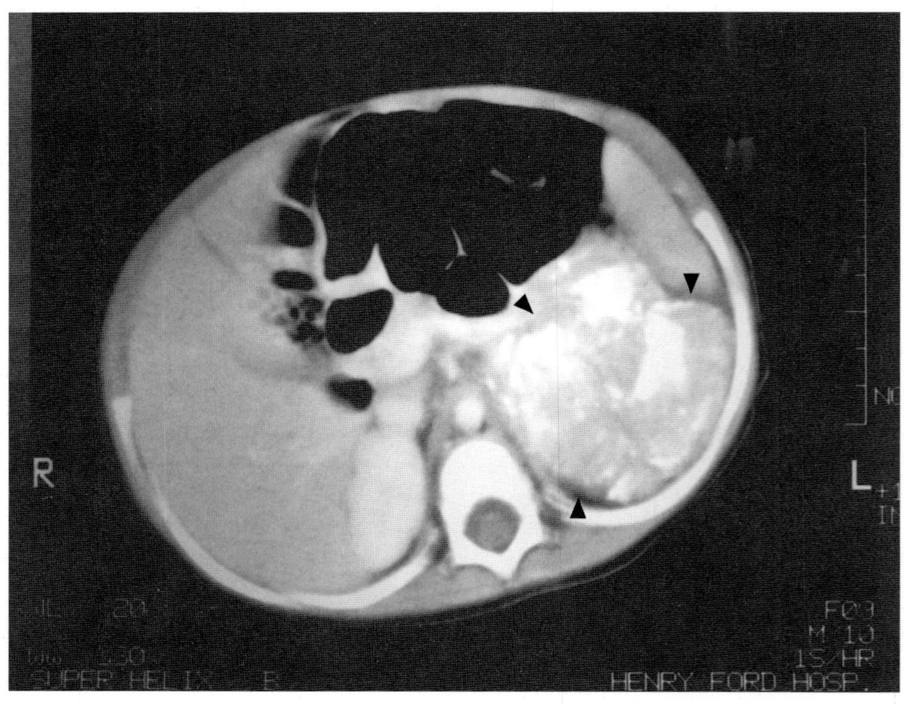

FIG. 3-10. A 3-year-old girl was diagnosed with stage IV neuroblastoma. **A:** Contrast-enhanced computed tomography showed a large, enhancing left suprarenal mass with extensive calcification (*arrowheads*). **B:** On bone scan, there was markedly abnormal uptake in the large left upper abdominal mass, as well as involvement of the skull base and sphenoid (*arrow*); there was residual activity in a right subclavian infusion catheter reservoir (*arrowhead*). **C:** Anterior iodine-131-metaiodobenzylguanidine scan of the chest and upper abdomen showed marked uptake in the left abdomen (*arrows*), consistent with neuroblastoma; physiologic uptake was seen in the heart (*H*) and liver (*L*).

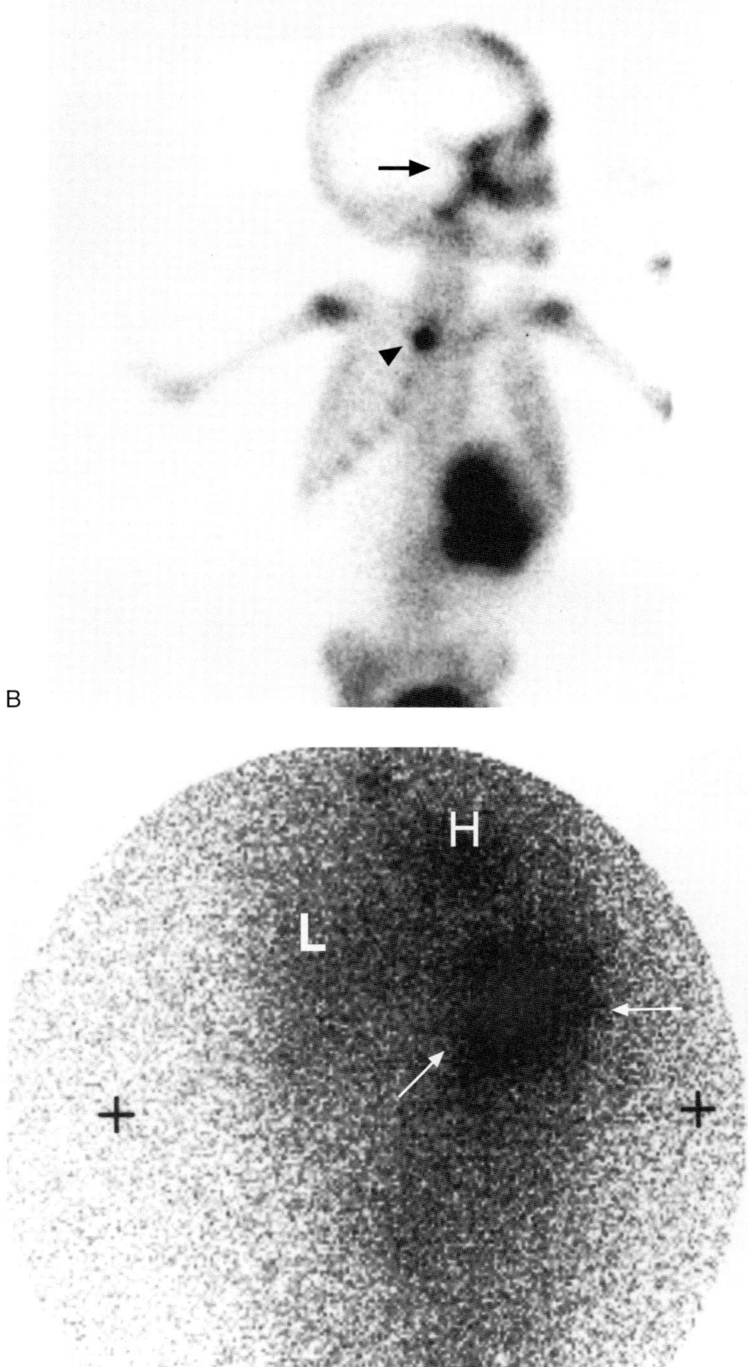

FIG. 3-10. *Continued.*

the preferred agent. MIBG and bone scintigraphy are both useful in the diagnosis of osseous involvement by neuroblastoma (38,39).

Hemorrhage

Adrenal hemorrhage is most commonly seen in the neonatal period, when it is the most frequent cause of an adrenal mass. It may occur with perinatal stress or hypoxia, sepsis, coagulopathy, renal vein thrombosis, and extracorporeal membrane oxygenation. It has been sonographically detected as early as in utero. Although radiographs may show a mass, the diagnosis is primarily made by sonography, which shows a round or adreniform mass that may be hypoechoic or cystic, heterogenous or hyperechoic, depending on the stage of hemorrhage. Increased echogenicity of the medulla may be the only sign of a small hemorrhage (Fig. 3-11). There are no pathognomonic sonographic findings in adrenal hemorrhage; hence, follow-up may be indicated to exclude an underlying mass such as a neuroblastoma. MRI can add specificity to equivocal sonographic findings. In the older child or adult, abdominal trauma may also cause hemorrhage.

In the adult, bilateral adrenal hemorrhage (apoplexy) is the most common cause of an acute addisonian crisis. Causes may be coagulopathy or anticoagulation, overwhelming sepsis (meningococcemia resulting in Waterhouse-Friderichsen syndrome), or metastases. The first line of evaluation involves CT, which shows enlarged, often hyperdense glands, a finding best appreciated on noncontrast scans (40). Traumatic hemorrhage more often involves the right adrenal gland. Acute hemorrhage is often focal and hyperechoic on US and presents as a hyperdense mass on CT. Late hemorrhage can become hypodense on CT (41) and hypoechoic, complex, or cystic on US. The appearance of adrenal hemorrhage on MRI varies as the blood components degrade and thus can be variable (Fig. 3-12). Acute hemorrhage can show decreased signal on both T1- and T2-weighted sequences; sub-

acute blood often has a high signal on T1-weighted images and may range from hypointense to hyperintense on T2-weighted images. Chronic changes from adrenal hemorrhage are typically of low signal as a result of hemosiderin deposition and calcification (31).

Other Tumors of the Adrenal

Metastatic Disease

The adrenal glands are a very common site of hematogenous metastasis and can also be involved by direct extension of retroperitoneal malignancies such as renal cell carcinoma. The most common tumors to metastasize to the adrenal are lung carcinoma and breast cancer; other common sources include melanoma, renal cell carcinoma, gastrointestinal tumors (especially gastric and pancreatic carcinoma), and thyroid cancer. Adrenal metastases are demonstrated by CT in more than 15% of patients with bronchogenic carcinoma (42). Normal-appearing adrenal glands on CT scan may still harbor microscopic metastases in a significant proportion of cases (43).

If a metastatic lesion is of sufficient size, it may be seen with virtually any imaging modality. Metastases are most often encountered with CT and tend to appear as soft tissue attenuation masses of variable size, which may be bilateral or unilateral. Depending on their size and type, they may contain areas of necrosis, calcification, or hemorrhage. The degree of contrast enhancement often depends on the vascularity of the primary tumor, although if a metastasis has undergone significant necrosis, it can appear quite different from the parent lesion. Large or necrotic masses suggest metastases; small lesions may appear indistinguishable from benign adenomas on CT. CT-guided biopsy is a common, accepted method for diagnosis, although scintigraphy and MRI can aid in determining the malignant or benign nature of adrenal lesions in a large proportion of patients (Fig. 3-13).

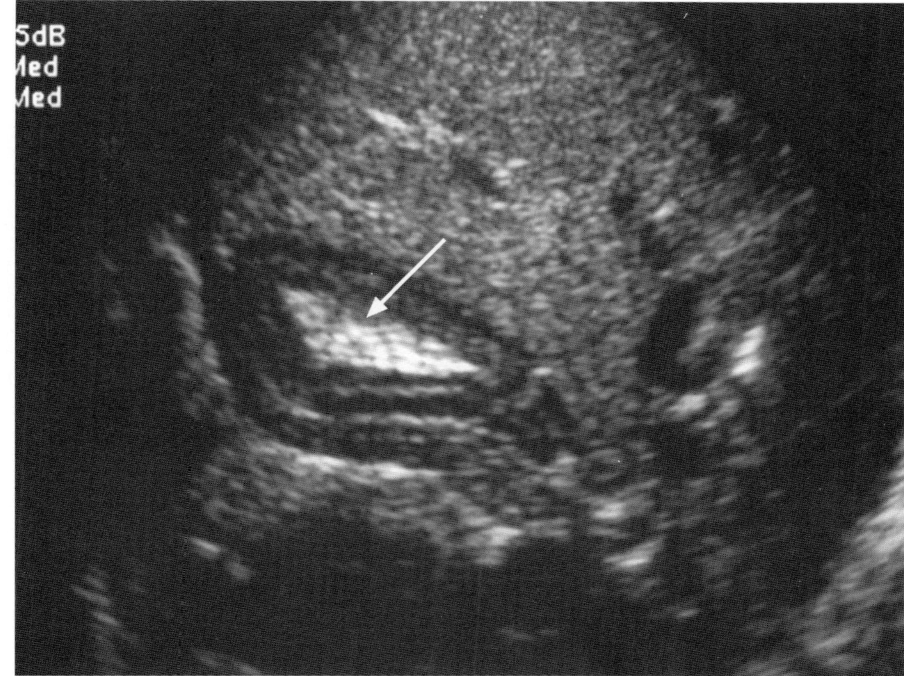

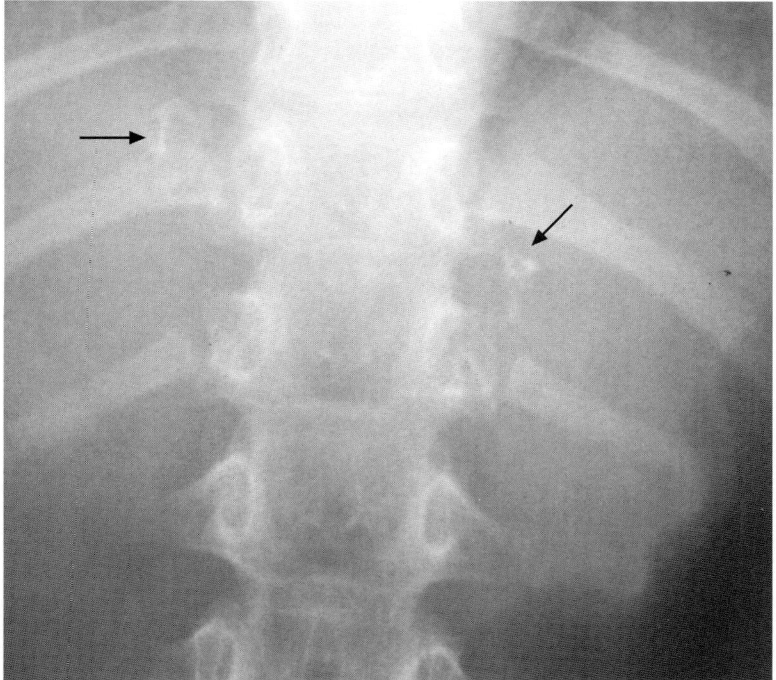

FIG. 3-11. A 1-day-old male infant was evaluated for possible renal anomaly resulting from the presence of a two-vessel cord. **A:** Abdominal ultrasonography revealed a prominent echogenic right adrenal medulla (*arrow*), consistent with hemorrhage. An abdominal radiograph **(B)** of a 7-year-old girl demonstrated incidental bilateral adrenal calcifications (*arrows*), consistent with previously unsuspected adrenal hemorrhages.

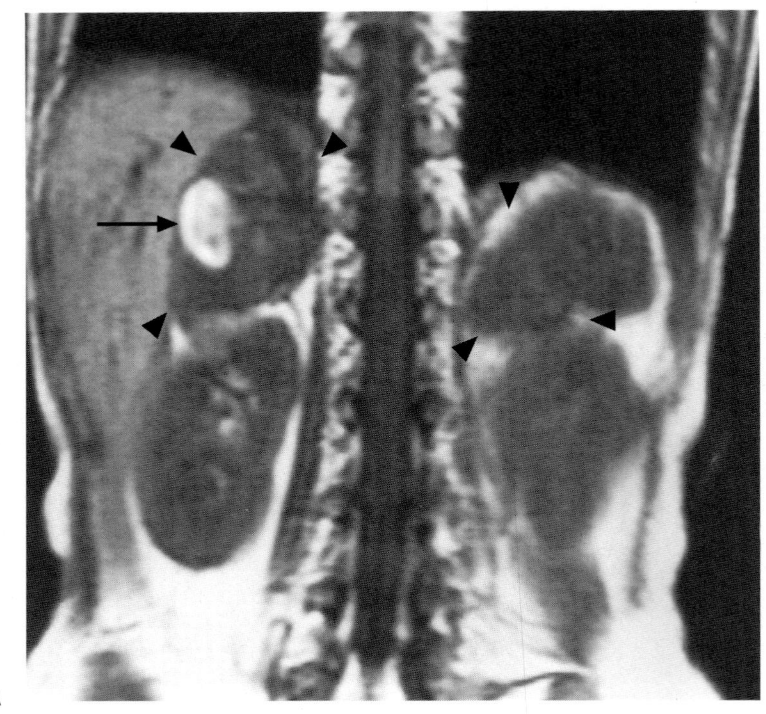

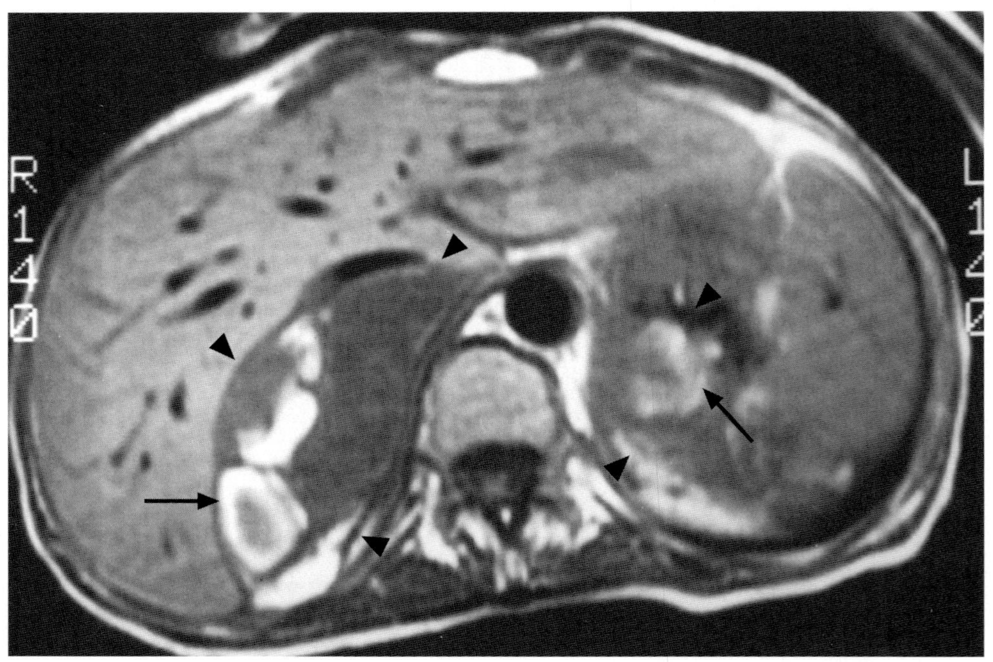

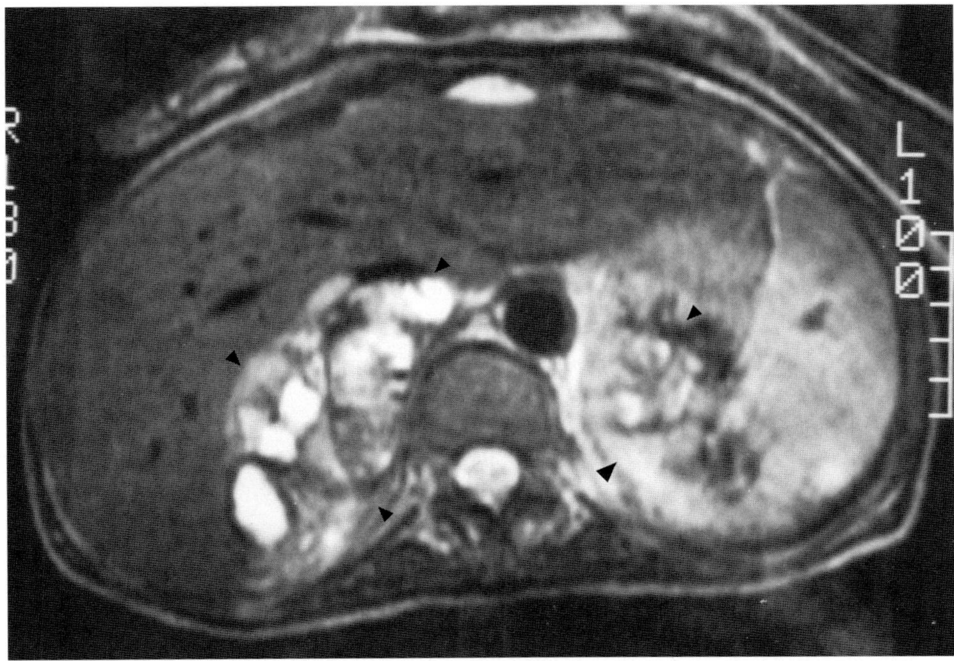

C

FIG. 3-12. A 50-year-old woman with metastatic melanoma to the brain. Coronal **(A)** and axial **(B)** T1-weighted magnetic resonance imaging (MRI) study showed bilateral large adrenal metastases (*arrowheads*) predominantly of lower signal than the liver, with high-signal hemorrhagic zones (*arrow*), more prominently on the right. **C:** Axial T2-weighted MRI showed heterogeneity of these metastases *(arrowheads),* with high- and low-signal changes resulting from hemorrhage.

On MRI, adrenal metastases are typically hypointense to liver on T1-weighted images and significantly hyperintense to liver on T2-weighted images. Heterogeneity may be produced by necrosis, and if there is hemorrhage there may be hyperintensity on T1-weighted images (see Fig. 3-12) (4,23,28). There is usually strong, early to mid-phase contrast enhancement on dynamic imaging after intravenous gadolinium chelate injection, followed by delayed washout of 15 minutes or more (16,29). There is generally no signal loss with opposed-phase chemical-shift gradient echo images (17).

Lymphoma

Most cases represent non-Hodgkin's lymphoma, primarily in patients who also have extraadrenal disease. Primary adrenal lymphoma is rare. Involvement of the adrenal glands by non-Hodgkin's lymphoma has been shown by CT as causing diffuse enlargement, which is round, oval, or triangular (44). MRI usually demonstrates bilateral masses, which are of low signal on T1-weighted images and show moderate hyperintensity on T2-weighted images, with abnormal enhancement akin to that of metastases. Lymphoma cannot be distinguished from metastasis or other malignant lesions on MRI (4,31).

Hemangioma

Hemangioma is an unusual neoplasm in the adrenal gland, with a number of cases having been reported in the imaging literature. The US appearance is variable and seems to be nonspecific. CT shows a low-attenuation mass, often heterogeneous, with peripheral, phlebolith-like calcification, which may also be visible on radiographs; there can be irregular calcification from previous hemorrhage as well. With contrast, there is heterogenous

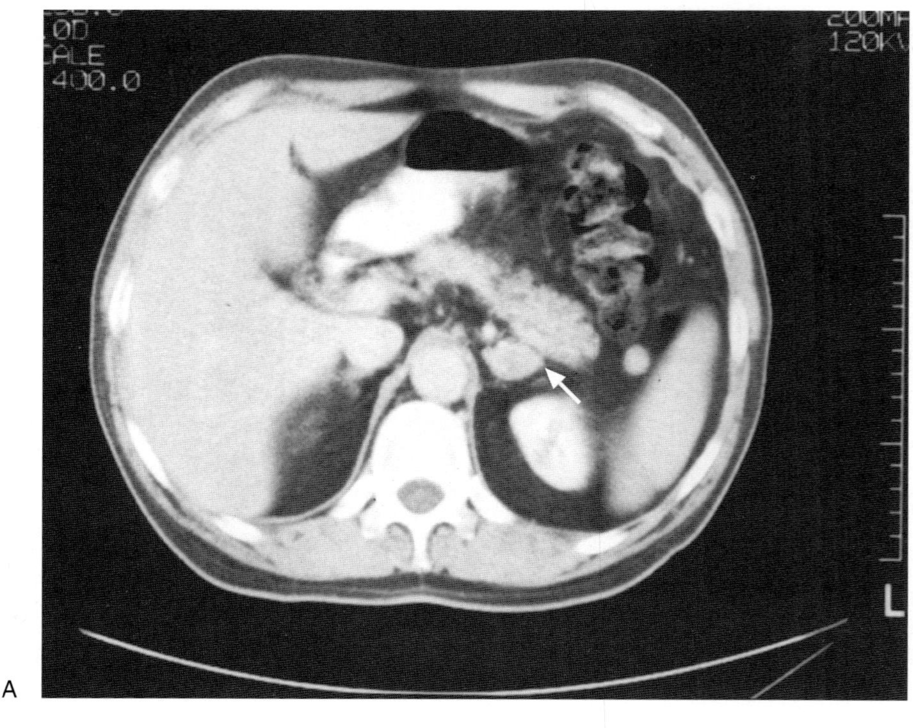

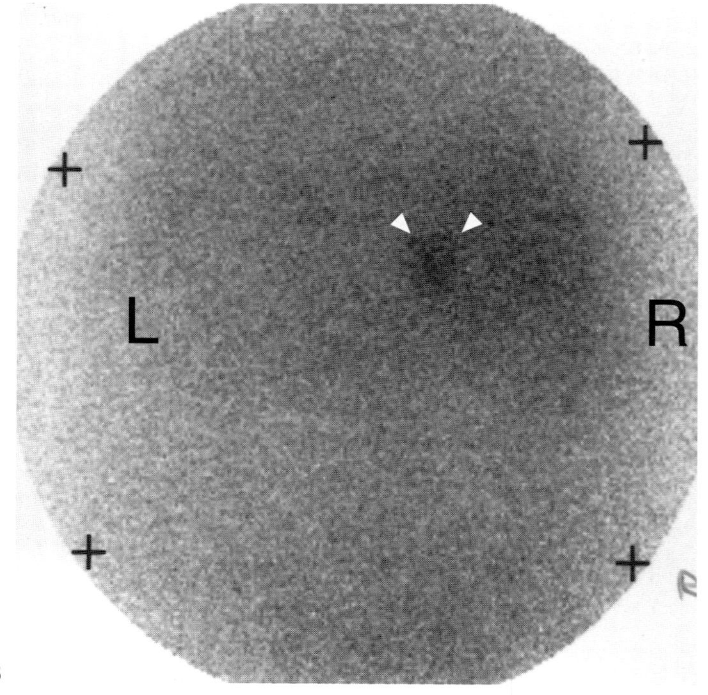

FIG. 3-13. A 55-year-old man with lung carcinoma had a 2-cm indeterminate left adrenal mass (*arrow*) on staging computed tomography study **(A)** and no biochemical abnormality. **B:** An iodine-131 iodocholesterol (NP-59) scan demonstrated discordant adrenal uptake, with visualization of only the right adrenal (*arrowheads*), excluding nonhyperfunctioning adenoma. Subsequent biopsy revealed metastasis to the left adrenal.

peripheral enhancement, which can progress toward the center of the lesion (45). MRI has shown hemangiomas to be heterogenous low-signal masses on T1-weighted images, which become hyperintense on T2-weighted images and show a somewhat hypointense, stellate central region of presumed fibrosis (45,46). On postgadolinium T1-weighted images, heterogenous peripheral enhancement can be seen.

Miscellaneous Lesions

Infection

Adrenal abscess may occur by bacterial seeding of a hematoma. The US appearance is generally that of a complex, hypoechoic cyst with internal debris and echoes, although it can appear as a solid mass. Differentiation from a necrotic tumor or pseudocyst can be difficult and may require aspiration. CT may show a heterogenous or hypodense mass with peripheral inflammatory stranding of retroperitoneal fat. A characteristic appearance on MRI has not been described.

Infection disseminated to the adrenal glands is most often granulomatous. Although infectious adrenalitis is not often seen in industrialized nations, it may occur more frequently in the immunocompromised patient. There are no specific imaging features; acutely, bilateral enlargement and variable necrosis and calcification may be seen. With longstanding granulomatous adrenalitis, the glands can appear atrophic and may have dense calcifications (47,48). Calcification is poorly distinguished on MRI, although it is clearly seen with CT. Limited descriptions in the literature suggest that tuberculous adrenalitis manifests with low-signal changes on T1-weighted images and increased signal on T2-weighted images (25). Generally, granulomatous infection of the adrenals is seen in patients who also have extraadrenal disease and causes a spectrum of CT findings, including small regions of calcification, mild enlargement with hypodense nodularity, and symmetric enlargement with prominent regions of necrosis or massive calcification; gland enlargement with maintained adreniform or cylindrical morphology is visible with US (46).

Cysts

Adrenal cysts are uncommon in the adult, have a female predominance, and are most often unilateral. The most common causes are simple lymphangiomatous endothelial cysts (45%), which are usually small (15 mm or less) and inflammatory, necrotic, or hemorrhage pseudocysts (39%); the latter are more frequently detected clinically, in that these cysts can become quite large (49). In the neonate, they most often occur as pseudocysts arising with resolving hemorrhage (Fig. 3-14). Neuroblastoma can present in a cystic form, much as pheochromocytoma can in the adult. True epithelial or endothelial cysts are rare in this age group. True epithelial cysts are less common (9%). Cysts are also seen in parasitic infections (7%), often with echinococcal disease (49).

Adrenal cysts are round, hypodense, nonenhancing masses on CT and urography and, if small, may be difficult to discriminate from adenomas by CT. Like other cysts, they are typically anechoic and transmissive on US, although they can contain low-level echoes or debris if complicated. Adrenal cysts may have perceptible or calcified walls, particularly if complicated or parasitic, which can show enhancement. Septations can be seen in pseudocysts on CT, US, and MRI. The MR features are typically those of any fluid lesion: homogenous, marked hypointensity on T1-weighted images, and marked hyperintensity on T2-weighted images. No enhancement of the cyst occurs with gadolinium administration. If there is complex (hemorrhagic or proteinaceous) fluid in the cyst, there can be a variable degree of hyperintensity with T1 weighting (27). This may have to be differentiated from fat by the use of fat saturation techniques. Symptomatic cysts can be aspirated for diagnosis and treatment.

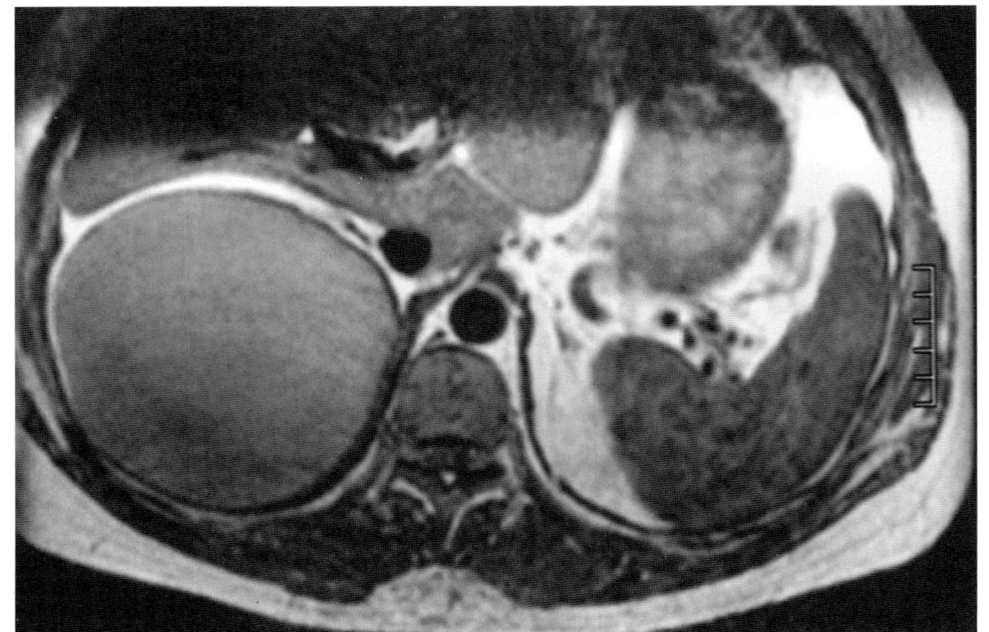

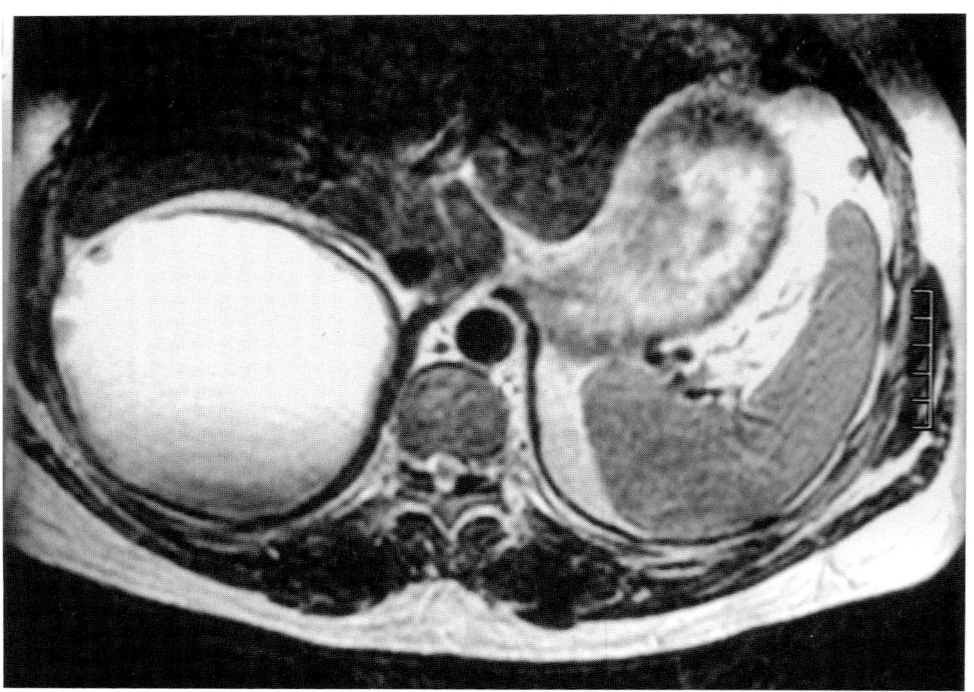

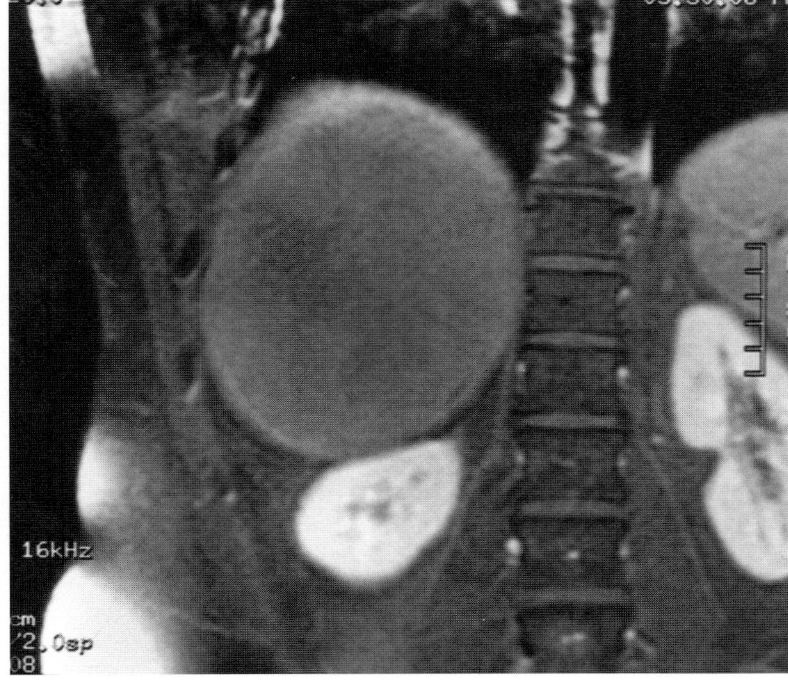

FIG. 3-14. A 38-year-old man with symptoms of upper abdominal mass. **A:** An axial T1-weighted magnetic resonance imaging study showed a homogenous, intermediate-signal, round right adrenal mass measuring 14 cm. **B:** An axial T2-weighted image showed the mass to be encapsulated, containing hyperintense, fluid-signal material, with papillary excrescences arising from the wall. **C:** A coronal postgadolinium contrast T1-weighted image showed only minimal enhancement along the wall. Pathologic examination following resection showed this to be a pseudocyst from prior hemorrhage.

The Incidental Adrenal Mass: Characterization as Benign or Malignant

Benign adrenal adenomas have an incidence of up to 9% and may be more common in hypertensive patients; hence, incidentally discovered adrenal masses by CT are commonly benign (50). Most malignant masses are metastases; however, a significant proportion of adrenal masses in oncologic patients are benign (51). The differentiation of benign from malignant adrenal masses is a common problem, particularly in the oncologic patient.

A number of methods using CT, MRI, and nuclear medicine techniques have been investigated as noninvasive solutions to this clinical conundrum. Simple morphologic analysis of the appearance of the lesion has proved insufficient. Increasing size, lesion heterogeneity, enhancement, and poor definition of margins favor malignancy; however, the overlap between benign and malignant lesions by size criteria alone is significant. Small masses (<3 cm) are generally benign in patients with no known primary malignancy, whereas up to 20% of similar masses may be metastases in oncologic patients.

As morphologic criteria have proven insufficiently specific, quantitative analyses of CT attenuation values, MRI T1 and T2 values, (4,23,27), and dynamic contrast enhancement patterns (16,29,52) have been attempted. Most recently, the promising chemical-shift MRI technique has been studied (17,53,54). Using this method, benign adenomas show a signal decrease on opposed-phase gradient-echo images because of their larger lipid content. The reported sensitivity of this method appears to approach 100% (Fig. 3-15). Nuclear medicine techniques use the functional

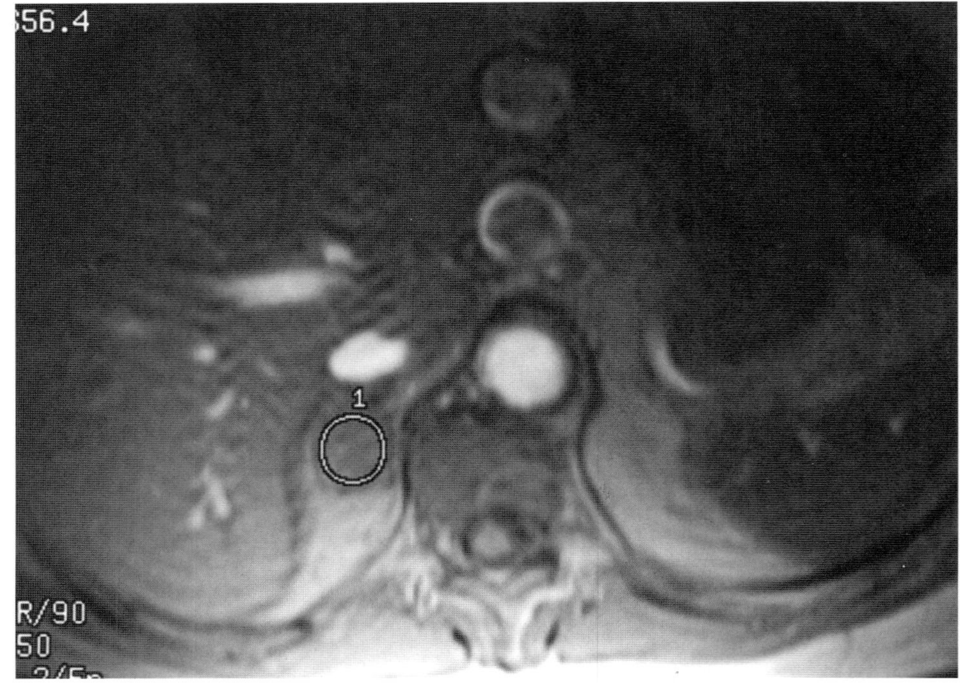

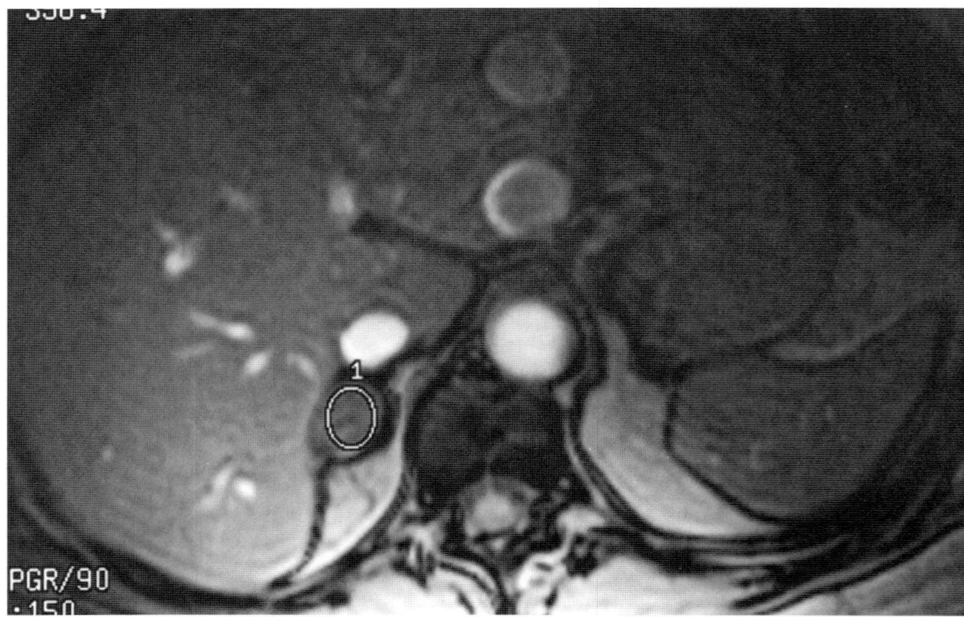

FIG. 3-15. A 70-year-old man was found to have a 3-cm right adrenal mass by computed tomography but no demonstrable biochemical abnormality. Gradient echo magnetic resonance imaging study obtained with fat and water in phase **(A)** and out of phase **(B)** showed homogenous low signal and significant signal loss of the mass on out-of-phase images. These findings were consistent with non-hyperfunctioning adenoma.

physiology of the benign adenoma and rely on detectable uptake within a lesion on adrenocortical scintigraphy as a determinant of benignity (see Fig. 3-13) (6,55). Recently, 2-[F-18]-fluoro-2-deoxy-D-glucose PET scanning has been shown to be useful in differentiating benign from malignant lesions (56).

The best current approach is to begin with CT. A lesion that has equivocal features but is large (5 cm or more) should be biopsied. Smaller lesions should be examined with chemical-shift MRI, especially if less than 2 cm in size, or with adrenocortical scintigraphy. Intermediate-sized (3–5 cm) lesions with otherwise benign features should be followed up and biopsied if they enlarge. An accurate direct comparison of the yield and costs of chemical-shift MRI versus iodocholesterol scintigraphy in this type of clinical scenario has not been performed to date; an analytic comparison by Dwamena and colleagues (57) favors adrenocortical scintigraphy but appears to be skewed by low NP-59 costs within their institution.

SUMMARY

CT is a mature modality and remains the mainstay of adrenal imaging. It is a rapid, accessible, and cost-effective technique for diagnosis, with continued improvements being made in speed and resolution. MRI is still rapidly being developed and has ever more to offer. Additionally, the lack of ionizing radiation makes it a desirable tool in the pediatric population. Application of surface-coil technology has improved its resolution in imaging of the adrenal glands, although CT remains superior in this regard. US is best exemplified by its ubiquitous role in pediatric imaging. Percutaneous image-guided biopsy methods have become widely accepted as safe and effective means of diagnosis, and angiographic and venous sampling techniques remain infrequently used but critical problem-solving tools.

MRI is being used with increasing success for characterization of adrenal masses, particularly since the advent of chemical-shift tech-

niques, and appears at least competitive with scintigraphic methods in this regard. In adrenocortical carcinoma and neuroblastoma, MRI is better able than CT to assess the origin, morphology, and potential vascular involvement by tumor. At present, the optimal role of MRI and adrenal scintigraphy is to supplement the diagnostic specificity of the initial evaluation by CT in many clinical situations. Adrenal cortical and medullary scintigraphy continue to offer invaluable physiologic information in addition to anatomic diagnosis. Although still not widely available, iodocholesterol adrenal cortical scintigraphy remains useful in the diagnosis of hyperaldosteronism, as well as in the diagnosis and preoperative assessment of patients with hypercortisolism. It can also be successfully used in the characterization of benign versus malignant solitary adrenal lesions. MIBG scintigraphy continues to be an effective tool in the diagnosis of pheochromocytoma and neuroblastoma.

REFERENCES

1. El-Sherief MA, Hemmingsson A, Lorelius LE. Computed tomography and angiography in the evaluation of adrenal diseases. *Acta Radiol Diagn (Stockh)* 1982;23: 625–637.
2. Abrams HL, Siegelman SS, Adams DF, et al. Computed tomography versus ultrasound of the adrenal gland: a prospective study. *Radiology* 1982;143:121–128.
3. Adams JE, Johnson RJ, Rickards D, et al. Computed tomography in adrenal disease. *Clin Radiol* 1983;34: 39–49.
4. Chang A, Glazer HS, Lee JK, et al. Adrenal gland: MR imaging. *Radiology* 1987;163:123–128.
5. Reschini E, Catania A. Clinical experience with the adrenal scanning agents iodine 131-19-iodocholesterol and selenium 75-6-selenomethylcholesterol. *Eur J Nucl Med* 1991;18:817–823.
6. Francis IR, Gross MD, Shapiro B, et al. Integrated imaging of adrenal disease. *Radiology* 1992;184:1–13.
7. Freitas JE: Adrenal cortical and medullary imaging. *Semin Nucl Med* 1995;25:235–230.
8. Krenning EP, Kwekkeboom DJ, Reubi JC, et al. 111 In-octreotide scintigraphy in oncology. *Metabolism* 1992; 41(9 suppl 2):83–86.
9. Shulkin BL, Mitchell DS, Ungar DR, et al. Neoplasms in a pediatric population: 2-[F-18]-fluoro-2-deoxy-D-glucose PET studies. *Radiology* 1995;194:495–500.
10. Glazer GM, Francis IR, Quint LE. Imaging of the adrenal glands. *Invest Radiol* 1988;23:3–11.
11. Doppman JL, Miller DL, Dwyer AJ, et al. Macronodular adrenal hyperplasia in Cushing disease. *Radiology* 1988;166:347–352.

12. Doppman JL. The dilemma of bilateral adrenocortical nodularity in Conn's and Cushing's syndromes. *Radiol Clin North Am* 1993;31:1039–1050.

13. Doppman JL, Nieman LK, Travis WD, et al. CT and MR imaging of massive macronodular adrenocortical disease: a rare cause of autonomous primary adrenal hypercortisolism. *J Comput Assist Tomogr* 1991;15:773–779.

14. Doppman JL, Travis WD, Nieman L, et al. Cushing's syndrome due to primary pigmented nodular adrenocortical disease: findings at CT and MR imaging. *Radiology* 1989;172:415–420.

15. Glazer GM. MR imaging of the liver, kidneys, and adrenal glands. *Radiology* 1988;166:303–312.

16. Krestin GP, Steinbrich W, Friedmann G. Adrenal masses: evaluation with fast gradient-echo MR imaging and Gd-DTPA-enhanced dynamic studies. *Radiology* 1989;171:675–680.

17. Mitchell DG, Crovello M, Matteucci T, et al. Benign adrenocortical masses: diagnosis with chemical shift MR imaging. *Radiology* 1992;185:345–351.

18. Dunnick NR. Adrenal carcinoma. *Radiol Clin North Am* 1994;32:99–108.

19. Hamper UM, Fishman EK, Hartman DS, et al. Primary adrenocortical carcinoma: sonographic evaluation with clinical and pathologic correlation in 26 patients. *Am J Roentgenol* 1987;148:915–919.

20. Schlund JF, Kenney PJ, Brown ED, et al. Adrenocortical carcinoma: MR imaging appearance with current techniques. *J Magn Reson Imaging* 1995;5:171–174.

21. Goldfarb DA, Novick AC, Lorig R, et al. Magnetic resonance imaging for assessment of vena caval tumor thrombi: a comparative study with venacavography and computerized tomography scanning. *J Urol* 1990;144:1100–1103.

22. Geisinger MA, Zelch MG, Bravo EL, et al. Primary hyperaldosteronism: comparison of CT, adrenal venography, and venous sampling. *Am J Roentgenol* 1983;141:299–302.

23. Reinig JW, Doppman JL, Dwyer AJ, et al. MRI of indeterminate adrenal masses. *Am J Roentgenol* 1986;147:493–496.

24. Bryan PJ, Caldamone AA, Morrison SC, et al. Ultrasound findings in the adrenogenital syndrome (congenital adrenal hyperplasia). *J Ultrasound Med* 1988;7:675–679.

25. Baker DE, Glazer GM, Francis IR. Adrenal magnetic resonance imaging in Addison's disease. *Urol Radiol* 1988;9:199–203.

26. Mitnick JS, Bosniak MA, Megibow AJ, et al. Non-functioning adrenal adenomas discovered incidentally on computed tomography. *Radiology* 1983;148:495–499.

27. Reinig JW, Doppman JL, Dwyer AJ, et al. Adrenal masses differentiated by MR. *Radiology* 1986;158:81–84.

28. Falke TH, te Strake L, Shaff MI, et al. MR imaging of the adrenals: correlation with computed tomography. *J Comput Assist Tomogr* 1986;10:242–253.

29. Ichikawa T, Ohtomo K, Uchiyama G, et al. Contrast-enhanced dynamic MRI of adrenal masses: classification of characteristic enhancement patterns. *Clin Radiol* 1995;50:295–300.

30. Gross MD, Shapiro B, Bouffard JA, et al. Distinguishing benign from malignant euadrenal masses. *Ann Intern Med* 1988;109:613–618.

31. Shady KL, Brown JJ. MR imaging of the adrenal glands. *Magn Reson Imaging Clin North Am* 1995;3:73–85.

32. Welch TJ, Sheedy PF, van Heerden JA, et al. Pheochromocytoma: value of computed tomography. *Radiology* 1983;148:501–503.

33. Bowerman RA, Silver TM, Jaffe MH, et al. Sonography of adrenal pheochromocytomas. *Am J Roentgenol* 1981;137:1227–1231.

34. Quint LE, Glazer GM, Francis IR, et al. Pheochromocytoma and paraganglioma: comparison of MR imaging with CT and I-131 MIBG scintigraphy. *Radiology* 1987;165:89–93.

35. Tenenbaum F, Lumbroso J, Schlumberger M, et al. Comparison of radiolabeled octreotide and metaiodobenzylguanidine (MIBG) scintigraphy in malignant pheochromocytoma. *J Nucl Med* 1995;36:1–6.

36. White SJ, Stuck KJ, Blane CE, et al. Sonography of neuroblastoma. *Am J Roentgenol* 1983;141:465–468.

37. Hoefnagel CA, Voute PA, de Kraker J, et al. Radionuclide diagnosis and therapy of neural crest tumors using iodine-131 metaiodobenzylguanidine. *J Nucl Med* 1987;28:308–314.

38. Gelfand MJ. Meta-iodobenzylguanidine in children. *Semin Nucl Med* 1993;23:231–242.

39. Shulkin BL, Shen SW, Sisson JC, et al. Iodine-131 MIBG scintigraphy of the extremities in metastatic pheochromocytoma and neuroblastoma. *J Nucl Med* 1987;28:315–318.

40. Wolverson MK, Kannegeisser H. CT of bilateral adrenal hemorrhage with acute adrenal insufficiency in the adult. *Am J Roentgenol* 1984;142:311–314.

41. Murphy BJ, Casillas J, Yrizarry JM. Traumatic adrenal hemorrhage: radiologic findings. *Radiology* 1988;169:701–703.

42. Nielsen MJ, Heaston DK, Dunnick NR, et al. Preoperative CT evaluation of adrenal glands in nonsmall cell bronchogenic carcinoma. *Am J Roentgenol* 1982;139:317–320.

43. Pagani JJ. Nonsmall-cell lung carcinoma adrenal metastases: computed tomography and percutaneous needle biopsy in their diagnosis. *Cancer* 1984;53:1058–1060.

44. Jafri SZ, Francis IR, Glazer GM, et al. CT detection of adrenal lymphoma. *J Comput Assist Tomogr* 1983;7:254–256.

45. Rieber A, Brambs HJ. CT and MR imaging of adrenal hemangioma: a case report. *Acta Radiol* 1995;36:659–661.

46. Hamrick-Turner JE, Abbitt PL, Allen BC, et al. Adrenal hemangioma: MR findings with pathologic correlation. *J Comput Assist Tomogr* 1993;17:503–505.

47. Doppman JL, Gill JJ, Nienhuis AW, et al. CT findings in Addison's disease. *J Comput Assist Tomogr* 1982;6:757–761.

48. Buxi TB, Vohra RB, Sujatha, et al. CT in adrenal enlargement due to tuberculosis: a review of literature with five new cases. *Clin Imaging* 1992;16:102–108.

49. Kearney GP, Mahoney EM, Maher E, et al. Functioning and nonfunctioning cysts of the adrenal cortex and medulla. *Am J Surg* 1977;134:363–368.

50. Glazer HS, Weyman PJ, Sagel SS, et al. Nonfunctioning adrenal masses: incidental discovery on computed tomography. *Am J Roentgenol* 1982;139:81–85.

51. Oliver TJ, Bernardino ME, Miller JI, et al. Isolated adrenal masses in nonsmall-cell bronchogenic carcinoma. *Radiology* 1984;153:217–218.

52. Krestin GP, Friedmann G, Fishbach R, et al. Evaluation of adrenal masses in oncologic patients: dynamic contrast-enhanced MR vs. CT. *J Comput Assist Tomogr* 1991;15:104–110.
53. Tsushima Y, Ishizaka H, Matsumoto M. Adrenal masses: differentiation with chemical shift, fast low-angle shot MR imaging. *Radiology* 1993;186:705–709.
54. Outwater EK, Siegelman ES, Radecki PD, et al. Distinction between benign and malignant adrenal masses: value of T1-weighted chemical-shift MR imaging. *Am J Roentgenol* 1995;165:579–583.
55. Kloos RT, Gross MD, Francis IR, et al. Incidentally discovered adrenal masses. *Endocrinol Rev* 1995;16:460–484.
56. Boland GW, Goldberg MA, Lee MJ, et al. Indeterminate adrenal mass in patients with cancer: evaluation at PET with 2-[F-18]-fluoro-2-deoxy-D-glucose. *Radiology* 1995;194:131–134.
57. Dwamena BA, Kloos RT, Fendrick AM, et al. Diagnostic evaluation of the adrenal incidentaloma: decision and cost-effectiveness analyses. *J Nucl Med* 1998;39:707–712.

*Medical and Surgical Management of
Adrenal Diseases,* edited by Joseph C. Cerny.
Lippincott Williams & Wilkins, Philadelphia © 1999.

4

Cushing's Syndrome

M. Saeed Zafar and Max Wisgerhof

Division of Endocrinology and Metabolism, Henry Ford Hospital, Detroit, Michigan 48202

CLINICAL MANIFESTATIONS

Harvey Cushing recognized the central role of the adrenal gland in what has come to be known as Cushing's syndrome, or the manifestations of excessive adrenal secretion of cortisol. In 1912, he described in his book, *The Pituitary Body and Its Disorders* (1), the patient, Minnie G., as a patient with a polyglandular syndrome. Cushing drew attention to clinical findings, similar to hers, in patients with adrenal tumors and wrote, "It will thus be seen that we may perchance be on the way toward the recognition of the consequences of hyperadrenalism." By 1932, he had recognized the trophic influence of the pituitary basophils on the adrenal glands and he had shown that basophil tumors of the pituitary can cause the same clinical syndrome as do tumors of the adrenal glands (2). Over subsequent decades, tumors other than of the adrenal or pituitary have been shown to produce hypercortisolism—the hallmark of Cushing's syndrome.

The symptoms and signs of Cushing's syndrome are due to the glucocorticoid action of cortisol, secreted in excess by one or both adrenal glands in this disorder. Early in the course of Cushing's syndrome there can be weight gain, but eventually the catabolic effect of excessive cortisol results in nitrogen wasting with muscle weakness, osteopenia, and fragile skin. The mood disturbance commonly encountered in patients with Cushing's syndrome is the manifestation of hypercortisolism in the brain. The disturbance in reproductive function and cycle can result from the effect of hyper-

cortisolism on hypothalamic-pituitary function or be the consequence of the catabolic effects of hypercortisolism. Metabolic disturbances of enhanced gluconeogenesis and insulin resistance result from the effects of hypercortisolism in the liver and in other insulin-responsive tissues. The global function of the immune system is also impaired by the excessive amount of cortisol. In some forms of Cushing's syndrome, sex steroid precursors as well as cortisol are produced in excess and lead to masculinization in women and feminization in men. Also, some forms of Cushing's syndrome are associated with a high production of nonaldosterone mineralocorticoids. Along with cortisol, these mineralocorticoids result in an increase in blood pressure and characteristic electrolyte abnormalities. When excessive adrenocorticotropic hormone (ACTH) is the cause of Cushing's syndrome, this can be signaled by the presence of dermomelanosis.

The fundamental clinical manifestation in Cushing's syndrome, the cushingoid appearance, can range from barely detectible to a florid, unmistakable facies and habitus. Color plate 16 (Fig. 4-1) shows a patient with florid Cushing's syndrome resulting from adrenal cancer.

PHYSIOLOGIC REGULATION OF CORTISOL SECRETION

The adrenal cortex secretes the steroid hormones cortisol and aldosterone and sex steroid precursors using cholesterol as substrate. ACTH is the stimulus to cortisol secretion and

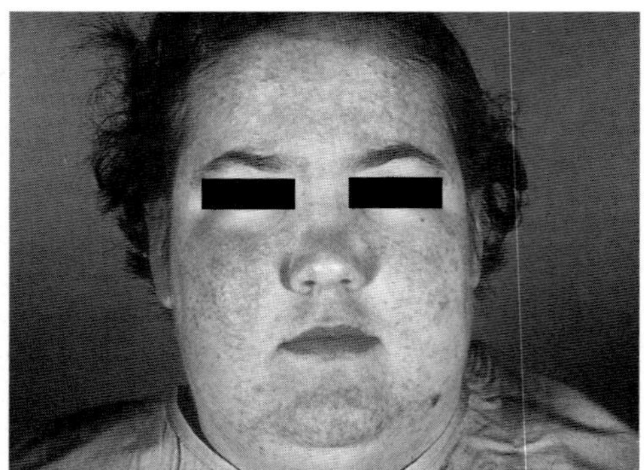

FIG. 4-1. Typical appearance of a patient with florid Cushing's syndrome.

to adrenal androgen production. The physiological synthesis and secretion of ACTH is stimulated by corticotropin-releasing hormone (CRH) from the hypothalamus. Circulating cortisol in the blood dampens the stimulation by CRH of ACTH secretion by the pituitary gland and the production of CRH by the hypothalamus. The secretion of ACTH and cortisol demonstrates a diurnal rhythm, which is highest upon awakening in the morning and lowest at onset of sleep in the night. The major determinant of this cycle appears to be the diurnal release of CRH from the hypothalamus.

In addition to CRH pulses from the hypothalamus, the secretion of ACTH is triggered by fever, hypoglycemia, stress, psychological disturbance, and a decrease in plasma cortisol. During stress, there is a twofold to tenfold increase in adrenal steroid secretion, particularly cortisol. An increase in cortisol concentration in the plasma decreases ACTH secretion by the pituitary, and a decrease in cortisol secretion into the plasma enhances the synthesis and release of ACTH. Thus, a feedback relationship exists between the secretion of cortisol by the adrenal gland and the secretion of ACTH by the pituitary (Fig. 4-2).

ETIOLOGY AND PATHOPHYSIOLOGY OF CUSHING'S SYNDROME

Excessive amounts of glucocorticoids in the circulation arise from an exogenous or an endogenous (adrenal) source. Endogenous hypercortisolism can develop from a variety of causes, either dependent upon, or independent of, ACTH. Classification of Cushing's syndrome is as follows:

- ACTH-independent disorders:
  Cortisol-secreting adrenal adenoma
  Cortisol-secreting adrenal carcinoma
  Primary cortisol-secreting hyperplasia
  Exogenous glucocorticoid excess
- ACTH-dependent disorders:
  Pituitary-origin (Cushing's disease)
  Ectopic ACTH syndrome

Adrenocorticotropic Hormone-Independent Disorders

Those causes of endogenous hypercortisolism that are independent of ACTH and are primary to one or both adrenal glands are cortisol-secreting adrenal adenoma, cortisol-secreting carcinoma, and primary cortisol-secreting hyperplasia. The excessive secretion of cortisol in these disorders suppresses the production of ACTH by the pituitary—a characteristic of these disorders.

Cortisol-Secreting Adrenal Adenoma

Cortisol-secreting adrenal adenomas secrete cortisol only, and the consequent suppression of ACTH by this hypercortisolism decreases the production by the adrenal of other ACTH-dependent steroids, androgens, and sex steroid precursors. These adenomas are intermediate in size, larger than aldosterone-secreting adrenal adenomas, and considerably smaller than adrenal cortical carcinomas.

Cortisol-Secreting Adrenal Carcinoma

Cancerous adrenal lesions presenting as Cushing's syndrome are usually large and can sometimes be palpated by abdominal examination. They are usually greater than 6 cm in diameter and readily detected by computed tomography. They usually secrete adrenal steroids other than cortisol in abundance, so that if Cushing's syndrome is accompanied by virilization, feminization, or mineralocorticoid excess, adrenal cancer is the likely cause (3).

Primary Cortisol-Secreting Hyperplasia

Primary cortisol-secreting hyperplasia, or micronodular adrenal hyperplasia, is a heterogenous disorder. In one form, yellow nodules can be seen in the adrenal cortex; in another form, the adrenal cortex contains numerous, small pigmented nodules laden with lipofuscin. The tissue between the nodules in these disorders is atrophied, reflecting low, suppressed ACTH secretion. There has been described a familial aggregation of patients with coexisting microlentigo and blue nevi, cutaneous myxomas, singular or multiple cardiac myxomas, large cell calcifying Sertoli cell tumors of the testes, and single or multiple mammary fibroadenomas (4–6). The pathophysiology also is heterogenous in this group of primary adrenal hyperplasia because the degree of autonomous cortisol production is variable. That is, in some cases, the ACTH concentration in the plasma is clearly low and fully suppressed whereas, in others, there is evidence of continued ACTH secretion. Autonomy of adrenal cortisol production in these cases, however, can be demonstrated when the ACTH production is either suppressed by exogenous glucocorticoid or removed by pituitary surgery. In the familial cases, adrenal autonomy is usually evident (4–8).

Adrenocorticotropic Hormone-Dependent Cushing's Syndrome

The causes of ACTH-dependent Cushing's syndrome are adrenocortical hyperplasia secondary to excess ACTH secretion from the pituitary (Cushing's disease); adrenal cortical hyperplasia produced by ACTH secretion from nonpituitary tumors, benign or malignant, such as a carcinoid tumor or small cell lung cancer (ectopic ACTH syndrome); and, rarely, CRH-secreting, nonhypothalamic tumors. A hypothalamic cause and an intermediate-lobe pituitary origin of ACTH-dependent Cushing's syndrome have been suggested. The ACTH-dependent types of hypercortisolism are characterized by excessive cortisol secretion dependent upon clearly high ACTH secretion or an apparently normal but inappropriately high degree of ACTH secretion.

Pituitary-Origin ACTH (Cushing's Disease)

A characteristic of pituitary-origin ACTH dependent Cushing's syndrome (Cushing's disease) is the maintenance of a degree of feedback relationship between cortisol and ACTH secretion. In Cushing's disease, it is as if the threshold concentration for glucocorticoid effect is higher in the tumorous tissue than in the normal pituitary. This is the explanation for the suppression of ACTH by a high dose of dexamethasone in Cushing's disease.

More than 80% of patients with ACTH-dependent Cushing's syndrome have a pituitary microadenoma. The consensus presently is that the adenoma is the primary site of the cause of Cushing's disease. A few patients with pituitary-origin ACTH-dependent Cushing's syndrome have hyperplasia of the ACTH-producing pituitary cells, or an intermediate lobe origin of the ACTH. This has led to the proposal that neurohypothalamic stimulation is the primary cause of excessive ACTH secretion in these instances.

Ectopic ACTH Syndrome

The ectopic ACTH syndrome, or extrapituitary-origin ACTH-dependent Cushing's syndrome, is caused by a variety of neoplasms, benign or malignant. More than 50% of these tumors are found in the lung. Other sites are the thymus and pancreas, and even adrenal medulla; these are usually carcinoid-type tumors with a variably aggressive course and prognosis. The ectopic production of CRH has been reported in metastatic prostatic cancer, medullary thyroid cancer, and bronchial carcinoid. This disorder is difficult to identify, but reported cases have had high ACTH concentrations and a short clinical course (9,10).

DIAGNOSIS AND TREATMENT OF PRIMARY ADRENAL CAUSES OF CUSHING'S SYNDROME (ACTH-INDEPENDENT)

Hypercortisolism

The first maneuver to diagnose a primary disorder of the adrenal that causes Cushing's syndrome is to confirm the clinical impression by demonstrating cortisol excess (Fig. 4-3). Hypercortisolism is convincingly shown by finding a higher than normal excretion of cortisol in a 24-hour urine collection; by the inappropriate concentration of plasma cortisol in the morning after 1 mg of dexamethasone by mouth 8 hours previously the night before; or, probably most sensitively, by the absence of a diurnal variation in cortisol concentration in the plasma. Convincing evidence of hypercortisolism is essential to have in hand before attempting further diagnostic maneuvers upon which to base treatment for suspected Cushing's syndrome. The intermittent secretion of cortisol over days or weeks can make difficult the clear demonstration of excessive cortisol secretion in a single measurement (11,12).

Adrenocorticotropic Hormone Assessment

The assessment of ACTH secretion in Cushing's syndrome is the next step after hypercortisolism has been convincingly shown. The plasma concentration of ACTH is characteristically below the reference range and usually undetectable in ACTH-independent hypercortisolism. In rare instances in which primary

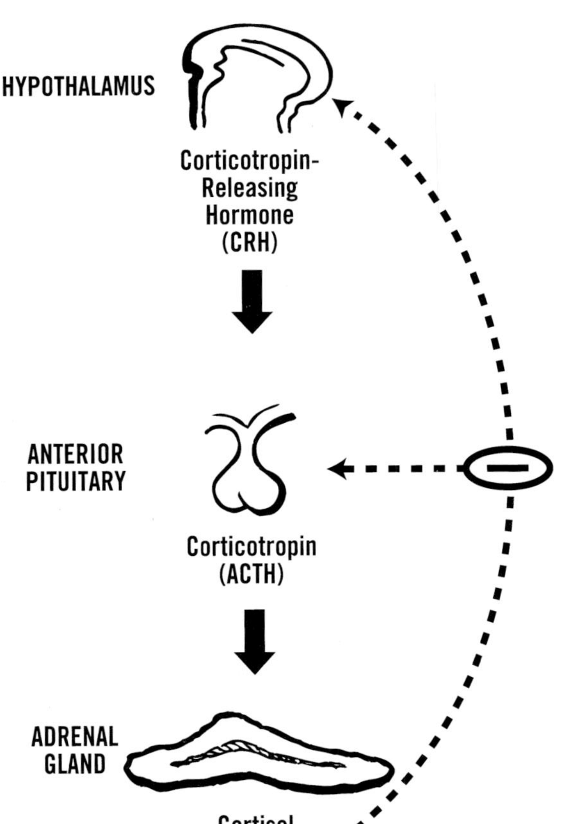

FIG. 4-2. Hypothalamic, pituitary, and adrenal feedback mechanism.

adrenal autonomy is developing after prolonged ACTH stimulation, ACTH may still be detectable. Thus, once hypercortisolism is established, the demonstration of low plasma concentration of ACTH identifies a primary adrenal cause of the hypercortisolism.

Localization Testing

The treatment goal for primary adrenal Cushing's syndrome is the removal of the adrenal tissue, which is the seat of the autonomy. This would restore physiologic cortisol secretion from the remaining normal adrenal gland, if the process is unilateral. Therefore, the next diagnostic maneuver after establishing that the hypercortisolism is independent of ACTH production is to identify whether the cause of hypertisolism is unilateral adrenal disease. This lateralization of the adrenal disease can be accomplished by adrenal cortical scintigraphy with (131-I)-iodomethyl-19-norcholesterol, computed tomography, magnetic resonance imaging, or adrenal vein sampling to measure cortisol concentration in the effluent venous blood. Ultrasound imaging is less sensitive for the adrenal. The frequency of nonsecretory adrenal cortical adenomas is sufficiently high, approaching 10%, that computed tomography or magnetic resonance imaging used alone to identify unilateral adrenal disease risks inaccurate localization. A unilateral image by scintigraphy is strong support for the presence of disease in the imaged gland. Primary hyperplasia, or a hyperplasia syndrome that had preceding ACTH dependency, is likely to show two scintigraphic images. Adrenal cancer is likely to yield a poor quality image by scintigraphy because of the size of most cancerous adrenal lesions and the inefficiency in concentrating the radioiodinated steroid precursor (13–16).

Treatment and Prognosis

Unilateral adrenalectomy is the effective therapy for cortisol-secreting adrenal adenoma, achieving a cure of the disorder after a temporary period of postoperative dependence on glucocorticoid replacement therapy. This occurs because of the prior suppression of the normal adrenal by the hypercortisolism from the adenoma. Recovery of function by the remaining adrenal might require months, and the tapered discontinuation of the replacement therapy is necessarily slow. The dose of replacement glucocorticoid therapy immediately after adrenalectomy and for some weeks afterward is considerably greater than physiologic replacement, because the previous exposure to high levels of cortisol leads to a dependence upon glucocorticoid which is difficult to relieve (17).

Unilateral adrenalectomy is desirable therapy for adrenal cancer; however, the prognostic prospect is poor. The cancer is usually aggressive, growing large and metastasizing early and frequently. Surgical removal of the cancerous adrenal lesion can lead to temporary remission. Radiation therapy to the adrenal bed and nonspecific chemotherapy have been, in general, effective only for palliation (18). Antiadrenal medications that block steroid hormone synthesis in the adrenal can ameliorate temporarily the adverse effects of the steroid hormone excess, particularly that of cortisol, by decreasing the amount of steroid produced. Metyrapone and ketoconazole decrease the 11-hydroxylase enzyme activity and thus impair cortisol synthesis. Mitotane is adrenolytic, that is, it can cause lysis of adrenal cells, normal or cancerous (19,20).

Bilateral adrenalectomy is the effective therapy for primary cortisol-secreting hyperplasia. This corrects the hypercortisolism and necessitates lifelong adrenal steroid replacement with glucocorticoid and mineralocorticoid.

DIAGNOSIS AND TREATMENT OF ACTH-DEPENDENT CUSHING'S SYNDROME

Hypercortisolism and Adrenocorticotropic Hormone Assessment

The recognition of a cushingoid appearance and of cortisol excess is approached and confirmed as described earlier (see Fig. 4-3). The plasma level of ACTH, in contrast to that in Cushing's syndrome caused by primary adrenal disease, is either higher than the reference normal range or is inappropriately in the reference range when the cortisol is high in urine or blood.

Localization Testing

The localization testing in ACTH-dependent Cushing's syndrome is different from that in primary adrenal disease. In ACTH-dependent Cushing's syndrome, the goal is to localize the origin or source of the excessive ACTH to either the pituitary gland or to another source, an ectopic tumor. Additionally, laboratory testing is used to obtain test results that point to the source, which can be further defined by imaging techniques.

Cushing's Disease

The laboratory test results that support the presence of pituitary-origin ACTH-dependent Cushing's syndrome are as follows:

1. At least 90% decrease in cortisol urinary excretion in response to dexamethasone given in high dose, 2 mg orally every 6 hours for 48 hours (21)
2. A greater than twofold increase in excretion of 17-hydroxycorticosteroids or a much greater than normal increase in plasma desoxycortisol concentration in response to metyrapone administration, either given in six divided doses of 750 mg every 4 hours or as one dose of 30 mg/kg 8 hours before blood sampling (22)
3. A convincing increase in plasma ACTH concentration in response to an injection of CRH (ovine) intravenously, 1 μg/kg (23)

These tests are at best 90% accurate, which is not optimal to direct surgical, curative treatment to the pituitary or to an ectopic source of ACTH. Therefore, localizing tests using imaging techniques and simultaneous blood sampling from each inferior petrosal sinus and a peripheral vein have been developed to maximize the accuracy of diagnosis of ACTH-dependent Cushing's syndrome. The imaging technique of choice to detect a pituitary microadenoma, the usual cause of ACTH-dependent Cushing's syndrome, is magnetic resonance imaging of the pituitary, particularly with gadolinium contrast. Computed tomography is less sensitive. However, about one-third of ACTH-secreting pituitary microadenomas are not visualized by magnetic resonance imaging. Furthermore, the prevalence of nonsecreting pituitary microadenomas might be as high as 10%.

Simultaneous bilateral inferior petrosal sinus sampling for measurement of ACTH concentrations in the samples appears to be the most accurate method to detect the pituitary origin of excessive ACTH in Cushing's syndrome (24). The higher concentration of plasma ACTH from the left or right sinus, obtained simultaneously, is compared to the ACTH concentration in also simultaneously obtained peripheral venous blood. Multiple simultaneous samplings and measurements enhance the discrimination. The use of CRH to stimulate ACTH production and thus an increase in petrosal sinus ACTH concentration is a great adjunct to the accuracy of this test. When the source of excessive ACTH is the pituitary, the petrosal sinus concentration is at least twice (threefold if CRH is used) that in the peripheral vein. An attempt has been made to lateralize the source of ACTH to one side of the pituitary or the other, to aid the surgeon in correctly approaching a microadenoma not visualized by magnetic resonance imaging (25).

Ectopic ACTH Syndrome

The identification or localization of an ectopic source of excess ACTH can be challenging. Magnetic resonance imaging is the most productive localizing maneuver to detect ectopic sources, such as lung cancer or carcinoid tumors of the lung, pancreas, thymus, adrenal, or other site. Pentetreotide (OctreoScan) nuclide scanning has promise for identifying ectopic ACTH-producing tumors that cannot be otherwise localized, and selective venous sampling for ACTH gradients around tumors or organs could be considered. The diagnosis can be elusive (26,27).

Treatment and Prognosis

Cushing's Disease

Removal of the ACTH-secreting pituitary adenoma by transsphenoidal surgery is the treatment of choice for patients with Cushing's disease, both in children and adults. A skilled surgeon achieves this cure in 90% of patients who have a demonstrated pituitary adenoma secreting ACTH. If the first attempt fails, but a pituitary origin of ACTH can be documented again, a second surgical attempt has a success rate of about 50% in most series. Even if a tumor is not detected by imaging techniques, surgical exploration of the pituitary gland is still in order, because a tumor can be found in approximately 90% of these patients also. Even if a tumor invades the dura, a total resection may still be possible in about half the cases. The advent of bilateral inferior petrosal sinus sampling for ACTH allows the surgeon the choice of hemihypophysectomy in the event that a pituitary tumor cannot be found. If the endocrine studies strongly support the diagnosis of Cushing's disease but the petrosal sinus sampling is not lateralizing and fertility is not an issue, a total hypophysectomy should be considered (28–30).

Transient diabetes insipidus may occur for a few weeks following surgery. Permanent diabetes insipidus, cerebral spinal fluid rhinorrhea, and meningitis are uncommon complications (31).

After selective pituitary adenomectomy, the patients who are cured experience transient secondary adrenal insufficiency for 6 to 18 months. In the perioperative period, patients with Cushing's syndrome are given 100 mg of hydrocortisone intravenously every 4 to 6 hours, maximally 300 mg per 24 hours, 60 mg of prednisolone, or 6 mg of dexamethasone in divided doses, daily. The dose is halved every other day until a maintenance dose of 10 mg of hydrocortisone is reached. During this period, the ACTH response to CRH is subnormal. If ACTH and cortisol do not decrease to low levels, recurrence is more likely. Within 6 to 18 months after surgery, recovery of hypothalamic-pituitary-adrenal function usually takes place. Glucocorticoid therapy can then be safely withdrawn. An ACTH test of cortisol secretion before the administration of a dose of glucocorticoid replacement therapy can help decide the timing of glucocorticoid withdrawal. The reported recurrence rate after transsphenoidal adenectomy is 5%.

If transsphenoidal surgery fails or surgery is not a therapeutic option, pituitary irradiation should be considered. High-voltage irradiation provided by cobalt-60 (60 Co) delivering 4,000 to 5,000 cGy produces favorable results in about 50% of patients. The best responses are observed in children. Combining the radiation therapy with mitotane (O-P-DDD) can increase the response rate to 85% (32). Radiation therapy has the advantage of preserving some pituitary adrenal function and recurrence is rare. A slow therapeutic response, however, is a major disadvantage. Six to 18 months may elapse before the therapeutic objective is achieved.

Heavy particle and Bragg peak proton irradiation therapy appears to be more effective than conventional irradiation, and remission rates of 80% can be achieved. Postirradiation panhypopituitarism is common, however. Gold-198 or yttrium-90 implantation can also result in complete or partial response in about 80% of patients with Cushing's disease. This mode of therapy, however, is complicated by hypopituitarism in about half the cases (33,34).

Recently, sophisticated evaluation of patients who have received irradiation has detected a higher incidence of postirradiation side effects, such as subtle cognitive dysfunction and postirradiation brain necrosis years after completion of therapy. Intracranial malignancies have also been reported (34).

Total bilateral adrenalectomy corrects the hypercortisolism of Cushing's disease. This procedure should receive due consideration in patients in whom transsphenoidal surgery has either failed or is not a therapeutic option. The development of Nelson's syndrome (invasive ACTH-secreting pituitary adenoma) in 10% of patients so treated remains a concern because the pituitary adenoma may become locally invasive and be difficult to control. Lifelong therapy with adrenal steroids is necessary after bilateral adrenalectomy, and growth of ectopic adrenal tissue may develop in 5% to 10% of patients as a result of continued ACTH hyperstimulation.

Many drugs have been tried in the management of Cushing's syndrome. These may inhibit ACTH secretion, block cortisol synthesis, or compete with cortisol at the receptor level. Adrenal enzyme inhibitors have the greatest utility.

Cyproheptadine, bromocriptine, and sodium valproate have been tried by various investigators to inhibit ACTH secretion, with mixed results. The mechanism of action of these agents is not fully established and there is limited enthusiasm for their use in the management of Cushing's disease (35,36).

Useful agents that block cortisol synthesis include aminoglutethimide, metyrapone, ketoconazole, and mitotane.

Aminoglutethimide acts by blocking the conversion of cholesterol to delta-5-pregnenolone. The synthesis of all three varieties of corticosteroids is inhibited. Side effects of aminoglutethimide include anorexia, nausea, vomiting, lethargy, and blurred vision. Hypothyroidism may occur infrequently, but transient skin rash is frequently observed. This agent may be useful in the management of adrenal carcinoma (37).

Metyrapone inhibits the conversion of desoxycortisol to cortisol. This agent can be used in adrenal carcinoma as well as ACTH-dependent Cushing's syndrome. Hypertension and hypokalemia may result from the accumulation of deoxycorticosterone. Hirsutism may worsen because of increased production of adrenal androgens, and nausea and vomiting may occur. Aminoglutethimide and metyrapone in lower doses have been used in combination (37,38).

Ketoconazole is an imidazole derivative. It inhibits the synthesis of ergosterol in fungi and cholesterol in mammalian cells. In normal men, ketoconazole in doses of 200 to 600 mg per day lowers testosterone production. Used in patients with Cushing's syndrome, the drug lowers cortisol production promptly, with disappearance of its clinical and metabolic effects within 4 to 6 weeks. Surprisingly, escape from its suppressive effect does not occur. Adverse reactions include nausea, vomiting, abdominal pain, and pruritus in up to 3% of patients. Hepatotoxicity, primarily of the hepatocellular type, has been reported (39,40).

Mitotane (O-P-DDD) is the only agent that inhibits biosynthesis of adrenal steroids and destroys adrenocortical cells. It inhibits the conversion of cholesterol to pregnenolone and blocks the final step in cortisol synthesis. The combination of mitotane with cobalt radiation is particularly effective, and patients so treated have shown a decrease in their cortisol levels within 4 months. Mitotane appears to have a partially suppressive effect on ACTH also. Mitotane is a selective inhibitor of zonae fasciculata and reticularis, so aldosterone secretion is usually spared. The side effects include anorexia, nausea, diarrhea, somnolence, pruritus, hypercholesterolemia, and hypouricemia. Alkaline phosphatase levels can increase and thyroxine levels may decline. Mitotane interferes with the binding of thyroxine to its binding globulin. Mitotane affects cortisol metabolism, so that the measurement of urinary metabolites of cortisol is not a reliable index. Urinary and plasma cortisol levels are measured to determine the therapeutic response (19,20).

Mifepristone or RU-486 is a glucocorticoid antagonist. It acts as an inhibitor at the receptor level. Patients demonstrate clinical improvement, but ACTH and cortisol levels remain unchanged. The ACTH secretion in patients with Cushing's disease may be enhanced, and this effect may make this agent ineffective. Experience with the drug is limited (41).

Ectopic ACTH Syndrome

Surgical resection of the primary tumor and the removal of the ectopic source of ACTH is the ideal treatment. When the source of ACTH cannot be localized or is too advanced for an effective surgical therapy, then inhibition of adrenal steroidogenesis is the treatment of choice. The availability of ketoconazole has considerably facilitated this approach. Aminoglutethimide and metyrapone can also be used, but the very high ACTH levels characteristic of this syndrome may overcome the blocking effect of these drugs. Alternatively, bilateral adrenalectomy can be undertaken. Although this can correct the hypercortisolism, it may not be a practical approach in patients with rapidly advancing metastatic disease.

INCIDENTALOMA OF THE ADRENAL

The prevalence of adrenal tumors discovered incidentally by computed tomography of the abdomen is reported at 5 to 10 per 100. Because the patient has no clinical disorder attributable to a hormonal secretion from these tumors, the label incidentaloma is appropriate. Yet, a highly sensitive evaluation can show that many of these apparently silent adrenal tumors secrete cortisol. Although very few (less than 10%) may be proven to demonstrate increased urinary cortisol, a greater percentage (15%) may show lack of diurnal variation of plasma cortisol. Close to 25% may demonstrate a blunted ACTH response to CRH, and close to 50% may show low plasma dehydroepiandrosterone (DHEAS) levels. In almost 25%, cortisol is not suppressed after overnight administration of dexamethasone (1 mg) (42).

An incidentaloma secreting cortisol may be shown to have autonomous function by a concordant, unilateral image by (131-I)-iodomethyl-19-norcholesterol adrenal cortical scintigraphy. Most clinics recommend careful follow-up of such tumors to detect the development of the clinical disorder of Cushing's syndrome before recommending their surgical removal.

ADRENAL INSUFFICIENCY

Adrenal insufficiency is the clinical syndrome resulting from impairment or absence of production of cortisol by the adrenal cortex. The disorder results from disease of the adrenals, primary adrenal insufficiency, and from disease of the hypothalamus or pituitary, secondary adrenal insufficiency and the impaired pituitary reserve for ACTH secretion. Impaired or absent production of aldosterone can occur in primary adrenal insufficiency, and plasma androgen concentrations can be low in primary or secondary adrenal insufficiency in the postmenopausal woman. Catecholamine secretion might be reduced in glucocorticoid deficiency, but it is not a prominent manifestation of adrenal insufficiency.

The disorders of the adrenals that cause primary adrenal insufficiency are (a) an autoimmune pathogenesis directed against adrenalcortical antigens (idiopathic), (b) infection, particularly associated with acquired immunodeficiency syndrome, and (c) hemorrhage during anticoagulation. Medications used to treat hypercortisolism can result in hypocortisolism. Heparinoids have caused primary aldosterone deficiency. Panhypopituitarism causes impaired ACTH secretion, important during stress, but does not produce as severe a deficiency of cortisol production as does primary adrenal insufficiency. Impaired hypothalamic (CRH) and pituitary (ACTH) function can result from intrasellar or suprasellar tumors and their treatment, sarcoidosis (hypothalamic infiltration), and hypophysitis (autoimmune pituitary lymphocytic infiltration). Exogenous glucocorticoid therapy for a week can suppress the hypothalamic-pituitary-adrenal axis for a prolonged time.

The syndrome of adrenal insufficiency is characterized by degrees of asthenia, nausea, and orthostatic hypotension. When primary

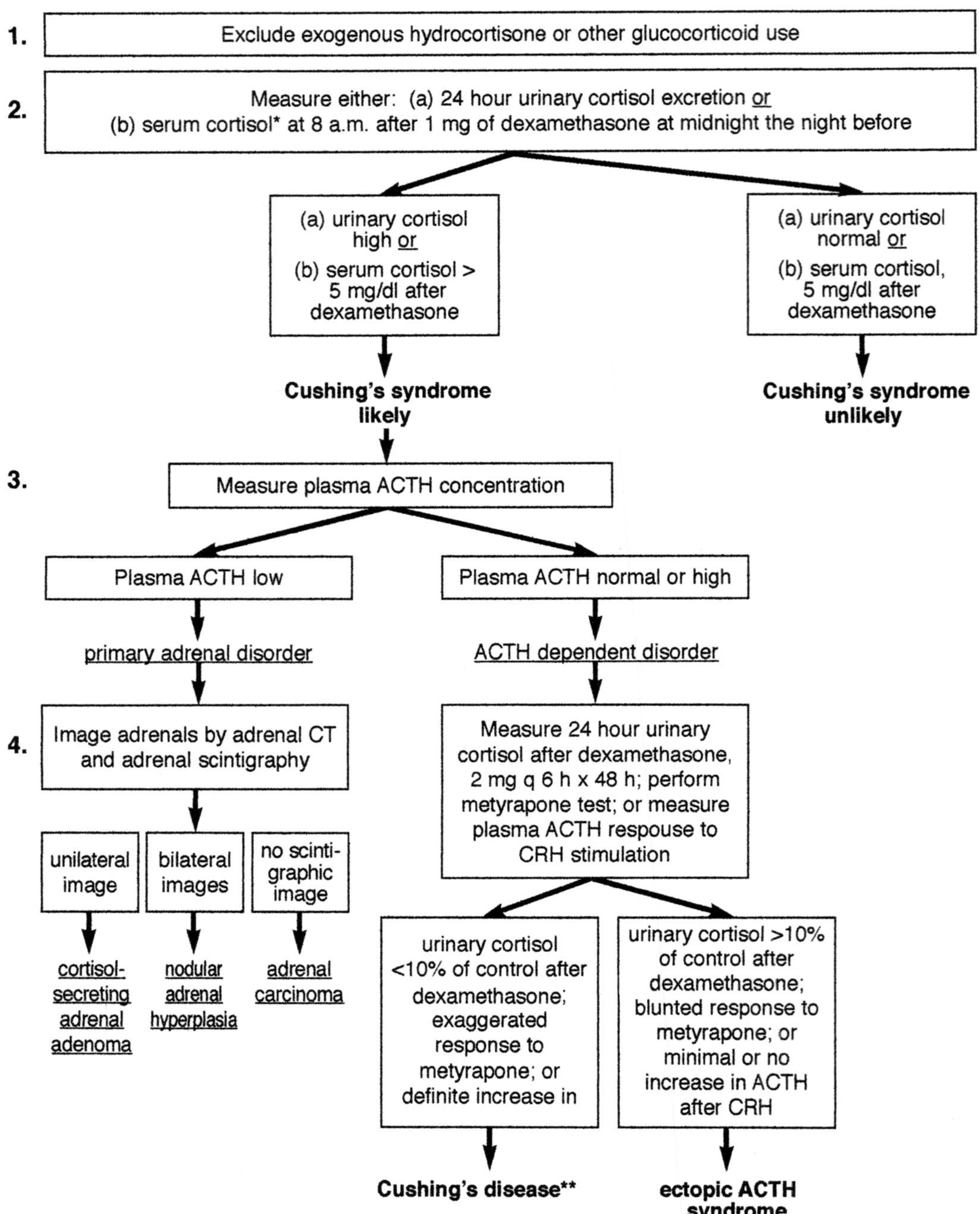

FIG 4-3. The differential diagnosis of suspected Cushing's syndrome. *Estrogen, as in oral contraceptives, increases serum but not urinary cortisol concentration. **This is confirmed by determining the ratio of plasma ACTH concentrations between simultaneous peripheral vein and bilateral petrosal sinus concentrations.

adrenal insufficiency is present, hyperpigmentation is present. In severe cases, vomiting and fever occur. Laboratory testing can show hyponatremia, hypoglycemia, hypercalcemia, eosinophilia, and lymphocytosis, and in primary adrenal insufficiency, hyperkalemia, acidosis, and high ACTH concentration. Plasma cortisol concentration and urinary excretion of cortisol are not sensitive indicators of impaired cortisol production. The failure of plasma cortisol concentration to achieve 18 μg/dL at 60 minutes after 250 μg of cosyntropin (synthetic ACTH) is given intravenously denotes some degree of adrenal insufficiency. Using smaller doses of cosyntropin might detect mild degrees of adrenal insufficiency. The use of cosyntropin stimulation of cortisol secretion is not intended to demonstrate the secondary adrenal insufficiency of hypothalamic-pituitary disease. Insulin-induced hypoglycemia stimulation of cerebral cortical-hypothalamic-pituitary-adrenal function is the certain method of showing secondary adrenal insufficiency. The adrenals must first be shown to be responsive to ACTH for this test to be diagnostic, and insulin-induced hypoglycemia has risks.

The treatment of adrenal insufficiency is medical—the replacement of glucocorticoid; when primary adrenal insufficiency is present, mineralocorticoid is given also. In some cases, androgen replacement is indicated. Surgical treatment of pituitary disease causing secondary adrenal insufficiency is not likely to restore cortisol secretion to normal. Replacement doses of glucocorticoid are difficult to assess. Overreplacement is a risk when well-being, pigmentation, and ACTH concentration are used to assess the glucocorticoid dose. The use of hydrocortisone as replacement and its measurement by urinary excretion as cortisol, and the effects of the glucocorticoid dose on bone mineral density are valid methods of assessing the appropriateness of the dose of glucocorticoid replacement. The measurement of serum potassium concentration assesses mineralocorticoid replacement with fludrocortisone (usually, 0.1 mg daily). Patients should have on their person a notification of the diagnosis "adrenal insufficiency" so that they may be given glucocorticoid therapy in an emergency.

The detection of acute or chronic adrenal insufficiency results from a degree of clinical suspicion of its presence. Prompt diagnosis and appropriate steroid replacement therapy restores the patient to well-being and to a prognosis not limited by corticosteroid deficiency.

REFERENCES

1. Cushing H. *The pituitary body and its disorders.* Philadelphia: JB Lippincott, 1912:219.
2. Cushing H. The basophil adenomas of the pituitary body and their clinical manifestations (pituitary basophilism). *Bull Johns Hopkins Hospital* 1932;50:137.
3. Hutter AM, Kayhoe DE. Adrenal cortical carcinoma: clinical features of 138 patients. *Am J Med* 1966;41:572.
4. Shenoy BV, Carpenter PC, Carney JA. Bilateral primary pigmented nodular adrenal cortical disease: rare cause of Cushing's syndrome. *Am J Surg Pathol* 1984;8:335.
5. Bohm N, Lippman-Grob B, Petrykowski WV. Familial Cushing's syndrome due to pigmented multinodular adrenocortical dysplasia. *Acta Endocrinol* 1983;102:428.
6. Schweizer-Caigianut M, Salomon F, Hedinger CE. Primary adrenocortical nodular dysplasia with Cushing's syndrome and cardiac myxomas. *Virchous Arch (Patsal Anta)* 1982;397:183.
7. Smals AG, Pieters GF, Van Haelst UJ. Macronodular adrenocortical hyperplasia in long standing Cushing's disease. *J Clin Endocrinol Metab* 1984;58:25.
8. Aron DC, Findling JW, Fitzgerald PA, et al. Pituitary ACTH dependency of nodular adrenal hyperplasia in Cushing's syndrome. *Am J Med* 1981;71:302.
9. Immura H. Ectopic hormone syndromes. *Clin Endocrinol Metab* 1980;9:235.
10. Schteingart DE, Lloyd RV, Akil H, et al. Cushing's syndrome secondary to ectopic CRH-ACTH secretion. *J Clin Endocrinol Metab* 1986;63:770.
11. Kaye TB, Crapo L. The Cushing syndrome: an update on diagnostic tests. *Ann Intern Med* 1990;112:434–444.
12. Glass AR, Zavadil AP, Halberg F. Circadian rhythm of serum cortisol in Cushing's disease. *J Clin Endocrinol Metab* 1984;59:161.
13. Van Slooten H, Schaberg A, Smeenk D, et al. Morphological characteristics of benign and malignant adrenocortical tumors. *Cancer* 1985;55:766.
14. Doppman JL, Reining JW, Dwyer AJ, et al. Differentiation of adrenal masses by magnetic resonance imaging. *Surgery* 1987;102:1018.
15. Anderson BG, Beierwaltes WH. Adrenal imaging with radioiodocholesterol in the diagnosis of adrenal disorders. *Adv Intern Med* 1974;19:327.
16. Smith SM, Patel SK, Turner DA, et al. Magnetic resonance imaging of adrenal cortical carcinoma. *Urol Radiol* 1989;11:1.
17. Delaney JP, Solomkin JS, Jacobson ME, et al. Surgical

management of Cushing's syndrome. *Surgery* 1978;84: 465.

18. Percarpio B, Knowlton AH. Radiation therapy of adrenal cortical carcinoma. *Acta Radiol Oncol Radiat Phys Biol* 1976;15:288.

19. Becker D, Schumacher OP. OP DDD therapy in invasive adrenocortical carcinoma. *Ann Intern Med* 1975;82: 677.

20. Hoffman DL, Mattox VL. Treatment of adrenocortical carcinoma with OP DDD. *Med Clin North Am* 1972; 50:999.

21. Flack MR, Oldfield EH, Cutler GB, et al. Urine-free cortisol in the high-dose dexamethasone suppression test for the differential diagnosis of the Cushing syndrome. *Ann Intern Med* 1992;116:211–217.

22. Merkle AW, Jubiz W, Hutchings MD, et al. A simplified metyrapone test with determination of plasma II-deoxy-cortisol (metyrapone test with plasmas). *J Clin Endocrinol Metab* 1969;29:985.

23. Nieman L, Chrousos G, Oldfield E, et al. The ovine CRF test and the dexamethasone suppression test in the differential diagnosis of Cushing's syndrome. *Ann Intern Med* 1986;105:862.

24. Snow RB, Patterson RH, Howith M, et al. Usefulness of preoperative inferior petrosal vein sampling in Cushing's disease. *Surg Neurol* 1988;29:17.

25. Oldfield EH, Chrousos GP, Schulte HM, et al. Preoperative lateralization of ACTH secreting pituitary microadenomas by bilateral and simultaneous inferior petrosal venous sinus sampling. *N Engl J Med* 1985;312: 100.

26. Philipponneau M, Nocaudie M, Epelbaum J, et al. Somatostatin analogs for the localization and preoperative treatment of adrenocorticotropin-secreting bronchial carcinoid tumor. *J Clin Endocrinol Metab* 1994;78:20.

27. Doppman JL, Loughlin T, Miller DL, et al. Identification of ACTH producing intrathoracic tumors by measuring ACTH levels in aspirated specimens. *Radiology* 1987;163:501.

28. Tyrrell JB, Brooks RM, Fitzgerald PA, et al. Cushing's disease: selective transsphenoidal resection of pituitary microadenomas. *N Engl J Med* 1978;298:753.

29. Styne DM, Grumbach MM, Kaplan SL, et al. Treatment of Cushing's disease in childhood and adolescence by transsphenoidal microadenomectomy. *N Engl J Med* 1984;310:889.

30. Boggan JE, Tywell JB, Wilson CB. Transsphenoidal microsurgical management of Cushing's disease: report of 100 cases. *J Neurosurg* 1983;59:195.

31. Nolan PM, Sheeler LR, Hahn JR. Therapeutic problems with transsphenoidal pituitary surgery for Cushing's disease. *Cleve Clin Q* 1982;49:199.

32. Schteingart DE, Tsao HS, Taylor CT, et al. Sustained remission of Cushing's disease with mitotane and pituitary irradiation. *Ann Intern Med* 1980;92:613.

33. Lawrence JH, Okerlund MD, Linfoot JE, et al. Heavy particle treatment of Cushing's disease. *N Engl J Med* 1971;285:1263.

34. Sharpe GF, Kendall-Taylor P, Prescott RWG, et al. Pituitary function following megavoltage therapy for Cushing's disease: long-term follow up. *Clin Endocrinol* 1985;22:169.

35. McKenna MJ, Linares M, Mellinger RC: Prolonged remission of Cushing's disease following bromocriptine therapy. *Henry Ford Hosp Med J* 1987;35:188–191.

36. Krieger DT. Physiopathology of Cushing's disease. *Endocrinol Rev* 1983;4:22–43.

37. Schteingart DE, Conn JW. Effects of aminoglutethimide upon adrenal function and cortisol metabolism in Cushing's syndrome. *J Clin Endocrinol Metab* 1967;27: 1657.

38. Thoren M, Adamson U, Sjoberg HE. Aminoglutethimide and metyrapone in the management of Cushing's syndrome. *Acta Endocrinol* 1985;109:45.

39. Pont A, Williams PL, Loose DS, et al. Ketoconazole blocks adrenal steroid synthesis. *Ann Intern Med* 1982; 97:370.

40. Feldman D. Ketoconazole and other imidazole derivatives as inhibitors of steroidogenesis. *Endocr Rev* 1986; 7:409.

41. Nieman LK, Chrousos GP, Kellner C, et al. Successful treatment of Cushing's syndrome with a glucocorticoid antagonist RU486. *J Clin Endocrinol Metab* 1985;71:536.

42. Osella G, Terzdo M, Corretta G, et al. Endocrine evaluation of individually discovered adrenal mass (incidentaloma). *J Clin Endocrinol Metab* 1994;79:1532.

Medical and Surgical Management of Adrenal Diseases, edited by Joseph C. Cerny. Lippincott Williams & Wilkins, Philadelphia © 1999.

5

Primary Aldosteronism

Orlin Sergev and Max Wisgerhof

Division of Endocrinology and Metabolism, Henry Ford Hospital, Detroit, Michigan 48202

Primary aldosteronism is the excessive adrenal secretion of the mineralocorticoid hormone aldosterone, independently of the renin-angiotensin system. It occurs in less than 1% of unselected patients with high blood pressure. Since the original description of the disorder as being due to a unilateral aldosterone-producing adrenal adenoma (Conn's syndrome) (1), other causes of primary aldosteronism have been identified. These are the bilateral adrenal disorders of idiopathic hyperaldosteronism (2) and glucocorticoid-remediable hyperaldosteronism (3), the unilateral or bilateral adrenal disorder of primary adrenal hyperplasia (4), and adrenocortical carcinoma (5). The diagnosis of primary aldosteronism is suspected in the hypertensive patient with unprovoked hypokalemia.

PHYSIOLOGY OF ALDOSTERONE

Biosynthesis of Aldosterone

Aldosterone is the final steroid in the mineralocorticoid biosynthetic pathway. This pathway uses enzymes common to the glucocorticoid pathway until the final enzymatic reaction converts corticosterone to aldosterone, which is unique to the glomerulosa zone of the adrenal cortex. This final reaction is the point at which angiotensin II stimulates aldosterone synthesis. Potassium and adrenocorticotropic hormone (ACTH) stimulate aldosterone synthesis at the earliest step in the steroid synthetic pathway; potassium can stimulate the final step in aldosterone synthesis also. The genes responsible for the enzymes involved in the latter steps of aldosterone biosynthesis are the genes for 11-β-hydroxylase and aldosterone synthase. They are 95% homologous and are found on chromosome 8. A unique crossover between the regulatory region of 11-β-hydroxylase and the coding region of the aldosterone synthase genes results in a hybrid gene that is under ACTH control and represents the molecular basis for glucocorticoid-remediable hyperaldosteronism (6). Currently, there are no known abnormalities in the aldosterone synthase gene in other forms of primary aldosteronism. Atrial natriuretic factor or peptide appears to have a direct suppressive effect on aldosterone synthesis, but its role in the physiologic or pathophysiologic regulation of aldosterone biosynthesis has not yet been established (7).

Regulation of Aldosterone Synthesis

Aldosterone secretion is regulated primarily by stimuli that increase its synthesis. The most potent stimulus is angiotensin II, which is the product of the action of the converting enzyme on angiotensin I. Angiotensin I is the product of the action of renin, an enzyme, on angiotensinogen, which is a large peptide synthesized in the liver. The activity of the enzyme renin is the rate-limiting factor in the generation of angiotensin II from angiotensinogen. Renin is produced by cells of the juxtaglomerular apparatus at the distal renal tubule in response to a decrease in pressure and sodium in the distal tubule luminal fluid. The pressure and sodium content in the distal tubule fluid reflect plasma volume and the sodium content of the body. Aldosterone stimulates sodium reabsorption from the distal nephron into the plasma; thus, the feedback of aldosterone action on the regulation of its synthesis is established. Plasma volume regulates aldosterone synthesis through the renin-angiotensin system, and aldosterone is a major determinant of plasma volume.

Potassium is a potent stimulus of aldosterone secretion, but its effect is direct on the aldosterone-producing cells of the adrenal glomerulosa. Aldosterone is the important physiologic determinant of the amount of potassium in the body. ACTH also is a stimulus of aldosterone secretion, but its effect is acute and transient. Longer exposure of aldosterone-secreting glomerulerosa cells to ACTH leads to a decrease in aldosterone synthesis by the cells. During pathophysiologic states of chronic sodium retention as in primary aldosteronism, the renal response to aldosterone escapes from the sodium-retaining effects of aldosterone. This suggests the presence of another factor that interacts with the action of aldosterone, a natriuretic factor such as atrial natriuretic peptide.

Effects of Aldosterone

The physiologic effects of aldosterone are those of a mineralocorticoid, causing sodium reabsorption and potassium excretion. These effects occur primarily in the distal nephron but also occur in the colon and salivary glands. There is suggestion that the vascular endothelium and the brain also respond to aldosterone as a corticoid having cellular membrane as well as intranuclear effects (8). Aldosterone exerts its mineralocorticoid action by entering target cells and binding to a specific corticoid receptor in the cytosol of the cells. The aldosterone-receptor complex then enters the nucleus of the cell, interacting with DNA in the nucleus and thereby initiating the synthesis of a protein, which is produced by the cell and leads to the reabsorption of sodium or excretion of potassium by the epithelial target cells. Aldosterone also enhances the excretion of hydrogen ion, particularly in the nephron. Sodium reabsorption is a major determinant of plasma volume because, as body sodium is increased, body water is increased concomitantly. This leads to an increase in plasma volume, and thereby in blood pressure. This does not lead to an increase in plasma or serum sodium concentration because of the parallel increase in water content of the blood. The stimulus by aldosterone to potassium excretion, however, leads to a decrease in plasma and total body potassium for which there is no physiologic compensation, such as a change in body or plasma water content, so that the plasma or serum potassium concentration responds directly to changes in aldosterone effect in the nephron, colon, sweat, or salivary glands.

The aldosterone or mineralocorticoid receptor complex in the distal nephron responds to cortisol, a glucocorticoid, also. The inappropriate activation of the mineralocorticoid receptor by cortisol is prevented by the conversion of cortisol to cortisone (which does not activate the receptor) by 11-β-hydroxysteroid dehydrogenase in the distal nephron cells containing the mineralocorticoid receptor. This is important physiologically because cortisol circulates in the plasma in an amount 1,000 times more than aldosterone, and the regulation of cortisol synthesis by ACTH is not responsive to the effects of activating the mineralocorticoid receptor (sodium retention, increase in plasma volume, and kaliuresis) as is the regulation of aldosterone synthesis. An insufficiency of this dehydrogenase in the distal nephron causes a pathologic syndrome of apparent mineralocorticoid excess, which is actually an excess in effect of a normal amount of cortisol on the mineralocorticoid receptor, which normally is protected from cortisol by the dehydrogenase (9).

Metabolism of Aldosterone

Aldosterone is weakly bound to plasma proteins so that there is not a large reservoir of aldosterone in the plasma as there is for cortisol or sex steroids. Aldosterone is metabolized by the liver and kidney by reduction to inactive reduced steroid metabolites. These metabolites are conjugated to a glucuronide for excretion into the urine. The measurement of aldosterone has relied on the measurement of these metabolites excreted into the urine, because there is a very small amount of nonmetabolized aldosterone excreted into the urine. Assays have been developed to measure aldosterone in the plasma; they represent primarily the effective concentration of aldosterone because there is little protein building of aldosterone in the plasma. Renal disease or hepatic disease decrease the excretion of aldosterone metabolites; to a lesser extent, they affect the active, plasma concentration of aldosterone.

PATHOPHYSIOLOGY OF PRIMARY ALDOSTERONISM

Primary aldosteronism is the nonregulated or autonomous production of aldosterone, which results in an increase in body sodium, plasma volume, and blood pressure, with a concomitant decrease in body potassium and plasma potassium. These consequences of a pathologically increased secretion of aldosterone in primary aldosteronism reflect the excess of its physiologic actions. These excessive effects of aldosterone directly suppress the renin-angiotensin system, the physiologic regulator of aldosterone secretion. Although there is a spectrum of severity of primary aldosteronism, the basic pathophysiology of the disorder is manifested by high blood pressure and hypokalemia.

Clinical Presentation of Primary Aldosteronism

Unlike most endocrine or hormonal disorders, primary aldosteronism does not have characteristic symptoms or signs. High blood pressure is consistently present, but high blood pressure is a common medical sign and not sufficiently specific to be a reliable clue to the presence of primary aldosteronism. Unprovoked hypokalemia, however, is a laboratory finding that is a strong clue to the presence of primary aldosteronism. Thus, the measurement of the serum potassium before prescribing therapy for high blood pressure is an important screening or diagnostic maneuver in medical practice. A reasonable threshold of serum potassium concentration that could set aside the diagnosis of primary aldosteronism is 4.0 mEq/L or greater. This threshold (except under circumstances such as spironolactone or amiloride therapy, which can increase serum potassium concentration even in the presence of primary aldosteronism, or extreme restriction of sodium intake) can guide the decision as to whether to pursue the diagnosis of surgically curable (unilateral) primary aldosteronism.

Thus, the clinical presentation of primary aldosteronism is most often asymptomatic, incidentally detected, unprovoked hypokalemia in the hypertensive patient.

Diagnosis of Primary Aldosteronism

The diagnosis of primary aldosteronism is established by demonstrating the presence of high blood pressure, unprovoked hypokalemia, inappropriate kaliuresis, low plasma renin activity, and high aldosterone secretion as shown by an abnormally high aldosterone excretion or plasma concentration (Fig. 5-1). The presence of high blood pressure, low serum potassium, and high urinary potassium (to exclude the presence of potassium loss from a gastrointestinal villous adenoma) is readily demonstrated. The presence of low renin activity and high aldosterone secretion has been cumbersome and difficult to readily accomplish, however. The generally accepted maneuvers to show low renin activity are either (a) stimulation of plasma renin activity with three doses of 40 mg of furosemide orally at 6-hour intervals followed by 4 hours

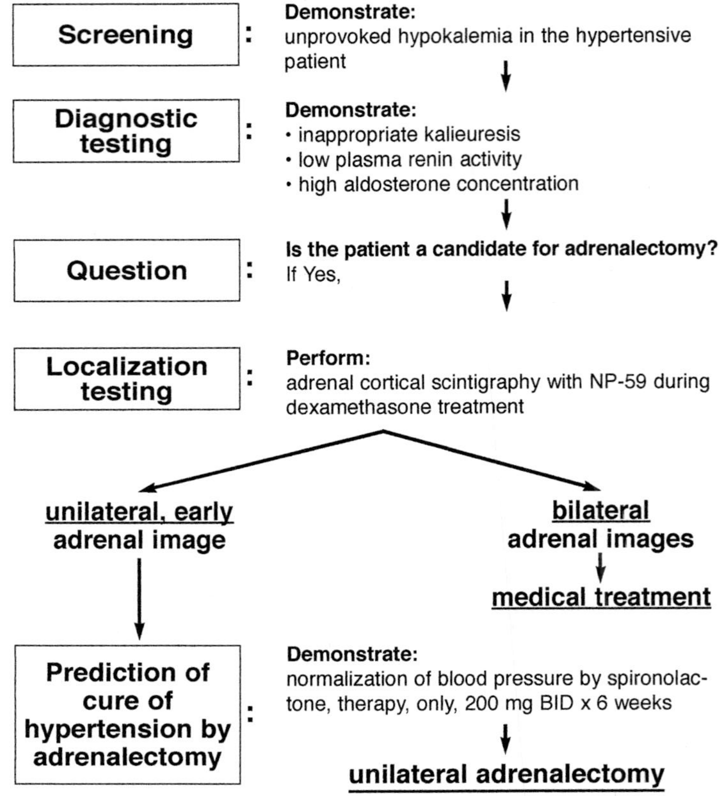

FIG. 5-1. Algorithm to detect a surgically curable aldosterone-producing adrenal adenoma.

of upright posture in the morning (the Carey test) (10) or (b) severe restriction of sodium intake or intravenous furosemide and upright ambulatory activity. Each test has a degree of potential adverse effects. Generally, each clinical laboratory would define the normal renin activity response to these maneuvers so that a low renin activity in response to these stimulations could be identified. Because of the differences in renin activity among segments of the population (e.g., effects of age, gender, and race on the response of renin activity to stimuli), the classification of any one person's result is somewhat difficult.

The assessment of aldosterone secretion to detect an inappropriate or nonsuppressible secretion has also been cumbersome. It has been necessary to show that aldosterone excretion does not appropriately decrease in response to a high intake of sodium orally (11) or to show that the plasma concentration of aldosterone does not appropriately decrease in response to an intravenous administration of sodium chloride (the Kem test) (12). As with plasma renin activity, most laboratories and clinics have a determined threshold of abnormality; however, the use of an excretion rate of 8 μg/24 hours or a plasma concentration of 8 ng/dcl is generally accepted as the upper limit of normal suppression of aldosterone concentrations by sodium administration. Researchers have attempted to identify patients with primary aldosteronism by relating the ratio of their plasma aldosterone concentration to their plasma renin activity to the plasma aldosterone concentration itself (13). The plasma aldosterone concentration is expressed in molar units. This method is convenient because it requires that one blood sample be obtained from the patient in a seated position, but without prior medication that might influence either plasma aldosterone concentration or plasma renin activity. This ratio appears to be useful, but further experience will determine its acceptability and utility.

When primary aldosteronism is suspected, the diagnosis can be demonstrated with attention to the accurate estimation of renin activity and aldosterone secretion. Once unprovoked hypokalemia and inappropriate kaliuresis have been shown, test procedures should be undertaken during potassium therapy to normalize serum potassium. Marked hypokalemia impairs aldosterone secretion and stimulates renin production.

Once the diagnosis of primary aldosteronism has been established, the goal is to determine whether the disorder resides in one or both adrenal glands. This question should be investigated early because, if adrenalectomy is not appropriate for the patient, then distinguishing between unilateral primary aldosterone (a surgically treatable disorder) and bilateral primary aldosteronism (a medically treatable disorder) would not be indicated. Most patients with primary aldosteronism, however, are otherwise well and within an age group and medical status that make a curative adrenalectomy an appropriate therapeutic prospect. Adrenal cortical scintigraphy using NP-59, a radioiodinated cholesterol-like precursor of steroid synthesis, during dexamethasone use is a reliable method of identifying and localizing unilateral primary aldosteronism (14). The use of imaging techniques such as computerized tomography and magnetic resonance imaging can be helpful, but the incidence of nonsecretory adrenal cortical adenoma is sufficiently high to risk a misleading result using these lateralizing procedures only. Adrenal vein sampling during ACTH infusion to measure aldosterone production has been a gold standard maneuver to show unilateral aldosteronism, but the risks of adrenal hemorrhage from the adrenal venography necessary for successful sampling and the difficulty of the procedure have considerably limited its utility (15). The plasma concentration of 18-hydroxycorticosterone has been used to signal the presence of an aldosterone-producing adrenal adenoma as the cause of primary aldosteronism (16). A concentration of 18-hydroxycorticosterone of 100 ng/dcl or higher has been associated with the presence of an adenoma and not with the presence of bilateral hyperplasia. The presence of an adenoma has been associated also with a decrease in plasma aldosterone concentration during upright posture in the morning from 8 a.m. until noon (17). This likely shows the responsiveness of adenomas to ACTH and to its circadian rhythm of a decrease of ACTH secretion during these morning hours. Adenomas are not responsive to upright posture, which might stimulate a very slight increase in activity of the renin-angiotensin system. The bilateral hyperplasia syndrome, however, appears to be responsive to the very slight increase in activity of the renin-angiotensin system during the upright posture in the morning and not to the decline in ACTH, so that plasma aldosterone concentration increases or does not change during this maneuver in idiopathic hyperaldosteronism. It is helpful to measure plasma cortisol concentrations in the blood samples to show that, in fact, the diurnal variation in ACTH has occurred.

The dexamethasone treatment in preparation for adrenal cortical scintigraphy with NP-59 can give a clue to the presence of glucocorticoid-remediable primary aldosteronism. If a blood sample for the measurement of plasma aldosterone, as well as for plasma cortisol, is obtained at the end of the 1-week of relatively high-dose dexamethasone administration, before the injection of the NP-59 radioiodinated isotope, the aldosterone concentration will be low in the presence of glucocorticoid-remediable hyperaldosteronism. The blood pressure does not respond as promptly as the aldosterone secretion to dexamethasone treatment so that the blood pressure response to dexamethasone is not a reliable indicator or clue to the presence of glucocorticoid-remediable primary aldosteronism. Because of the characteristic corticoid metabolites in the glucocorticoid-remediable syndrome (18) and of the presence of specific gene characteristics, there has been a more specific diagnostic approach to this disorder, particularly when a cohort of family members has been detected with severe hypertension at early age, without severe hypokalemia (19).

An unusual subset of primary aldosteronism is primary adrenal hyperplasia, in which the pathologic finding is hyperplasia, but in which the testing responses of aldosterone hypersecretion are those of the adenomatous type of primary aldosteronism. Unilateral or bilateral forms have been described, and in contrast to idiopathic hyperaldosteronism, have been treated successfully by unilateral or subtotal adrenalectomy. The bilateral subset of primary adrenal hyperplasia is suspected when testing maneuvers suggest unilateral adenomatous disease, but adrenal cortical scintigraphy shows bilateral images. A subset of renin-responsive, unilateral, adenomatous primary aldosteronism has been observed also.

In summary, the diagnosis of primary aldosteronism rests on the presence of high blood pressure, unprovoked hypokalemia, inappropriate kaliuresis, and demonstration of high aldosterone secretion and its effect, a low plasma renin activity. The therapeutic intervention is primarily determined by whether the primary aldosteronism is due to unilateral or bilateral disease as shown by adrenal cortical scintigraphy during dexamethasone use, and perhaps supplemented by the measurement of the aldosterone response to upright posture in the morning or the measurement of the 18-hydroxycorticosterone plasma connection. Glucocorticoid-remediable hyperaldosteronism is shown by the personal and family hypertension history, the response of plasma aldosterone to the dexamethasone preparation for NP-59 adrenal scintigraphy, gene studies, measurements of aldosterone metabolites, and the subacute response of the high blood pressure to dexamethasone replacement therapy. A precise diagnosis of primary aldosteronism, an unusual disorder, can be made using these diagnostic maneuvers.

Treatment

Primary aldosteronism has the morbidity of high blood pressure and the additional morbidity of chronic hypokalemia, which can impair renal function and predispose the patient to cardiac arrhythmias. Appropriate adrenalectomy for unilateral primary aldosteronism is curative of the hypokalemia and ameliorative, if not curative, of the high blood pressure. Thus, the goal of diagnosis of primary aldosteronism is to detect an aldosterone-producing adenoma, the removal of which will be curative. A prediction of the blood pressure response to adrenalectomy for unilateral primary aldosteronism can be estimated by the response of the blood pressure to high-dose (400 mg daily in divided doses) spironolactone treatment for 6 weeks as the sole antihypertensive therapy (20). This medical blockade of aldosterone effect consistently normalizes the serum potassium, and it normalizes the blood pressure in patients who respond to adrenalectomy. Thus, if there is particular medical reason to be more predictive about the benefits of adrenalectomy, the response to high-dose spironolactone can be used to aid in that prediction. If the disorder is bilateral or if the response to high-dose spironolactone is not satisfactory, antihypertensive medication therapy and medication to prevent kaliuresis are reasonable alternatives to adrenalectomy, even if the prospect for their use in the patient is lifelong. Calcium channel blockers have been successfully used to control the blood pressure, and spironolactone or amiloride to control the hypokalemia in primary aldosteronism. Spironolactone is more effective than amiloride in decreasing the blood pressure but has the adverse effects of disruption of menstrual periods and causing tender gynecomastia. Amiloride has little, if any, antihypertensive effect but is usually well tolerated and does not have the potential for urinary stone disease as does triamterene therapy for the same purpose. Thus, if surgical cure by unilateral adrenalectomy is not a reasonable prospect, successful medical therapy can usually be achieved.

After adrenalectomy for primary aldosteronism, there may well be a prolonged period of suppressed aldosterone secretion from the contralateral, remaining adrenal, resulting in a degree of hyperkalemia or susceptibility to hyperkalemia. This, in time, remits and there is no easy way to prevent it in advance. Bilateral adrenalectomy in an attempt to successfully treat bilateral aldosteronism does not ameliorate the hypertension, inexplicably, and leads to another medical problem, adrenal insufficiency. Appropriate treatment that is most likely to be successful for primary aldosteronism depends on precise diagnosis (21).

ALDOSTERONE-PRODUCING ADRENAL CANCER

Aldosterone-producing adrenal cancers are rare. Adrenal cancers presenting with hypokalemia are usually due to the excessive production of other mineralocorticoids such as deoxycorticosterone. The approach to a cancerous adrenal lesion secreting aldosterone is surgical removal and control of the effects of excess aldosterone by antihypertensive and antikaliuretic medication.

SURGICAL CONSIDERATIONS IN THE TREATMENT OF PRIMARY ALDOSTERONISM

Preoperative preparation of these hypertensive hypokalemic patients with spironolactone, 100 to 300 mg/d for 4 to 6 weeks, safely reduces blood pressure and restores normal electrolytes in most cases. Occasionally, potassium supplementation or additional antihypertensive therapy is required in patients with very large tumors producing hyperaldosteronism. In these cases, continued close collaboration with the endocrinologist and preoperative consultation with the anesthesiologist is appropriate (see Chapter 10).

As described in Chapters 12 and 13, laparoscopic total uniadrenalectomy or partial adrenalectomy is safe and effective for most patients with adenoma. In those cases in which open adrenalectomy is appropriate, we prefer a posterior surgical incision, although an extraperitoneal flank approach can also be used. An anterior incision for adenoma is usually not indicated, because it is associated with greater morbidity, except in those rare instances of hyperaldosteronism in which adrenal carcinoma is a genuine diagnostic concern. The traditional bilateral posterior approach for simultaneous exploration of both adrenals is no longer necessary, because precise preoperative localization of adenoma has become routine.

SUMMARY

Primary aldosteronism is the least common of the identifiable causes of secondary hypertension that present as high blood pressure. The best clue to its presence is that of unprovoked hypokalemia. The diagnosis can be established by demonstrating the presence of inappropriate kaliuresis, low plasma renin activity, and high aldosterone concentration. Therapy is best directed by adrenal cortical scintigraphy with dexamethasone to determine whether the disorder resides in one or in both adrenal glands. Unilateral primary aldosteronism is optimally treated by unilateral adrenalectomy; bilateral primary aldosteronism is optimally treated medically. The beneficial effects of unilateral adrenalectomy can be reasonably predicted by assessing the response of the blood pressure to high-dose spironolactone therapy only for 6 weeks. An unusual form of primary aldosteronism, which is remediable by glucocorticoid treatment and which produces severe hypertension without severe hypokalemia, is present primarily in families and is suggested by the unexpected decrease of plasma aldosterone in response to dexamethasone administration, such as in the preparation for adrenal cortical scintigraphy.

Conn's demonstration of primary aldosteronism resulting from an aldosterone-producing adrenal adenoma clearly showed the presence of a newly discovered cause of high blood pressure, stimulating much advance in the understanding of the influence of mineralocorticoid activity on the blood pressure and potassium balance physiologically, and in persons with forms of hypertension other than primary aldosteronism.

REFERENCES

1. Conn JW. Presidential address: primary aldosteronism, a new clinical syndrome. *J Lab Clin Med* 1955;45(pt 2): 6–17.
2. Laragh JH, Ledingham JGG, Sommers SC. Secondary aldosteronism and reduced plasma renin in hypertensive disease (Liddle GW, in discussion). *Trans Assoc Am Physicians* 1967;80:168–182.
3. Sutherland DJA, Ruse JL, Laidlow JC. Hypertension, increased aldosterone secretion, and low plasma renin activity relieved by dexamethasone. *Can Med Assoc J* 1966;95:1109–1119.
4. Ganguly A, Zager PG, Luetscher JA. Primary aldosteronism due to unilateral adrenal hyperplasia. *J Clin Endocrinol Metab* 1980;51:1190–1194.
5. Revach M, Shilo S, Cabili S, et al. Hyperaldosteronism caused by adrenal cortical carcinoma. *Isr J Med Sci* 1977;13:1123–1128.
6. Lifton, Dluhy RG, Powers M, et al. A chimaeric 11 beta-hydroxylase/aldosterone synthase gene causes glucocorticoid-remediable aldosteronism and human hypertension. *Nature* 1992;355:262–265.
7. Sergev O, Racz K, Varga I, et al. Dissociation of plasma atrial natriuretic peptide responses to upright posture and furosemide administration in patients with normal, low-renin essential hypertension, and primary aldosteronism. *Clin Exp Hypertens* 1991;13:409–423.
8. Wehling M. Non-genomic aldosterone effects: the cell membrane as a specific target of mineralocorticoid action. *Steroids* 1995;60:153–156.
9. Ulick S, Levine LS, Gunczler P, et al. A syndrome of apparent mineralocorticoid excess associated with defects in the peripheral metabolism of cortisol. *J Clin Endocrinol Metab* 1979;49:757–764.
10. Carey RM, Douglas JG, Schweikert R, et al. The syndrome of essential hypertension and suppressed plasma renin activity: normalization of blood pressure with spironolactone. *Arch Intern Med* 1972;130:849–854.
11. Brown RD, Wisgerhof M. Radioimmunoassay of aldosterone. In Duarte CG: *Renal Function Tests*, 1st ed. Boston: Little, Brown, 1980:174.
12. Kem DC, Weinberger MH, Mayes DM, et al. Saline suppression of plasma aldosterone in hypertension. *Arch Intern Med* 1971;128:380–386.
13. McKenna TJ, Sequira SJ, Heffernan A, et al. Diagnosis under random conditions of all disorders of the renin-angiotensin-aldosterone axis, including primary aldosteronism. *J Clin Endocrinol Metab* 1991;73:952–957.
14. Gross MD, Thrall JH, Beierwaltes WH. The adrenal scan: a current status report on radiotracers, dosimetry, and clinical utility. In: Freeman LM, Weissman HS, eds. *Nuclear Medicine Annual 1980*. New York: Raven Press, 1980;142–150.
15. Weinberger MH, Grim CE, Hollifield JW, et al. Primary aldosteronism: diagnosis, localization, and treatment. *Ann Intern Med* 1979;90:388–390.
16. Biglieri EG, Schambelan M, Hirari J, et al. The significance of elevated levels of plasma 18-hydroxycorticosterone in patients with primary aldosteronism. *J Clin Endocrinol Metab* 1979;49:87–91.
17. Ganguly A, Dowdy AJ, Luetscher JA, et al. Anomalous postural response of plasma aldosterone concentration in patients with aldosterone-producing adrenal adenoma. *J Clin Endocrinol Metab* 1973;36:401–404.
18. Gomez-Sanchez CE, Montgomery M, Ganguly A, et al. Elevated urinary excretion of 18-oxocortisol in glucocorticoid-suppressible aldosteronism. *J Clin Endocrinol Metab* 1984;59:1022–1024.
19. Rich GM, Ulick S, Cook S, et al. Glucocorticoid-remediable aldosteronism in a large kindred: clinical spectrum and diagnosis using a characteristic biochemical phenotype. *Ann Intern Med* 1992;116:813–820.
20. Herf SM, Teates DC, Tegtmeyer CJ, et al. Identification and differentiation of surgically correctable hypertension due to primary aldosteronism. *Am J Med* 1979;67: 397–402.
21. Wisgerhof M. Primary aldosteronism at Henry Ford Hospital in the 1980s. *Henry Ford Hosp Med J* 1987;35: 226–233.

*Medical and Surgical Management of
Adrenal Diseases*, edited by Joseph C. Cerny.
Lippincott Williams & Wilkins, Philadelphia © 1999.

6

Adrenal Cortical Carcinoma

James O. Peabody and Joseph C. Cerny

Department of Urology, Henry Ford Hospital, Detroit, Michigan 48202

EPIDEMIOLOGY

Adrenal cortical carcinomas are rare, occurring in 1 to 2 per million individuals, with about 100 new cases per year in the United States (1–4). They account for less than 0.05% of new cancers diagnosed. There is a bimodal occurrence, with tumors developing in children younger than 5 years of age and in adults in the fifth to seventh decades of life. The male-to-female ratio is 2:1, with functional tumors being more common in women. These tumors can occur as part of a hereditary cancer syndrome (Li-Frameni), with 9% to 11% of adrenal cancer patients having a second tumor (sarcoma, breast, lung, brain, leukemia, lymphoma). Up to 3% of patients with hereditary cancers have an adrenal cancer. Almost all patients in reported series are Caucasian (1–11). The left adrenal is involved slightly more often than the right (53% versus 47%), and bilateral tumors are rare (2%). A variety of genetic abnormalities have been documented in adrenal cortical carcinomas, including 17p, 11p, and 13q deletions. Mutant p53 has been found in 20% of cancers, and Ras overactivity appears uncommon. To date, a predictive marker has not been identified (1,12).

PATHOLOGIC FEATURES

There is considerable overlap between the features of benign and malignant adrenal cortical tumors, making the diagnosis of adrenal cortical carcinoma difficult. Several sets of histologic criteria have been proposed to refine the diagnosis (Table 6-1) (12).

A variety of clinical and pathologic features have been evaluated for their prognostic significance. These include stage, age, mitotic activity, tumor grade, presence of vascular invasion, various cytologic features, tumor size, DNA index, and functional status (1,12). Only stage, age, and possibly tumor size and mitotic index seem particularly useful. No independently predictive factor has been identified.

STAGING

The staging system in common use is presented in Table 6-2, and survival data are given in Table 6-3. Up to 70% of patients in reported series have advanced disease at the time of diagnosis, with a median survival in this group of less than 1 year. The Cleveland Clinic reviewed 82 patients and reported a

TABLE 6–1. *Pathologic criteria
for adrenal cortical cancer:
diffuse growth pattern*

Vascular invasion
Necrosis
Broad fibrous bands
Capsular invasion
High mitotic index (1/10 high-power fields)
High nuclear grade
Tumor size >100 g
Abnormal nucleoli

TABLE 6–2. *Staging of adrenal cortical cancer*

Stage	Size	Nodes	Local invasion	Metastasis	TNM
1	<5 cm	–	–	–	T1N0M0
2	>5 cm	–	–	–	T2N0M0
3	Any size		+	–	T3N0M0
		+	–	–	T1-2N1M0
		+	+	–	T3N1M0
		+/–	+ (adjacent organ)	+/–	T4N0-1M0-1
4	Any size	+/–	+/–	+	M1

3.8-year median survival in patients with stage I and II cancers, with median survival of 0.6 year in stage III and IV patients (1,4). Overall survival rate at 3 and 5 years was 37.5% and 25%, respectively. Patients who had localized tumors treated with apparently complete surgical excision had a 44% 5-year overall survival rate.

Nadler and colleagues reported the M.D. Anderson experience of 77 patients receiving treatment from 1950 to 1981 (6). They found a 50% 2-year overall survival rate and a 30% 5-year overall survival rate. Only 5 of 35 patients with apparently complete surgical resection remained with no evidence of disease (NED). Recurrences were seen up to 10 years after initial surgical treatment.

Icard and colleagues reported on 156 patients undergoing treatment from 1978 to 1991 by the French Association of Endocrine Surgery (7). The 5-year survival rate was 34% overall, with 53% in those with localized (stages I and II) cancers and 24% in those with regional (stage III) cancers. Twenty-seven percent of patients operated on for recurrence survived for 5 years. Median survival for stage IV patients was 6 months, with a 9% 1-year survival rate.

Pommier and Brennan reported the Memorial Sloan-Kettering Cancer Center (MSKCC) experience with 73 patients undergoing treat-

TABLE 6–3. *Survival with adrenal cortical carcinoma*

3 yr	37%
5 yr	22%–47%
Mean/median	28 mo to 3.8 yr
Metastatic	6–9 mo

ment from 1980 to 1991 (8). In patients with 53 resectable tumors, the mean survival was 28 months, the 5-year survival rate was 47%, and 45 tumors (85%) recurred. The 5- and 10-year overall survival rates were 35% and 21%, respectively. The mean survival was 35 months for stage I and II tumors, 26 months for stage III, and 9 months for stage IV.

Luton and colleagues reported on 105 patients receiving treatment from 1963 to 1987 (9). Only 30% had advanced disease at presentation, although metastasis developed in 82%. The median survival was 14.5 months, and the 5-year survival rate was 22%.

Mendonca and colleagues from Brazil reported on 38 patients, with functional adrenal tumors in 18 pediatric and 20 adult patients (6 male patients, 32 female patients) (10). Tumor size ranged from 1.5 to 21 cm. All patients underwent complete surgical excision of the tumor, with concurrent nephrectomy required in seven. Sixteen of 18 children had NED at 24 to 114 months' follow-up. All surviving patients had stage I disease with two deaths occurring at 6 and 12 months in children with stage III disease. Sixteen of 20 adults had NED at 18 to 132 months' follow-up, with four deaths occurring 2 to 5 years after diagnosis. Nineteen of 20 patients had stage I disease. Five of six patients with Cushing's syndrome associated with excessive androgen secretion died of their disease. Early diagnosis, perhaps as a result of functional status and low clinical stage, was thought to be the cause of better survival results in this group of patients.

Metastatic sites in adrenal cortical carcinoma are listed in Table 6-4.

Classification of adrenal cortical tumors is based on functional status, with functional tu-

TABLE 6–4. *Metastatic sites in adrenal cortical carcinoma*

Liver
Lung
Peritoneum
Pleura
Kidney
Vena cava
Bone
Pancreas
Brain

TABLE 6–6. *Presenting symptoms of nonfunctional adrenal tumors*

Abdominal pain
Mass
Fatigue
Gastrointestinal symptoms
Weight loss
Hematuria
Fever
Asymptomatic

mors occurring in approximately 60% of patients in reported series (1–10). The symptoms and signs associated with functional tumors (Table 6-5) are the result of excess production of corticosteroids, androgens, estrogens, and mineralocorticoids. Clinical symptoms are related to excess production of these steroids. Functional tumors produce cortisol alone in 50% to 70% of cases, androgens in 10% to 20%, and a mixture in 20% to 30%. Isolated mineralocorticoid production is rare. Cushing's syndrome with virilization is generally caused by adrenal carcinoma. Pure testosterone-secreting tumors are more often smaller than 6 cm, localized, and usually detected in women (1–4). Feminizing tumors are seen in 20- to 50-year-old men and are often larger and malignant. They secrete androstenedione, which is converted to estrogen.

TABLE 6–5. *Presenting symptoms of functional adrenal tumors*

Cortisol excess
  Truncal obesity
  Rounded facies
  Striae
  Hypertension
  Osteoporosis
Virilization
  Precocious puberty in boys
  Clitoromegaly
  Temporal balding
  Breast atrophy
  Oligomenorrhea
  Hirsutism
Feminization
  Gynecomastia
  Testicular atrophy
  Decreased libido in boys
  Precocious puberty in girls

The classification of a tumor as functional is generally based on clinical signs and symptoms; however, nonfunctional tumors may produce steroid precursors with less biologic activity. Nonfunctional tumors are more likely to grow and spread silently, to be more advanced at the time of diagnosis, and therefore to have a poorer prognosis. Nonfunctional tumors should be evaluated with catecholamine and metanephrine levels to rule out pheochromocytoma.

Presenting signs and symptoms of nonfunctional adrenal tumors include abdominal pain or mass, fatigue, gastrointestinal (GI) symptoms, weight loss, hematuria, and fever (Table 6-6) (1–9). Symptoms caused by cortisol excess include truncal obesity, rounded facies, striae, acne, hypertension, and osteoporosis. Androgen excess causes precocious puberty in prepubertal boys and clitoromegaly, temporal balding, breast atrophy, oligomenorrhea, and hirsutism in girls. Estrogen excess causes gynecomastia, testicular atrophy, and decreased libido in boys and precocious puberty in prepubertal girls.

DIAGNOSIS

The diagnosis of a functioning adrenal tumor can be suspected on the clinical grounds noted earlier. It can be confirmed by various biochemical tests, including elevated levels of urinary free cortisol or steroid precursors, serum cortisol levels showing loss of normal circadian rhythm, low serum adrenocorticotropic hormone, an abnormal dexamethasone suppression test, and elevated serum testosterone, estradiol, or aldosterone levels

(1,4,13). The decision to perform a particular test depends on the clinical presentation and the clinician's judgment.

The radiographic evaluation should include images of the adrenal glands as well as of suspected metastatic sites for purposes of staging and operative planning (1–4). Computed tomography (CT) and magnetic resonance imaging (MRI) of the abdomen can demonstrate the presence of visceral metastasis and the local tumor extent, although it can be difficult to show definitively invasion of the adjacent organs. MR images of adrenal tumors are isodense to the liver on T1-weighted images and hyperdense on T2-weighted images. MRI more accurately gauges the extent of any intracaval tumor thrombus and can give coronal and sagittal images. The role of fine needle aspiration for the diagnosis of small adrenal lesions is unclear. It can accurately distinguish metastasis from adrenal tumors but may not reliably distinguish adenoma from carcinoma, which can at times be difficult even on histopathologic section.

INCIDENTALLY DISCOVERED ADRENAL MASSES

With the increased use of cross-sectional imaging for a variety of purposes, more unsuspected adrenal tumors are being discovered (1,13,14). Series have reported that between 0.6% and 4.3% of abdominal scans show incidental tumors, and autopsy series report clinically silent adrenal tumors in 1.4% to 8.7% of individuals. Because adrenal cancers are diagnosed in only 1 to 2 per 1 million individuals, the majority of these lesions are adenomas. Differential diagnosis includes adrenal cortical neoplasms, metastatic tumors, pheochromocytoma, myelolipoma, and adrenal cysts (see Chapter 2). The incidental lesions tend to be small, with most being less than 3 cm. Belldegrun and colleagues found

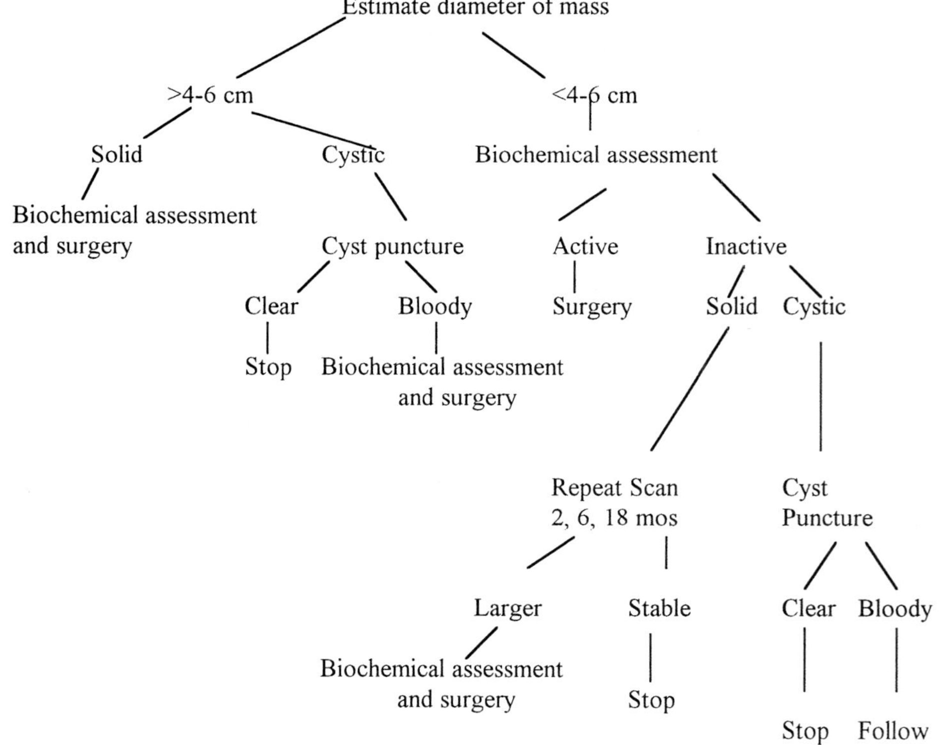

FIG. 6-1. Approach to the incidentally discovered adrenal mass.

that 105 of 114 adrenal cancers were larger than 6 cm (15). Mendonca and colleagues found 2 of 20 adult tumors and 6 of 18 pediatric tumors to be less than 3 cm (10).

All solid adrenal masses should undergo biochemical evaluation and, if functioning, should be removed. If lesions are nonfunctioning and less than 3 cm in diameter, serial CT scans every 3 to 6 months for 2 years should be done to demonstrate stability. Nonfunctioning lesions that are 3 to 5 cm in size are controversial. Some authors recommend exploration for lesions greater than 3 or 4 cm (16); others have estimated that only 1 in 4,000 tumors between 3 and 6 cm are cancers. In patients younger than 40 years old in whom adenomas are less common, a more aggressive approach to the smaller lesions may be warranted (Fig. 6-1).

TREATMENT

Complete surgical removal of the primary lesion and any resectable metastatic sites has been the mainstay of treatment. En bloc excision of the adrenal and kidney together with splenectomy and partial pancreatic or hepatic resection is sometimes necessary for total extirpation of the neoplasm (see Chapter 13) (1–11,17,18). Survival prognosis in patients requiring more extensive resection is generally poor.

The surgical approach can involve a subcostal, chevron, or thoracoabdominal incision. Early vascular control and thorough abdominal exploration for metastasis are important surgical principles. Patients with functioning tumors require corticosteroid and mineralocorticoid replacement postoperatively because of contralateral adrenal suppression. Patients should be followed up with periodic physical examinations, chest radiographs, abdominal CT scans, and biochemical testing when clinically indicated (1–4). Resection of recurrent disease has occasionally been successful in prolonging survival and providing palliation but has not produced long-term survival.

Chemotherapy has been used in patients with advanced adrenocortical cancers to control symptoms caused by excess steroid production and in an attempt to eradicate or palliate metastatic or residual disease (Table 6-7).

Mitotane (O-P-DDD) was originally noted to cause adrenal atrophy in dogs. It inhibits several enzyme systems, including delta-5-pregnenolone, 11-β-hydroxylation, and 18-hydroxylation, as well as inhibiting extraadrenal steroid metabolism. Bergenstal and colleagues showed regression of some metastatic lesions and normalization of steroid production in some patients (19). Overall, 70% to 90% of patients receiving mitotane have a greater than 50% decrease in steroid levels, with objective tumor regression in 10% to 61% (average 24%) of patients (1,4). Time to response is 1 to 2.5 months, with a duration of response of 9 to 12 months. Occasional responses of greater than 2 years have been noted. Adjuvant use in lower stage disease has not been shown to improve survival. The dose used ranges from 6 to 12 g/day; higher doses are less tolerable. A serum level of more than 14 µg/mL increases the response rate.

Side effects of mitotane include nausea, vomiting, anorexia, diarrhea, lethargy, dizziness, confusion, myalgias, headaches, and skin rashes. Because of the effective decrease in steroid production, concomitant use of corticosteroids and mineralocorticoids is needed.

Aminoglutethimide inhibits several steps in steroid biosynthesis. It decreases cortisol levels by 50% and temporarily reverses cushingoid features in some patients with adrenal cancer, but it does not affect tumor progression. Adrenal insufficiency can develop, and replacement therapy is warranted.

TABLE 6–7. *Chemotherapy for advanced adrenal cortical cancer*

Mitotane
Aminoglutethimide
Metyrapone
Platinum
VP-16
Doxyrubicin
Suramin

Metyrapone inhibits 11-β-hydroxylation and may be a useful adjunct to control symptoms of steroid excess.

Cytotoxic chemotherapy has been used in several small series (1,4). Most regimens are platinum based, with the addition of mitotane, doxorubicin, VP-16, or suramin. A 28% response rate was reported in a total of 10 series, with the numbers of patients ranging from 1 to 37. There were five complete and 34 partial responses in the 141 patients. Duration of response ranged from 2 to 78 months, with most responses lasting less than 1 year.

Radiation therapy has some utility in the palliation of metastatic lesions but no role in the treatment of primary lesions.

SUMMARY

Adrenal cortical carcinoma is a rare tumor. In addition to the usual constitutional symptoms associated with cancers, it produces a variety of clinical signs and symptoms through excess production of steroid hormones.

Surgical treatment with adrenalectomy remains the mainstay of treatment. Good survival rate is reported in patients with tumors confined to the adrenal. Patients with more extensive tumor achieve only temporary partial remission with currently available chemotherapeutic agents.

REFERENCES

1. Bukowski RM, Klein EA. Management of adrenal neoplasms. In: Vogelzang NJ, Scardino PT, Shipley WU, Coffey D, eds. *Comprehensive textbook of genitourinary oncology.* Baltimore: Williams & Wilkins, 1996:125–153.
2. Vaughn ED Jr, Carey RM. Adrenal carcinoma. In: Vaughn ED Jr, Carey RM, eds. *Adrenal disorders.* New York: Thieme Medical Publishers, Inc., 1996:231–242.
3. McDougal WS. Adrenal cortical carcinoma. In: Scott HW JR, ed. *Surgery of the adrenal glands.* Philadelphia: J.B. Lippincott, 1990:241–250.
4. Barzilay JI, Pazianos AG. Adrenocortical carcinoma in adrenal surgery. *Urologic Clinics of North America* 1989;16(3):457–468.
5. Wooten MD, King DK. Adrenal cortical carcinoma: epidemiology and treatment with mitotane and a review of the literature. *Cancer* 1993;72:3145–3155.
6. Nadler S, Hickery RC, Sellin RV, et al. Adrenal cortical carcinoma; a study of 77 cases. *Cancer* 1983;52:707–711.
7. Icard P, Chapuis Y, Andreassian B, et al. Adrenocortical carcinoma in surgically treated patients: a retrospective study on 156 cases by the French Association of Endocrine Surgery. *Surgery* 1992;112(6):973–980.
8. Pommier RF, Brennan MR. An eleven-year experience with adrenocortical carcinoma. *Surgery* 1992;112(6): 973–980.
9. Luton JP, Cerdas S, Billaud L, et al. Clinical features of adrenocortical carcinoma, prognostic factors, and the effect of mitotane therapy. *N Engl J Med* 1990;322(17): 1195–1201.
10. Mendonca BB, Lucon AM, Menezes CA, et al. Clinical, hormonal, and pathological findings in a comparative study of adrenocortical neoplasms in childhood and adulthood. *J Urol* 1995;154:2004–2009.
11. Richie JP, Gittes RF. Carcinoma of the adrenal cortex. *Cancer* 1980;45[suppl]:1957–1964.
12. Medeiros LJ, Weiss LM. New developments in the pathologic diagnosis of adrenal cortical neoplasms: a review. *AJCP* 1992;97(1):73–83.
13. Ross NS, Aron DC. Hormonal evaluation of the patient with an incidentally discovered adrenal mass. *N Engl J Med* 1990;323(20):1401–1405.
14. Herrera MF, Grant CS, Van Heerden JA, et al. Incidentally discovered adrenal tumors: an institutional perspective. *Surgery* 1991;110(6):1014–1021.
15. Belldegrun A, Hussain S, Seltzer SE, et al. Incidentally discovered mass of the adrenal gland. *Surgery, Gynecology and Obstetrics* 1986;163:203–208.
16. Cerfolio RJ, Vaughn ED Jr, Brennan TG, et al. Accuracy of computed tomography in predicting adrenal tumor size. *Surgery, Gynecology and Obstetrics* 1993;176(14): 307–309.
17. Javadpour N, Woltering EA, McIntosh CL. Thoracoabdominal median sternotomy for resection of primary adrenal carcinoma extending into the inferior vena cava and hepatic vein. *Urology* 1978;12:626–627.
18. Jensen JC, Pass HI, Sindelar WF, et al. Recurrent or metastatic disease in select patients with adrenocortical carcinoma. *Arch Surg* 1991;126:457–461.
19. Bergenstal DM, Hertz R, LipseH MB, et al. Chemotherapy of adrenocortical cancer with O, P, DDD. *Ann Intern Med* 1960;53:672–682.
20. Potter DA, Strolt CA, Javidpour N, et al. Prolonged survival following SN pulmonary resections for metastatic adrenal cortical carcinoma: a case report. *J Surg Oncol* 1984;25:273–277.

*Medical and Surgical Management of
Adrenal Diseases,* edited by Joseph C. Cerny.
Lippincott Williams & Wilkins, Philadelphia © 1999.

7

Adrenocortical Neoplasms in Childhood

Charles M. Keoleian, *David C. Leach, and Joseph C. Cerny

*Department of Urology, Henry Ford Hospital, Detroit, Michigan 48202; *Executive Director,
ACGME, 515 North State Street, Suite 2000, Chicago, Illinois 60610*

Adrenocortical neoplasms are rare in childhood and are potentially fatal. The differentiation of benign from malignant adrenocortical tumors is difficult, and reports in the literature often have not clearly categorized patients. Prompt diagnosis and careful perioperative management are necessary to achieve improved mortality rates for patients with this disease. Clinicians must be aware of presenting signs and symptoms that suggest the diagnostic consideration of adrenocortical neoplasm in children. Presenting characteristics and prognoses differ in childhood and adulthood adrenocortical neoplasms.

INCIDENCE

Adrenocortical neoplasms account for less than 0.5% of all malignancies in childhood. Cortical tumors comprise only 6% of all childhood adrenal tumors, with neuroblastoma being the most common adrenal malignancy (1). In Brazil, a much higher percentage of childhood neoplasms, 1% to 3%, are adrenocortical tumors (2). Hayles and colleagues added a 12-patient series to their literature review consisting of 222 cases in 1965 (3). Approximately 300 cases were described in the literature prior to 1989 (4). The literature mainly consists of isolated case reports or small series of children combined with larger numbers of adult patients.

Neblett and colleagues, in a literature review of 209 pediatric patients with adrenocor-

tical neoplasms, demonstrated a mean age at presentation of 4.63 years (range, 5 days to 16.5 years). These patients had a female-to-male ratio of 2.2:1, although other series suggest an even greater female predominance (1–3,5–9).

ETIOLOGY

The etiology of adrenocortical neoplasms in childhood has not been elucidated. Many associations with other disease processes have been reported, however. Fraumeni and Miller reported adrenocortical neoplasms in association with hemihypertrophy, brain tumors, and other disorders. They also noted an increased incidence of these tumors in children with hamartomous lesions such as vascular malformations and pigmented nevi (10). The association with hemihypertrophy, which may be an isolated condition or associated with the Beckwith-Wiedemann syndrome (omphalocele, macroglossia, visceromegaly), has been reported by several authors (5,10–14).

Although a specific chromosomal abnormality has not been isolated, a genetic predisposition to development of adrenocortical neoplasms and other tumors is postulated in children. Other primary tumors have been identified in pediatric patients with adrenocortical neoplasms (10,15,16). A renal cell cancer developed in a child who received treatment with irradiation of the adrenal bed after resection of an adrenocortical cancer

(17). Siblings have been diagnosed with these tumors, also supporting this concept (10,18). At least four patients with bilateral adrenocortical neoplasms have been reported (5). Thus, surveillance of patients with adrenocortical neoplasm for the development of other neoplasms has been recommended (19).

CLINICAL FEATURES

In contrast to adult adrenocortical neoplasms, approximately 95% of pediatric patients have a hormonally functional tumor (20). Nonfunctioning tumors may present as a palpable abdominal mass in about half of these patients. These nonfunctioning tumors may also present as metastases to lung, liver, lymph nodes, and, less commonly, to brain or bone (21). The adrenal gland produces glucocorticoids, mineralocorticoids, androgens, and, to a lesser extent, estrogens. These are produced individually or, more commonly, in combination by adrenocortical neoplasms (3).

Virilizing Tumors

Virilization, either alone or combined with features of Cushing's syndrome, accounts for the majority of clinical presentations in children (5,20). Androgen excess is manifested as acne, deepening of the voice, muscular appearance, hirsutism, pubic hair, enlarged penis or clitoris, rapid statural growth, and development of body odor (Figs. 7-1 and 7-2) (7). Aggressive behavior has also been observed. Secretion of dehydroepiandrostendione, dehydroepiandrosterone sulfate (DHEA-S), androstenedione, and testosterone can be identified as elevations on serologic tests. Increased 11-deoxycortisol secretion may be due to autonomous adrenal overproduction or, in these virilizing tumors, can be related to testosterone inhibition of 11-β-hydroxylase (22,23).

Cushing's Syndrome

The features of Cushing's syndrome are present in approximately one-third of the children with adrenocortical neoplasms. These features include obesity, muscle wasting, plethora, round moon facies, striae, and short stature. Endogenous Cushing's syndrome in children is usually due to an adrenal tumor; however, older children have an increased incidence of adrenal hyperplasia. If associated virilization is present, linear growth may be normal and hirsutism may be present. Hypertension and impaired glucose metabolism may be present (7). Plasma cortisol concentrations are elevated, with loss of the diurnal variation in production.

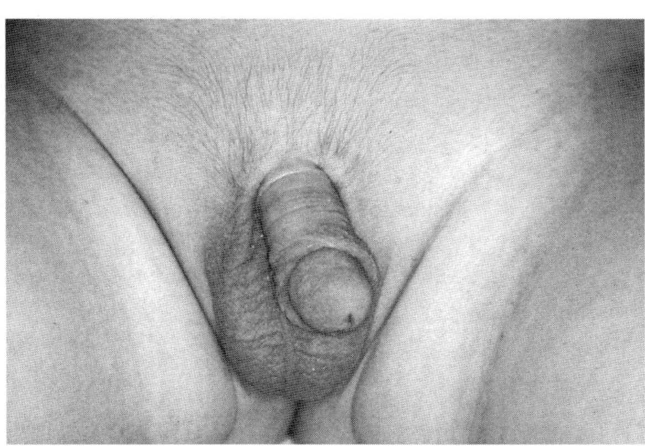

FIG. 7-1. Phallomegaly and pubic hair in a 16-month-old boy with a virilizing adrenal tumor.

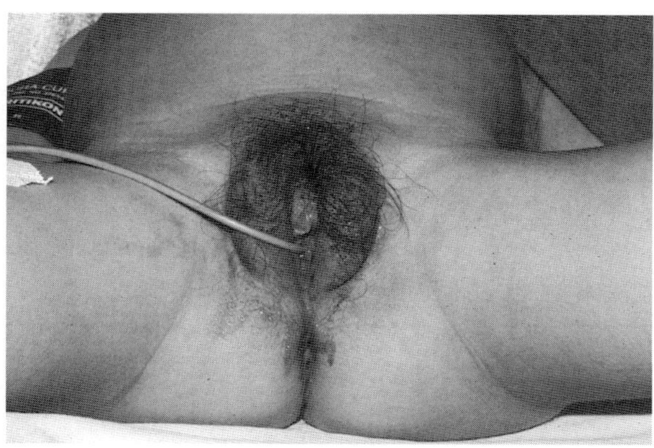

FIG. 7-2. A 20-month-old girl with virilization including clitoromegaly. A 4-cm adrenal neoplasm was removed.

Feminizing Tumors

Feminizing tumors in boys are rare, with fewer than 15 cases documented in the literature (24–34). Estrogen-producing tumors in girls may also occur, causing isosexual precocious puberty (35,36). Normal adrenal glands make little estrogen; however, tumors producing estradiol, estrogen, or estrone can produce the following features: bilateral gynecomastia, accelerated growth rate, female hair distribution, advanced bone age, and, in girls, vaginal bleeding (Fig. 7-3).

Aldosteronoma

Aldosterone-producing tumors are also rare in childhood. Most pediatric patients with aldosteronism have either bilateral adrenocortical hyperplasia or nodular hyperplasia. A child with the clinical symptoms of hypertension, muscle cramps, headaches, and weakness in association with hypokalemia is at risk. Almost all of these neoplasms are benign (Table 7-1) (37).

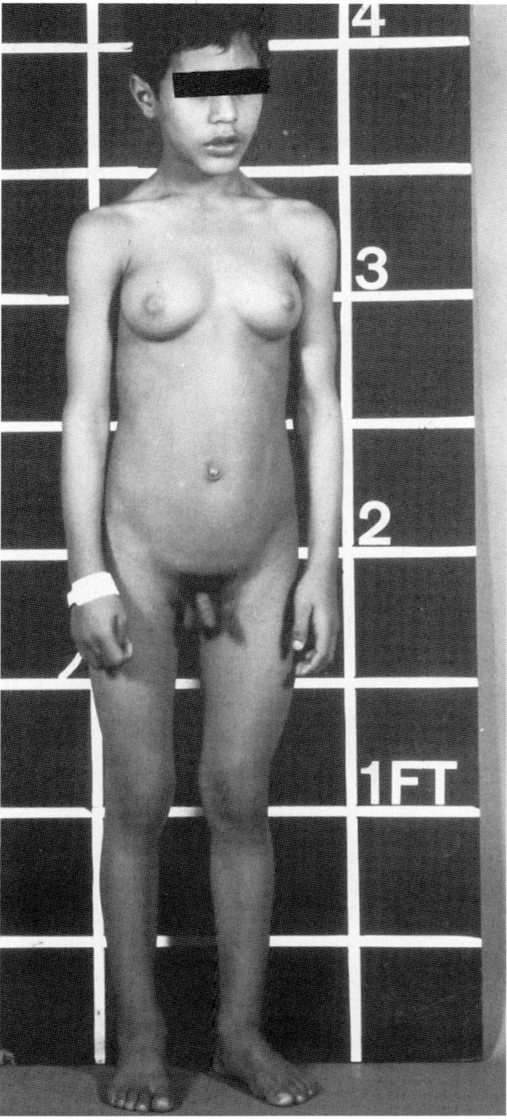

FIG. 7-3. A 6-year-old boy with bilateral gynecomastia who was later found to have a feminizing adrenal neoplasm.

TABLE 7–1. *Clinical features of functional adrenal neoplasms of childhood*

Virilizing	Feminizing	Cushing's	Aldosteronism
Hirsutism	Female hair distribution	Plethora	Hypertension
Pubic hair	Precocious puberty	Obesity	Muscle cramps
Rapid statural growth	Rapid statural growth	Short stature	Headaches
Muscularity	Gynecomastia	Muscle wasting	Weakness
Enlarged phallus	Advanced bone age	Striae	
Deep voice	Vaginal bleeding	Round facies	
Acne	Nipple discharge	Hypertension	
Body odor		Impaired glucose metabolism	

DIAGNOSIS

The differential diagnosis of the various hormonally functional adrenocortical neoplasms in children challenges the clinician. Congenital adrenal hyperplasia is the most common cause of virilization in infants. Neonatal physical findings including labial fusion and clitoromegaly, suggesting this diagnosis (21). When the onset of virilization occurs later in life, diagnostic possibilities include Leydig cell tumors, ovarian tumors, true isosexual precocity, human chorionic gonadotropin-producing tumors, and adrenal lesions. The use of appropriate laboratory and radiologic studies allows localization of the lesions in a timely fashion.

Biochemical Studies

Patients with clinical signs of virilization should have serum testosterone, dehydroepiandrosterone (DHEA), DHEA-S, and androstenedione levels assessed for abnormal elevation. Urinary 17-ketosteroids testing provides a measure of androgenic metabolites. Urinary 17-ketosteroids are usually markedly elevated in malignancy and are less so in benign adrenal lesions (5–7). Unlike adrenal neoplasms, ovarian tumors rarely produce cortisol excess or elevations in urinary 17-ketosteroids (38).

Patients with Cushing's syndrome have increased serum cortisol levels and high levels of urinary excretion of free cortisol and 17-hydroxycorticosteroids. Dexamethasone suppression usually has no effect on urinary steroid excretion in these patients (4). Plasma adrenocorticotropic hormone (ACTH) may help discern the various causes of Cushing's syndrome. Although nonfunctioning adrenal tumors do not produce active hormones, specific elevations in steroid precursors may be found and used as markers for tumor recurrence (21).

In children with feminization, serum estradiol, estrone, follicle-stimulating hormone, and luteinizing hormone should be included in the evaluation. Peripheral conversion of precursors, as opposed to endogenous adrenal production of estrogen, has been contemplated (36).

Imaging Studies

Intravenous pyelography has been replaced as the imaging study of choice for adrenocortical tumors in children. More recent studies have used ultrasound and computed tomography to readily identify the lesions and inspect the contralateral gland. Computed tomography, although more sensitive for very small lesions, is invasive and exposes children to ionizing radiation (Fig. 7-4). Magnetic resonance imaging may prove to be even more sensitive and specific while eliminating ionizing radiation exposure.

Plain radiographs may detect soft-tissue masses and calcifications in the area of the adrenal bed, suggesting adrenocortical neoplasm. These films may also detect lung and bone metastases. Advanced bone age, according to the criteria of Greulich and Pyle (39), may also be documented. The growth patterns of children with adrenocortical neoplasms before and after treatment have been studied. A

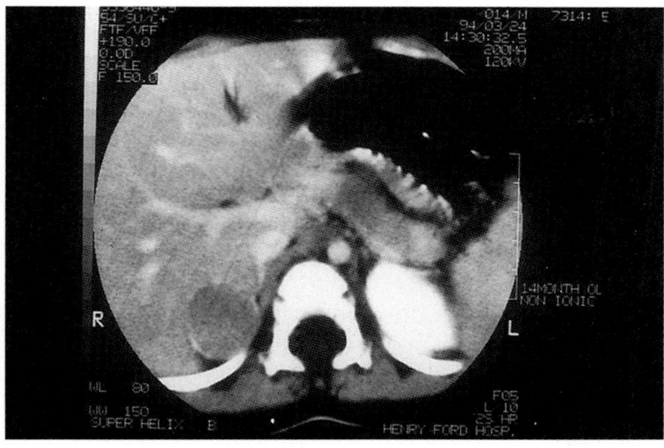

FIG. 7-4. The abdominal computed tomography scan of a 16-month-old boy with clinical virilization demonstrating a homogeneous, well-defined mass arising from the right adrenal gland.

period of growth deceleration after treatment has been described (40,41).

Arteriography and venography should be reserved for those cases in which a suspected functional tumor cannot be localized by less invasive means. Experience with adrenal scintigraphy in children to discern hyperplasia, adenoma, and carcinoma is limited (7).

PATHOLOGY AND PROGNOSIS

In previous reports, the majority of childhood adrenocortical neoplasms were classified as malignant (1,3). The prognosis in early reviews of these patients was poor. The comorbidities of infection and postoperative adrenal insufficiency were not clearly separated from deaths from malignant growth. In Hayles and colleagues' review of 222 childhood cases in 1966, only 34 patients (15%) were documented to have died of metastatic disease. Seventy of the patients died postoperatively from sepsis and other causes. Many of the patients in this series were either lost to follow-up or were followed up for less than 2 years (3). With antibiotic and postoperative adrenal hormone replacement therapy, overall survival rate has improved. However, the classification of benign versus malignant adrenocortical neoplasms in children remains difficult. Only the presence of metastasis is an absolute criterion for malignancy.

Histology and Morphology

Similar pathologic prognostic parameters are applied to children and adults. Cagle and colleagues (6) compared the morphologic features in children and adults. Only 6 of 23 (26%) childhood tumors behaved in a malignant manner. The authors reported that benign pediatric tumors are more likely to have mitoses, necrosis, broad fibrous band, and moderate to severe pleomorphism than benign adult tumors (6). Lack and colleagues, however, noted that increased numbers of mitoses, extensive tumor necrosis ($\geq$25%), and vascular invasion are more common in the clinically malignant adrenocortical neoplasms of children than in clinically benign tumors (42). Weatherby and Carney noted necrosis, capsular or vascular invasion, and increased mitotic activity to be much more frequent in nine tumors in the pediatric age group classified as adrenocortical carcinoma (20). Thus, even if certain histologic criteria are more frequent in patients with a poor outcome, their presence in some pediatric patients with good outcomes makes them ineffective for assessing malignancy in individual pediatric patients (Fig. 7-5).

Tumor weight was suggested by Cagle and colleagues as a useful predictor of malignancy in pediatric adrenocortical neoplasms. Benign behavior was observed in tumors weighing less than 150 g; with increasing size, malignant behavior increased. All of

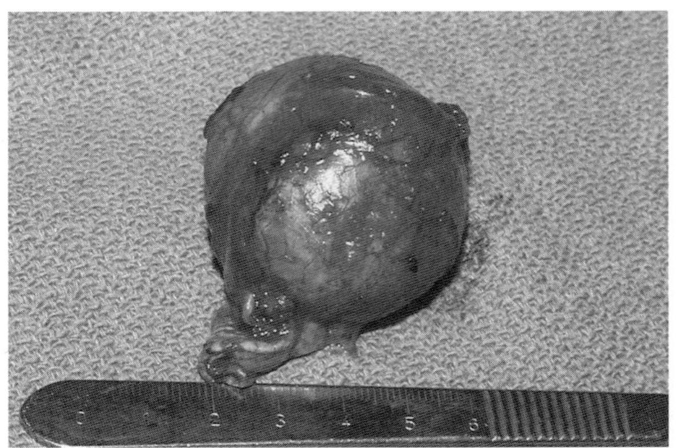

FIG. 7-5. A 4-cm, 35-g pediatric virilizing adrenal tumor. The presence of calcification, necrosis, vascular invasion, and abnormal mitoses was noted on microscopic examination. Postoperatively, serum hormones normalized, with no evidence of recurrence during 4 years of follow-up.

their pediatric tumors weighing more than 500 g behaved in a malignant fashion (6). Lefevre and colleagues described tumors weighing 180 g or less that were clinically malignant (43). Using a tumor weight-to-body weight ratio, Hayles and colleagues reported fewer metastases in children whose ratio was less than 0.7 g of tumor per 100 g of body weight (3). Humphrey and colleagues, in an overview of 114 childhood tumors, could not demonstrate such a correlation of tumor weight-to-body weight ratio and malignant potential. However, they did not use each child's actual weight; instead, the fiftieth percentile for each age was obtained from standard growth charts (44).

TREATMENT

Surgical Approach and Steroid Support

Attempts at complete surgical excision of adrenocortical neoplasm in children is suggested. Proponents of an anterior approach cite access to the contralateral adrenal for intraoperative inspection as an advantage. Improved imaging studies have decreased this need. A posterior retroperitoneal approach has been advocated for small lesions consistent with adenoma (5). Large tumors with suspected malignant potential are best approached anteriorly. A transabdominal approach allows optimal exposure for possible excision of lymph nodes, cava, or adjacent organs involved with disease (21). Survival of children with malignant adrenocortical tumors with no treatment, chemotherapy, or radiation therapy has been poor; thus, surgical excision has been attempted even in patients with extensive tumor involvement. The low incidence of adrenocortical neoplasms in children has prevented randomized trials from determining the best treatment protocol. However, nonrandomized series suggest that total excision of tumor is the most important prognostic factor (45).

Perioperative steroid support is necessary when tumor steroid production suppresses ACTH secretion (5). Prolonged steroid maintenance (3 to 4 months) is required when the remaining adrenal gland is atrophic (7). When the abnormal hormone production involves only sex steroids, this supplementation is not necessary.

Adjuvant Therapy

Adjuvant chemotherapy has shown poor results. O-P-DDD, or mitotane, has been reported to control symptoms of hormonal excess in patients with malignant adrenocortical tumors (1,5,8). The side effects include gastrointestinal distress (83%), neurotoxicity (41%), and skin rash (14%) (46). Improvements in dosing and administration have lessened these effects. The ability of mitotane to cure or even prolong survival is unclear. Anecdotal reports are hampered by the limited ability to accurately assess the remaining tumor burden after resection.

Adjuvant chemotherapy and radiotherapy have also been administered with limited efficacy. A consensus that controlled trials are needed to examine potential benefits in patients with or at increased risk for metastases has been reached (5).

SUMMARY

Adrenocortical neoplasms are rare in childhood and are potentially fatal. Clinicians must be aware of presenting signs and symptoms that suggest the diagnostic consideration of adrenocortical neoplasm in children so that prompt surgical extirpation can be accomplished. Presenting characteristics and prognoses differ in pediatric and adult adrenocortical neoplasms. Morphologic and histologic parameters cannot clearly differentiate benign from malignant neoplasms. For the indeterminate tumors, ultimately clinical follow-up is required.

REFERENCES

1. Stewart DR, Jones PH, Jolleys A. Carcinoma of the adrenal gland in children. *J Pediatr Surg* 1974;9:59–67.
2. Mendonca BB, Lucon AM, Menezes CAV, et al. Clinical, hormonal, and pathological findings in a comparative study of adrenocortical neoplasms in childhood and adulthood. *J Urol* 1995;154:2004–2009.
3. Hayles AB, Hahn HB, Sprague RG, et al. Hormone-secreting tumors of the adrenal cortex in children. *Pediatrics* 1966;37:19–25.
4. Federici S, Ceccarelli PL, Ferrari M. Adrenocortical tumors in children: a report of 12 cases. *Eur J Pediatr Surg* 1994;4:21–25.
5. Neblett WW, Frexes-Steed M, Scott HW. Experience with adrenocortical neoplasms in childhood. *Am Surg* 1987;53:117–125.
6. Cagle PT, Hough AJ, Pysher TJ, et al. Comparison of adrenocortical tumors in children and adults. *Cancer* 1986;57:2235–2237.
7. Holcombe JH, Pysher TJ, Kirkland RT. Functional adrenocortical tumors in childhood. In: Humphrey GB, Grindey GB, Dehner LP, et al, eds. *Adrenal and endocrine tumors in children*. Boston: Martinus Nijhoff, 1983:281.
8. Zaitoon MM, Mackie GG. Adrenal cortical tumors in children. *Urology* 1978;12:645–649.
9. Bergada I, Venara M, Maglio S, et al. Functional adrenal cortical tumors in pediatric patients: a clinicopathologic and immunohistochemical study of a long term follow-up series. *Cancer* 1996;77:771–777.
10. Fraumeni JF Jr, Miller RW. Adrenocortical neoplasms with hemihypertrophy, brain tumors, and other disorders. *J Pediatr* 1967;70:129–138.
11. Benson PF, Vulliamy DG, Taubman JO. Congenital hemihypertrophy and malignancy. *Lancet* 1963;1:468–469.
12. Tank ES, Kay R. Neoplasms associated with hemihypertrophy, Beckwith-Wiedemann syndrome, and aniridia. *J Urol* 1980;124:266–268.
13. Haicken BN, Schulman HH, Schneider KM. Adrenocortical carcinoma and congenital hemihypertrophy. *J Pediatr* 1973;83:284–285.
14. Groff DB, Buchino JJ. A child with hemihypertrophy and right flank mass. *J Pediatr* 1982;100:500–504.
15. Levine GW. Adrenocortical carcinoma in two children with subsequent primary tumors. *Am J Dis Child* 1978;132:238–240.
16. Gershanik JJ, Elmore M, Levkoff AH. Congenital concurrence of adrenal cortical tumor, ganglioneuroma, and toxoplasmosis. *Pediatrics* 1973;51:705–709.
17. Andler W, Havers W, Stambolis C, et al. Renal cell carcinoma following radiation therapy for an adrenal cortical carcinoma. *J Pediatr* 1978;93:634–638.
18. Maloudji M, Ronaghy H, Dutz W. Virilizing adrenal carcinoma in two sibs. *J Med Genet* 1971;8:160–163.
19. Kay R, Schumaker OP, Tank ES. Adrenocortical carcinoma in children. *J Urol* 1983;130:1130–1132.
20. Weatherby RP, Carney JA. Pathological features of childhood adrenocortical tumors. In: Humphrey GB, Grindey GB, Dehner LP, et al, eds. *Adrenal and endocrine tumors in children*. Boston: Martinus Nijhoff, 1983.
21. Chudler RM, Kay R. Adrenocortical carcinoma in children. *Urol Clin North Am* 1989;16:469–479.
22. Doerr HG, Sippell WG, Drop SL, et al. Evidence of 11-beta hydroxylase deficiency in childhood adrenocortical tumors: the plasma corticosterone/11-deoxycorticosterone ratio as a possible marker for malignancy. *Cancer* 1987;60:1625.
23. Lipsett MB, Hertz R, Ross GT. Clinical and pathophysiologic aspects of adrenocortical carcinoma. *Am J Med* 1963;35:374–383.
24. Wilkins L. A feminizing adrenal tumor causing gynecomastia in a boy of five years contrasted with a virilizing tumor in a five-year-old girl. *J Clin Endocrinol* 1948;8:111–131.
25. Landau RL, Stimmel BF, Humphreys E, et al. Gynecomastia and retard sexual development resulting from a long-standing estrogen-secreting adrenal tumor. *J Clin Endocrinol Metab* 1954;14:1097–1112.
26. Bhettay E, Bonnici F. Pure estrogen secreting feminizing adrenocortical adenoma. *Arch Dis Child* 1977;52:241–243.
27. Mosier HD, Goodwin WE. Feminizing adrenal adenoma in a 7-year-old boy. *Pediatrics* 1961;27:1016.
28. Bacon GE, Lowrey GH. Feminizing adrenal tumor in a 6-year-old boy. *J Clin Endocrinol Metab* 1965;25:1403–1406.
29. Leditschke JF, Arden F. Feminizing adrenal adenoma in a 5-year-old boy. *Aust Paediatr J* 1974;10:217.
30. Desai MB, Kapadia SN. Feminizing adrenocortical tumors in male patients: adenoma versus carcinoma. *J Urol* 1989;139:101–103.
31. Howard CP, Takahashi H, Hayles AB. Feminizing adrenal adenoma in a boy. *Mayo Clin Proc* 1977;52:354–357.
32. Sultan C, Descomps B, Garandeau P, et al. Pubertal gynecomastia due to an estrogen-producing adrenal adenoma. *J Pediatr* 1979;95:774–776.

33. Itami RM, Amundson GM, Kaplan SA, et al. Prepubertal gynecomastia caused by adrenal tumor. *Am J Dis Child* 1982;136:584.
34. Gabrilove JL, Shannon DC, Wotiz HH, et al. Feminizing adrenocortical tumors in the male. *Medicine* 1965;44:37–79.
35. Snaith AH. A case of feminizing adrenal tumor in a girl. *J Clin Endocrinol* 1958;14:318.
36. Comite F, Schiebinger RJ, Albertson BD, et al. Isosexual precocious pseudopuberty secondary to a feminizing adrenal tumor. *J Clin Endocrinol Metab* 1984;58:435–440.
37. Telander RL, Wolf SA, Simmons PS, et al. Endocrine disorders of the pancreas and adrenal cortex in pediatric patients. *Mayo Clin Proc* 1986;61:459–466.
38. Ritchie JP, Gittes RF. Carcinoma of the adrenal cortex. *Cancer* 1980;45:1957–1964.
39. Greulich WW, Pyle SI. *Radiologic atlas of skeletal development of the hand and wrist*, 2nd ed. Stanford, CA: Stanford University Press, 1959.
40. Hauffa BP, Roll C, Muhlenberg R, et al. Growth in children with adrenocortical tumors. *Klin Padiatr* 1991;203:83–87.
41. Salt AT, Savage MO, Grant DB. Growth patterns after surgery for virilizing adrenocortical adenoma. *Arch Dis Child* 1992;67:234–236.
42. Lack EE, Mulvihill JJ, Travis WD, et al. Adrenal cortical neoplasms in the pediatric and adolescent age group: clinicopathologic study of 30 cases with emphasis on epidemiological and prognostic factors. *Pathol Annu* 1992;27:1–51.
43. LeFevre M, Gerard-Marchant R, Gubler JP, et al. Adrenal cortical carcinoma in children: 42 patients treated from 1958–1980 at Villejuif. In: Humphrey GB, Grindey GB, Dehner LP, et al, eds. *Adrenal and endocrine tumors in children*. Boston: Martinus Nijhoff, 1983.
44. Humphrey GB, Pysher T, Holcombe J, et al. Overview on the management of adrenocortical carcinoma. In: Humphrey GB, Grindey GB, Dehner LP, et al, eds. *Adrenal and endocrine tumors in children*. Boston: Martinus Nijhoff, 1983.
45. Sabbaga CC, Avilla SG, Schulz C, et al. Adrenocortical carcinoma in children: clinical aspects and prognosis. *J Pediatr Surg* 1993;28:841–843.
46. Hutter AM Jr, Kayhoe DE. Adrenal cortical carcinoma: results of treatment with O,P DDD in 138 patients. *Am J Med* 1966;41:581–592.

*Medical and Surgical Management of
Adrenal Diseases,* edited by Joseph C. Cerny.
Lippincott Williams & Wilkins, Philadelphia © 1999.

8

Congenital Adrenal Hyperplasia

David C. Leach and *Joseph C. Cerny

*Executive Director, ACGME, 515 North State Street, Suite 2000, Chicago, Illinois 60610;
Department of Urology, Henry Ford Hospital, Detroit, Michigan 48202

Appreciation of congenital adrenal hyperplasia (CAH) requires that the clinician be capable of recognizing a much broader array of patterns than was the case a few years ago. In addition to the classic story of ambiguous genitalia with or without salt loss, this family of disorders may present as a normal-appearing male infant with an abnormal screening test, sudden death, a testicular mass, precocious puberty, mild virilization and hypertension during adolescence, hirsutism in adult females, a syndrome similar to sclerocystic ovaries, or infertility responsive to glucocorticoid in adult men. Prenatal diagnosis and treatment is possible. Once thought to be relatively rare, 21-hydroxylase deficiency has come to be considered the most common autosomal recessive disorder in humans (1).

Enhanced understanding of these disorders represents the fruit of both reductionistic and synthetic approaches to knowledge, that is, the elegant molecular analyses of classic biomedical research (2–9) and the contributions from traditional public health approaches of epidemiology and population screening (10,11). This chapter presents a pragmatic approach to these disorders, based on their pathophysiology, and promotes diagnostic pattern recognition and management of commonly encountered therapeutic dilemmas.

HISTORY

Brown-Séquard underscored Thomas Addison's clinical observations (12) with simple but persuasive experiments demonstrating that adrenalectomy is followed by death (13). Lacking effective replacement therapy, the next 100 years of observations were limited to hypothesizing how the adrenal cortex maintains life, purifying and injecting various extracts, and measuring circulating or excreted adrenal products using bioassay. Eventually, 21 steroid substances were isolated and crystallized from the adrenal, six of which could maintain life (14,15). However, it was not until the mid-1950s that all of the major adrenal steroids were isolated and characterized (16).

De Crecchio, a contemporary of Addison and Brown-Séquard, performed an autopsy on an apparent male patient only to find a uterus, ovaries, and enlarged adrenal glands (17). This was the first clinical description of what was almost certainly CAH. Almost 100 years later, Lawson Wilkins, in 1951, demonstrated that treatment of CAH with cortisone could suppress the excess androgen production associated with this syndrome. This observation and the increasing availability of glucocorticoid for treatment were milestones in the history of CAH.

Coupled with progressively more sophisticated measurement abilities (bioassay, chemical methods, radioimmunoassay), the ensuing clinical experiences yielded an appreciation that CAH was characterized by a failure of certain enzymes, a resultant inability to make cortisol, and consequent chronic stimulation by adrenocorticotropic hormone (ACTH), which in turn caused the adrenal to overproduce a variety of products (18–20). These discoveries took about 20 years.

The next 20 years increased understanding of CAH exponentially. Genes producing the enzymes were isolated (21,22), the crucial P450 enzyme system was elucidated (22), and intracellular biology clarified the mechanisms by which ACTH promotes gene expression, transcription, translation, and packaging and secretion of the resultant steroids (23). Likewise, the transport, mechanism of action, and metabolism of glucocorticoid were defined (23–25).

As exciting and pivotal as these clarifications were, clinicians were still confronted with more variability than "on/off" mechanisms could explain, and CAH was an analog rather than a digital phenomenon. Some patients seemed to fit "classic" patterns whereas others presented an attenuated or "nonclassic" picture. Likewise, patients within the classic category did not respond uniformly to treatment. Understanding the mechanisms supporting this variability constitutes current efforts in this field. Gene alleles account for some of the variability (26,27), but the range of virilization in patients with similar levels of androgens and the difficulty in achieving standardized optimal treatment programs have continued to call for further research.

PHYSIOLOGY

Several processes, some enzymatic and some not, complete the conversion of cholesterol to cortisol. Even though the adrenal can synthesize cholesterol, it usually depends on dietary sources to provide substrate cholesterol transported in the form of low-density lipoproteins (LDL) (28). ACTH stimulates adrenal uptake of LDL and the generation of free cholesterol, as well as promoting conversion of that cholesterol to cortisol.

The P450 enzyme system (so named because all of these enzymes have a single heme molecule and absorb light at 450 nm when reduced with carbon monoxide) is capable of catalyzing a wide array of substrates, that is,

each enzyme can oxidize several substances. Some of the enzymes are found in the endoplasmic reticulum and some on the inner surface of the mitochondria. Therefore, transportation of steroid-in-formation is a necessary prerequisite for steroidogenesis.

Four P450 enzymes and one non-P450 enzyme are needed for cortisol synthesis. Fig. 8-1 clarifies the role of each of these enzymes in the synthesis of cortisol, mineralocorticoids, and androgens.

An understanding of the physiology involved in the action of these enzymes is helpful in explaining some of the clinical variability observed in enzyme deficiency states. Although it is tempting to think that a gene either is or is not present, the facts describe a more graduated phenomenon:

1. Time. A single gene located on the long arm of chromosome 10 codes for the P450c17 enzyme. The 17,20 lyase activity of this gene product, which is expressed in the fetal adrenal and after adrenarche in childhood, is a different function than the 17-hydroxylase activity needed to form cortisol, but both activities result from the same enzymatic structure and gene. The 17-hydroxylase activity occurs more readily than the 17,20 lyase activity and may simply reflect the length of time the steroid occupies the enzymatic site. When substrate concentration increases, as 17-hydroxyprogesterone does in the 21-hydroxylase form of CAH, the 17,20 lyase function is more fully expressed and androgen formation is favored.

2. Pseudogenes and gene conversions. P450c21 is a single enzyme that can hydroxylase either 17-hydroxyprogesterone or progesterone, yielding 11-deoxycortisol (compound S) or deoxycorticosterone (DOC), respectively. Failure of the 21-hydroxylation function is the most common form of CAH. Some patients have significant salt loss, causing speculation that two enzymes were involved. However, there is only one P450c21 enzyme and its

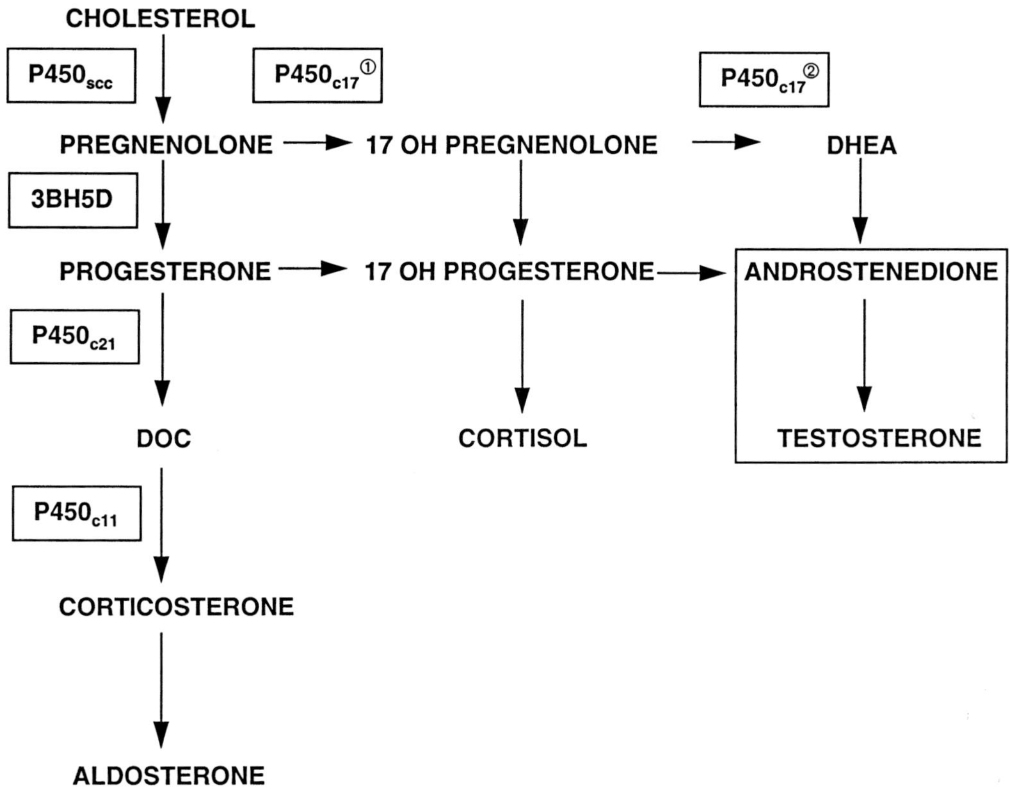

$P450_{c17}$ ① - 17 hydroxylone function of $P450_{c17}$ enzyme.
$P450_{c17}$ ② - 17, 20 lyase function of $P450_{c17}$ enzyme.

FIG. 8-1. Adrenal steroid synthesis.

gene is on the short arm of chromosome 6, between the HLA-B and HLA-DR loci of the HLA complex. There is an associated pseudogene that shares 98% homology with the functional gene. Whereas only one gene is functional, gene conversions, in which small exchanges of sequences occur between homologous genes, may account for some of the variability in this form of CAH. Four gene conversions of the P450c21 gene have been described (29–32); all were associated with the classic form of 21-hydroxylase deficiency. One of these conversions, in which a nonsense mutation in the pseudogene is incorporated into the functional gene, was always associated with salt loss (29), whereas another conversion, in which isoleucine-172 is changed into asparagine, preserved the ability to convert progesterone to DOC and hence to retain salt (30).

3. Deletions. In addition to gene conversions, straightforward deletions may at-

tenuate but not extinguish the P450c21 gene. The situation is further complicated by the fact that extraadrenal 21-hydroxylase activity exists and is not regulated by the P450c21 gene. Some patients, homozygous for classic 21-hydroxylase deficiency, have been able to synthesize some 21-hydroxylated steroids via this mechanism (33).

4. Location. The enzyme P450c11 has multiple functions. It can convert compound S to cortisol, and it performs three operations on DOC (11-hydroxylase, 18-hydroxylase, and 18-oxidase), converting it to aldosterone. Cortisol is made primarily in the zona fasciculata, and aldosterone is made primarily in the zona glomerulosa.

Intact 450c11-mitochondrial complexes extracted from zona fasciculata are unable to make aldosterone, but if P450c11 enzyme is removed from those mitochondria, they can (28). P450c11 is coded for by a gene or possibly duplicated genes in tandem on chromosome 8.

For practical purposes, the only adrenal steroid recognized by the pituitary-hypothalamic mechanism regulating ACTH is cortisol. Hence, deficiencies in P450scc, 3-β-hydroxysteroid dehydrogenase (HSD), P450c17, P450c21, or P450c11 cause failure of cortisol production and elevated ACTH levels. The ACTH, in turn, causes adrenal hyperplasia and overproduction of those steroids in the remaining functional pathways. The clinical syndrome is defined by the type of steroid that can be produced.

PATTERNS OF CONGENITAL ADRENAL HYPERPLASIA

A mechanism as complex as that outlined herein offers many chances for things to go wrong. In addition to failure to make particular enzymes, the functional aspects of existing enzymes may be modified or attenuated, resulting in variations on classic patterns of disease. Nonetheless, it is useful for clinicians to be familiar with established presentations of the various enzyme-deficient states. This section describes these patterns (Table 8-1). The various enzyme-deficient states are described in order of their frequency.

TABLE 8–1. *Clinical patterns associated with enzyme deficiency*

21-Hydroxylase	11-Hydroxylase	3-BHSD	17-Hydroxylase	Cholesterol desmolase
Classic				
Ambiguous genitalia in girls	Virilization of female, acne, hirsutism, irregular periods, and frontal balding	Death soon after birth	Males ambiguous genitalia	Hyperpigmented at birth
Precocious puberty and accelerated growth in boys	Hypertension	Females slightly virilized	Females normal at birth but fail to feminize at puberty	Usually fatal
± Salt loss	Rapid growth in boys	Males incompletely masculinized	Hypertension	Severe salt wasting
Positive neonatal screening	Gynecomastia	Nonclassic form		Males not masculinized
Nonclassic		Virilization at puberty		
Precocious adrenarche		Hirsutism and oligomenorrhea		
Cystic acne in adolescence		Acne and infertility		
Mildly accelerated growth in childhood		PCO pattern		
Short adult stature				
Hirsutism in adult women				
Polycystic ovarian syndrome				
Infertility in men				

21-Hydroxylase Deficiency

The syndromes associated with deficient or impaired 21-hydroxylase are the most common forms of CAH. The two commonly described forms are (a) *classic 21-hydroxylase deficiency*—presenting with virilization (ambiguous genitalia in newborn girls; precocious puberty and accelerated growth in boys) and salt loss in three-fourths of cases (hyponatremia, hyperkalemia, acidosis, low aldosterone, and high renin) and (b) *nonclassic 21-hydroxylase deficiency*, an allelic variant in which the manifestations are delayed and milder and include precocious adrenarche, cystic acne in adolescence, mildly accelerated growth, and premature closure of the epiphyseal plates, hirsutism in adult women, polycystic ovarian syndrome, and infertility in men.

Epidemiology

Approximately 1 in 61 persons is heterozygous for the classic form of this disease (1). Worldwide screening programs have derived an overall incidence of 1 in 14,500 live births (34), with much variation between populations.

Two populations have an especially high incidence—the Yupik population of Alaska, with an incidence of 1 in 280 live births, and the island population of LaReunion, with an incidence of 1 in 3,000 live births. The lowest incidence is 1 in 21,000 live births in New Zealand.

Nonclassic 21-hydroxylase deficiency is more frequent than any other autosomal recessive disease. The incidence varies by ethnic group from 1 in 27 Ashkenazi Jews, 1 in 53 Hispanics, 1 in 333 Italians, and 1 in 100 in a heterogeneous population (35). Children selected because of precocious pubarche have a 30% incidence of nonclassic 21-hydroxylase activity (36).

The prevalence of nonclassic 21-hydroxylase deficiency in hirsute women ranges from 1.2% to 30% (37). Women with the nonclassic form of this disease frequently have polycystic ovaries (38). Men with infertility may have this syndrome and may respond to glucocorticoid replacement (39). The linkage of the HLA complex and the 21-hydroxylase gene permitted discovery that the nonclassic gene is an allele of the classic gene (40). Thus, some of the nonclassic patients are heterozygotes with one classic gene and one nonclassic, whereas others are homozygous nonclassic and are asymptomatic but have abnormal stimulated levels of 17-hydroxyprogesterone.

Pattern Recognition of Classic 21-Hydroxylase Deficiency

Neonatal Screening

The most frequent presentation of classic 21-hydroxylase deficiency, in a state that conducts neonatal screening, is a positive screening test. Since 1977, it has been possible to measure 17-hydroxyprogesterone in samples of blood placed on filter paper (41).

Screening has been conducted in several million babies at birth and is more sensitive than clinical diagnosis, especially in boys. Mild virilization in girls may be overlooked; 50% of girls who were found to have a positive screening test were thought on reconsideration to have some degree of sexual ambiguity (42). Four girls with positive screening tests had been assigned a male sex, decisions that were reversed once the test results became available. However, in general, the major reason for screening is to detect the deficiency in male infants, who, because they appear normal, are subject to sudden and catastrophic salt loss, resulting in death. This incidence of this phenomenon has been reduced in areas where screening is offered.

Nonetheless, a positive screening test, in our experience, is usually falsely positive. This may reflect the fact that normal results were established on blood samples obtained at 72 hours of life, whereas most newborns go home before 72 hours and are screened at 1 to 2 days of age. The level of 17-hydroxyprogesterone is higher on the first day of life than on the third. Preterm babies and sick and low birth weight babies also have a high incidence of false-positive results. Neonates who do have a positive test and do have the disease may appear normal, yet their condition may abruptly deteriorate because of salt loss and hyperkalemia. Therefore, vigilance must be maintained despite the frequency of false-positive test results. All patients should be recalled and retested and have electrolytes measured.

Ambiguous Genitalia with or without Salt Loss

Ambiguous genitalia is the second most frequent way that classic 21-hydroxylase deficiency presents. The fetal adrenal in this disorder overproduces androgens in response to ACTH stimulation. This has no apparent untoward effect on boys, but it does virilize the female fetus. The degree of virilization is variable and ranges from mild clitoromegaly through varying degrees of labioscrotal fusion to the rare but described phallic urethra.

The karyotype, gonads, and internal sexual organs are all female. The wolffian structures are rarely masculinized, even in cases with severe virilization of the external genitalia. This may reflect that the local concentration of androgens is not sufficient to stimulate wolffian development.

Ambiguous genitalia in girls is frequently due to 21-hydroxylase deficiency and its presence warrants confirmation of the diagnosis with a 17-hydroxyprogesterone level, which is usually unequivocally elevated, and a search for salt loss. Sex assignment should be female. Most of these patients will be fertile as adults (43). If surgery is required, it is done in two stages.

The glans and neurovascular bundle of the clitoris is preserved and the corporal bodies resected at an early age, usually between 3 and 18 months. Successful intercourse is more likely if vaginoplasty is delayed until adolescence (44). Stress doses of cortisol are required for surgery.

Salt Loss in Infancy

Most girls in whom salt loss is caused by 21-hydroxylase deficiency also have ambiguous genitalia. Boys, however, frequently present have hyponatremia, hyperkalemia, acidosis, high renin, and low aldosterone levels, and this complex of features should trigger measurement of 17-hydroxyprogesterone levels.

The most frequent differential diagnosis is pseudohypoaldosteronism, which is usually seen in low birth weight or premature babies and is caused by transient resistance to aldosterone. However, aldosterone levels are elevated in this latter condition.

True salt loss in an infant is a medical emergency and warrants saline replacement and mineralocorticoid administration. As youngsters get older, they sometimes seem to have less salt loss and may not require mineralocorticoid except on very hot days or with vigorous exercise. This may simply reflect that they eat more salt as they get older.

Precocious Puberty

Because boys with 21-hydroxylase deficiency appear normal at birth, those who are not salt losers usually are seen in childhood with accelerated grow, advanced bone age, premature sexual hair, and what appears to be precocious puberty. A clue that distinguishes this from true precocious puberty may be that the testes are not enlarged.

However, the presence of adrenal rest tissue in testes may lead to some testicular enlargement, and if the pseudopuberty has progressed long enough that the bone age is extremely advanced, the child may, in fact, enter true puberty and testicular enlargement may develop. Although tall for their age, these patients are destined to be short as adults because of the premature closure of the epiphyses, unless this syndrome is recognized and treated.

Treatment

Prenatal Treatment

First trimester diagnosis of 21-hydroxylase deficiency can be accomplished using polymerase chain reaction amplification of fetal DNA obtained via amniocentesis or chorionic villus sampling. Earlier attempts to use HLA typing or amniotic fluid 17-hydroxyprogesterone levels have not proven totally accurate or interpretable. Treatment is suggested only for female fetuses in an attempt to prevent virilization.

Time is of the essence because fetal adrenal overproduction of androgens and virilization of developing external genitalia begins at 6 to 8 weeks of gestation. Prenatal diagnosis cannot usually be confirmed until about 10 weeks of gestation.

Accordingly, in a family at risk, dexamethasone 20 µg/kg/day is administered to the mother from about 4 weeks of gestation, as soon as pregnancy is established, and is discontinued if the fetus is proven either male or unaffected (45). Dexamethasone is not inactivated by the placenta. Side effects include a cushingoid response of the mother. To date, teratogenicity, although theoretically possible, has not been reported.

Postnatal Treatment

The goals of treatment in classic 21-hydroxylase deficiency are to replace essential and deficient hormones, to promote normal growth and development, and to suppress inappropriate androgen formation. If an infant is in a salt-losing crisis or an acute adrenal crisis, the immediate goals become intravenous hydration with saline, correction of electrolyte abnormalities, and supplementation with intravenous hydrocortisone (1.5 to 2.0 mg/kg). It is usually possible to switch to oral glucocorticoid and mineralocorticoid replacement fairly rapidly. Fludrocortisone acetate is given in doses that range from 0.1 to 0.3 mg/day. As the child becomes older, it is common for the dose of fludrocortisone to be reduced, probably because the child has free access to salt; however, in the salt-losing variant, lifelong replacement is needed. Electrolytes and renin levels are of use in monitoring replacement.

Glucocorticoid replacement should be started with hydrocortisone, 12 to 15 mg/m²/day in two or three divided doses. Many youngsters do well with this, but others require more individualized protocols. Undertreatment results in rapid growth, acceleration of the bone age, and virilization; overtreatment results in slower growth than normal and cushingoid features. In general, it is difficult to suppress the 17-hydroxyprogesterone level to normal without overtreating; however, the testosterone and sometimes the androstenedione can be brought to normal.

Some youngsters require 25 mg/m²/day of hydrocortisone and some require the use of longer acting steroids such as prednisone or dexamethasone to achieve adequate suppression, although use of the latter two agents requires especially close monitoring to avoid growth suppression.

Some patients have a secondary true central precocious puberty by the time the diagnosis is made or such develops as a result noncompliance. Such patients respond well to luteinizing hormone-releasing hormone analogues, which may be administered along with replacement therapy.

Some cases are very difficult to treat, seeming to bounce forever between undertreatment and overtreatment.

A recent report by Laue and Rennert (46) describe the use of a protocol of hydrocortisone 8 mg/m²/day coupled with an antiandrogen (flutamide) and an aromatase inhibitor (testolactone) in 12 children with good result. This approach may offer help for especially difficult cases.

Pattern Recognition of Nonclassic 21-Hydroxylase Deficiency

Nonclassic 21-hydroxylase deficiency presents in five main ways:

1. Premature pubarche. Pubic hair occurring in children as young as 6 months old has been a clue to the presence of this disorder. In one study (47), 30% of children with premature pubarche were reported to have nonclassical 21-hydroxylase deficiency. Even without confirmation, it is

clear that the disease and this manifestation are linked.

2. Cystic acne. Severe acne in adolescence that is refractory to usual treatment should provoke consideration that the patient may have the nonclassical form of this disease (48). Likewise, development of hirsutism in adolescence or adult life, or male pattern balding in a woman may be the presenting manifestation of this disorder.

3. Polycystic ovarian syndrome. The combination of hirsutism, oligomenorrhea, and polycystic ovaries on ultrasound examination may be caused by nonclassic 21-hydroxylase deficiency in as many as 30% of cases, although other series put that figure closer to 14% (38). It may be necessary to measure the 17-hydroxyprogesterone response to ACTH in order to distinguish this disease from other causes of polycystic ovarian syndrome.

4. Short adult stature. Children who are growing rapidly and have an advanced bone age but no clear sign of precocious puberty may have the nonclassic form of this disease. Often, the growth pattern is subtle enough to be unnoticed, but may result in adult short stature.

5. Infertility. Male or female infertility may be the presenting feature of nonclassic 21-hydroxylase deficiency (49). The excess adrenal androgens suppress gonadotropin release, and glucocorticoid treatment may restore fertility. The frequency of this phenomenon is probably low, but may be higher in those ethnic groups with a high incidence of nonclassic disease.

Diagnosis and Treatment of Nonclassic 21-Hydroxylase Deficiency

When one of the aforementioned patterns is present, or whenever unexplained excess androgen is apparent, measurement of 17-hydroxyprogesterone can be undertaken.

Some patients have elevated unstimulated values; however, it may be necessary to compare 17-OHP levels before and 60 minutes after 0.25 mg of intravenous Cortrosyn is given. A published nomogram (50) is helpful in confirming the diagnosis; an exaggerated response between normal values and the classic variant is obtained.

11-β-Hydroxylase Deficiency

The second most common form of CAH is due to deficiency of 11-β-hydroxylase. This autosomal recessive disorder accounts for 5% to 8% of cases of CAH (51). It is relatively rare, occurring once in about 100,000 births (52); however, the incidence in Israel and in Turkish Jews is much higher. There is an attenuated nonclassic form that is milder and occurs later in life. Two distinct isoenzymes of P450c11 operate in humans. They share 93% homology and are coded for by two genes on chromosome 8.

It would appear that one gene is expressed under the control of ACTH, operates in the zona fasciculata, and is better at 11-hydroxylation than 18-hydroxylation, that is, its primary function is to produce cortisol. A second gene, which is less responsive to ACTH, may be responsive to angiotensin II, operates in the zona glomerulosa, and is very good at 18-hydroxylation, that is, its primary function is to make aldosterone. Deficiencies of the first gene impair cortisol production and increase ACTH, resulting in increases in adrenal androgens and compound S. A parallel inability to form corticosterone from DOC may also exist. Because DOC is a mineralocorticoid, elevated DOC levels may provoke hypertension, hypokalemia, and alkalosis, even though aldosterone production is impaired.

Clinical Pattern Recognition of 11-β-Hydroxylase Deficiency

Virilization

The excess androgen production associated with this disorder is apparent in the female newborn, although it varies from mild to severe. Some patients with a penile urethra have been described.

The hypertension associated with this disease is not uniformly present at birth and its omission should not dissuade one from measuring compound S in suspicious cases.

A milder, nonclassic form of the disease may present in adolescence or adult life with acne, hirsutism, irregular periods, and male pattern balding. Boys may have rapid growth and gynecomastia may develop before puberty, presumably because of aromatization of adrenal androgens.

Hypertension

Hypertension develops in two-thirds of cases and is thought to be due to DOC; however, correlation with DOC levels has not been established. Usually, renin is suppressed, hypokalemia often but not always exists, and aldosterone is low. Thus, this is a form of low renin hypertension. In some patients, glucocorticoid treatment suppresses DOC, restores renin to normal, and then aldosterone returns to normal, suggesting that the enzyme in the zona glomerulosa is functional and that DOC in those cases is made in the zona fasciculata. Many patients become normotensive with glucocorticoid replacement.

Diagnosis and Treatment of 11-β-Hydroxylase Deficiency

Diagnosis is established by measurement of compound S and DOC. Several mutations of the gene have been described, and further elucidation of this syndrome may await clear distinction of which gene is abnormal and how it is abnormal.

Treatment of 11-β-hydroxylase deficiency is with standard replacement doses of glucocorticoid. Prenatal diagnosis and treatment have been described.

18-Hydroxylase Deficiency

18-Hydroxylase deficiency is not technically a form of CAH, because cortisol can be made and the adrenals are not hyperplastic. Defects in the 11-hydroxylase/18-hydroxy-lase gene located in the zona glomerulosa can occur and are associated with salt loss. In this case, DOC levels are not elevated and the protective effect of that mineralocorticoid is lacking. Aldosterone production is impaired. Treatment is with fludrocortisone or salt supplementation.

3-β-Hydroxysteroid Dehydrogenase Deficiency

This syndrome in its severe form is rare and fatal. However, an attenuated nonclassic form may be much more common than is generally appreciated. Complete absence of the 3-β-HSD enzyme substantially limits steroid synthesis. Neither glucocorticoid nor mineralocorticoids may be made, and the most potent androgen that can be made is dehydroepiandrosterone (DHEA). This latter substance may be acted upon outside the adrenal to produce small amounts of testosterone.

The gene for 3-β-HSD has been cloned. The enzyme is deficient in both adrenal and gonads; however, a different 3-β-HSD exists in the liver and may act on substrate provided by the adrenal.

Clinical Pattern Recognition in 3-β-HSD Deficiency

In the classic form of this disease, the infant may die at or soon after birth. Female infants are slightly virilized, because of the high DHEA levels, some of which is converted to testosterone peripherally. Male infants, on the other hand, are incompletely masculinized and have ambiguous genitalia and hypospadias. Either sex may have salt loss.

The nonclassic form of this disease is probably much more common. It presents with virilization in girls at the time of adrenarche or puberty. In one series, 16% of adult women with signs of androgen excess had evidence of a partial 3-β-HSD deficiency (53). Hence, hirsutism, oligomenorrhea, acne, and infertility may be presenting features. When sought in particular, polycystic ovaries were found in 50% of women with the nonclassic form of this disease. Men with the nonclassic form of this disease have not been described in large numbers, but presumably they would have impaired androgen synthesis.

Diagnosis and Treatment of 3-β-HSD Deficiency

Elevated levels of pregnenolone, 17-hydroxypregnenolone, and DHEA characterize this syndrome. Exaggerated responses of these hormones to ACTH characterize the nonclassic form of this disorder. Treatment consists of glucocorticoid replacement and, in cases of salt loss, mineralocorticoid replacement.

17-Hydroxylase Deficiency

One hundred and twenty cases of 17-hydroxylase deficiency have been described (54). Cortisol or sex steroids are not made in these patients, but DOC and corticosterone are. Male infants have ambiguous genitalia and are unable to completely masculinize. Female infants appear normal at birth, but they fail to feminize at the time of puberty and have primary amenorrhea. At the time of puberty, gonadotropin levels are high in both sexes. Both sexes have hypertension. The deficiency manifests as a low renin hypertension relieved with glucocorticoid treatment. A mild form of this disorder may be responsible for more cases of low renin hypertension than is currently appreciated.

17,20 Lyase Deficiency

This is a deficiency in the same enzyme, but the 17-hydroxylase function of the enzyme is preserved. Hence, it is not technically a form of CAH, because cortisol production is normal. Boys have hypospadias or more severe forms of failure to masculinize, and girls have amenorrhea and failure of secondary sexual characteristics to develop. Treatment requires sex hormone replacement.

Cholesterol Desmolase Deficiency

This disorder, also known as lipoid adrenal hyperplasia because the adrenal is full of cholesterol at autopsy, is severe and usually fatal. No adrenal steroids can be made. Patients are hyperpigmented, boys do not masculinize, and severe salt wasting is present. Thirty-two cases have been reported, mostly from Japan and Europe.

SURGICAL MANAGEMENT

Recent advances in establishing a rapid and precise diagnosis of CAH allow earlier reconstructive surgery in female infants with external genital masculinization. The goal of surgery in these patients is to establish functional capacity and an acceptable cosmetic appearance. The timing of surgical correction is important for normal psychosexual development of the patient, while minimizing emotional trauma to the parents, allowing them to raise the child in an unequivocal manner. Clitoroplasty and, if necessary, vaginoplasty should be undertaken as soon as the female infant is under good replacement hormonal control and is endocrinologically stable, preferably between 3 and 18 months of age.

The spectrum of masculinization of the female external genitalia in CAH ranges from clitoral enlargement alone, which is most

---

FIG. 8-2. Surgical technique for clitoroplasty and vaginoplasty in female infant with masculinized external genitalia and common urogenital sinus. **A:** Lines of incision for clitoroplasty and vaginoplasty are shown. A suture suspending the glans dorsally is helpful in developing glandular and corporal incisions. **B:** A portion of the ventral glans, or alternatively its lateral margins, and the entire corporal bodies are excised. Care is taken to preserve the dorsal neurovascular bundle, ventral frenular blood supply, and foreskin. The posteriorly based inverted U flap is developed, maintaining a well-vascularized pedicle, and sutured into an introital and posterior vaginal wall incision. A urethral Foley catheter in place during the dissection facilitates proper anatomic orientation. **C:** The incisions are closed, demonstrating a normal-sized, innervated and vascularized clitoris, absence of the corpora, and adequate vaginal introitus. (Redrawn from ref. 71.) *Continued on following pages.*

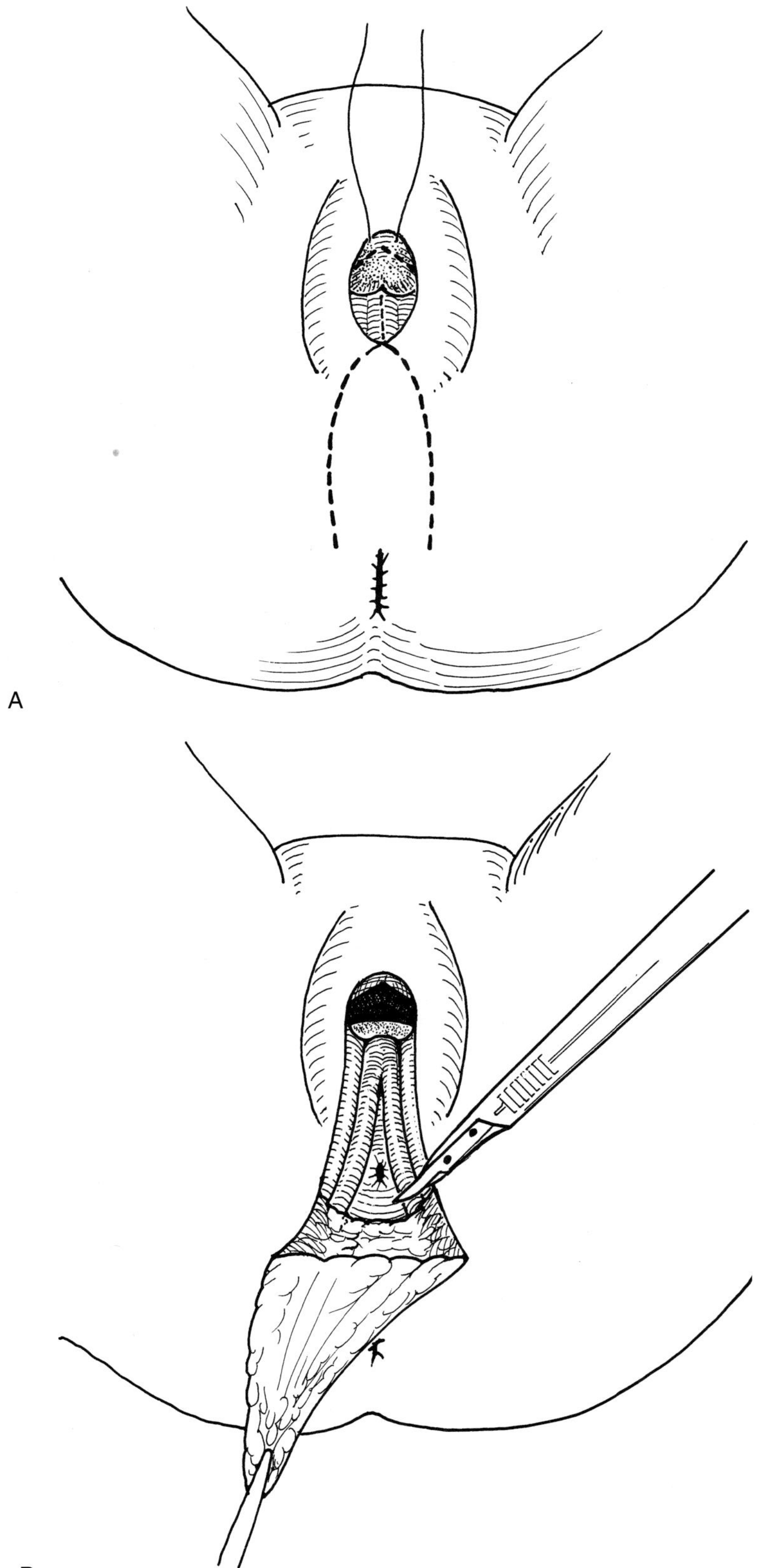

A
B

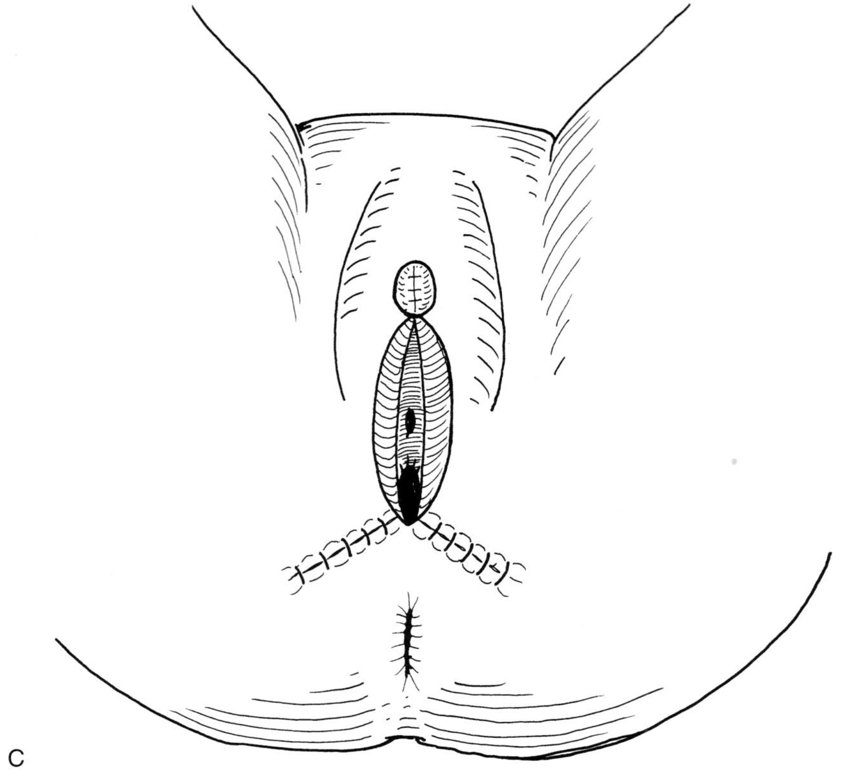

FIG. 8-2.C *(Continued from previous page.)*

common, to varying degrees of vaginal stenosis and a common urogenital sinus. Correction of clitoromegaly is optimally undertaken at 3 to 6 months of age. A variety of techniques have been used: clitoridectomy, clitoral recession, and clitoral plication (55–62). Although each has its advocates in certain clinical situations, clitoroplasty with resection of the corporal bodies, preservation of all or most of the glans, its foreskin, and the dorsal neurovascular bundle and ventral blood supply is the preferred technique (Fig. 8-2) (63–67).

In female infants in whom there is a common urogenital sinus, vaginoplasty may be performed at the time of clitoroplasty (67–70). A posteriorly based inverted U flap is developed, maintaining a well-vascularized pedicle, and is sutured into an incision made in the posterior vaginal wall (see Fig. 8-2). When performed in infants, vaginoplasty may require periodic vaginal dilation or revision at a later date. For this reason, in patients with only a minor degree of vaginal stenosis, vaginoplasty should be performed when the female child approaches puberty and appropriate size of the vaginal orifice is best determined.

As discussed previously, patients undergoing surgical correction require supplementation of their steroid replacement regimen. In these children, adrenal function is suppressed and unable to respond normally to perioperative stress. A regimen of administering ten times the usual daily dose of glucocorticoid parenterally on the day of surgery, with one-third being given immediately preoperatively and an additional one-third being given every 8 hours, is recommended (71). This dose may be halved each day until the maintenance dose level is reached. Replacing intravenous with oral dosing is begun as soon as oral intake is resumed. In children also receiving mineralo-corticoids, dosage is continued at its usual maintenance levels throughout surgery and hospitalization.

Optimal care of children with CAH requires close collaboration between the pediatrician, endocrinologist, and surgeon at all times.

CONCLUSION

CAH was once thought to be a rare and relatively stereotypic disease, but a much broader range of clinical and pathophysiologic phenomena fit under the rubric of CAH than was previously thought. This family of disorders affects adults as well as children, has attenuated and severe forms, and, when sought, is much more frequent than anticipated. The pathophysiologic mechanisms are also more interesting than simple enzyme deficiencies, and they include multifunctional enzymes that have greater or lesser degrees of impairment in one but not all functions, enzymes that function in one zone but not another, gene conversions and other pseudogene-gene interactions, and other phenomena that contribute to clinical variability. The disorders remain important primarily because knowledge of their manifestations can be life-saving and because so many stigmatized patients can be helped if their condition is recognized and treated.

REFERENCES

1. New MI, White PC, Dupont B, et al. The adrenal hyperplasia. In: Scriver CR, Beaudet AL, Sly WS, et al. *The metabolic basis of inherited disease*, 6th ed. New York: McGraw-Hill, 1989.
2. Kominami S, Ochi H, Kobayashi Y, et al. Studies on the steroid hydroxylation system in adrenal cortex microsomes. *J Biol Chem* 1980;259:3386.
3. John ME, John MC, Simpson ER, et al. Regulation of cytochrome P-45011B gene expression by adrenocorticotropin. *J Biol Chem* 1985;260:5760.
4. Nebert DW, Gonzalez FJ. P450 genes: structure, evolution, and regulation. *Annu Rev Biochem* 1987;56:945.
5. Chung BC, Matteson KJ, Voutilainen R, et al. Human cholesterol side-chain cleavage enzyme, P450scc: cDNA cloning assignment of the gene to chromosome 15, and expression in the placenta. *Proc Natl Acad Sci U S A* 1986;83:8962.
6. Chua SC, Szabo P, Vitek A, et al. Cloning of cDNA encoding steroid 11B-hydroxylase (P450c11). *Proc Natl Acad Sci U S A* 1987;84:7193.
7. White PC, New MI, Dupont B. Cloning and expression of cDNA encoding a bovine adrenal cytochrome P-450 specific for steroid 21-hydroxylation. *Proc Natl Acad Sci U S A* 1984;81:1986.
8. Matteson KJ, Picado-Leonard J, Chung B-C, et al. Assignment of the gene for adrenal P450c17 (steroid 17-alpha-hydoxylase/17,20-lyase) to human chromosome 10. *J Clin Endocrinol Metab* 1986;63:789.
9. White PC, New MI, Dupont B. Structure of the human steroid 21-hydroxylase genes. *Proc Natl Acad Sci U S A* 1986;83:5111.
10. Pang S, Spence DA, New MI. Newborn screening for congenital adrenal hyperplasia with special reference to screening in Alaska. *Ann N Y Acad Sci* 1985;458:90.
11. Cicognani A. The experience of neonatal screening for congenital adrenal hyperplasia. *Hormone Research* 1992;37[suppl 3]:34–38.
12. Addison T. *On the constitutional and local effects of disease of the suprarenal capsules.* London: Highley, 1855.
13. Brown-Séquard CE. Recherches experimentales sur la physiologie et al pathologie des capsules surrenales. *Comp Rendu* 1856;43:422–425.
14. Kendall EC. A chemical and physiological investigation of the suprarenal cortex. *Cold Springs Harb Symp Quant Biol* 1937;5:299–326.
15. Reichstein T, Shoppee CW. The hormones of the adrenal cortex. *Vitam Horm* 1945;1:345–413.
16. Nelson DH. A historical overview of the adrenal cortex. In: DeGroot LJ, ed. *Endocrinology*, 3rd ed, vol 2. Philadelphia: WB Saunders, 1995.
17. De Crecchio L. Sopra un caso di apparenze virile in una donna. *Morgagni* 1865;7:1951.
18. Nelson DH. *The adrenal cortex: physiological function and disease.* Philadelphia: WB Saunders, 1980.
19. Christy NP, ed. *The human adrenal cortex.* New York: Harper & Row, 1971.
20. Cope CL. *Adrenal Steroids and Disease.* Philadelphia: JB Lippincott, 1964.
21. White PC, New MI, Dupont B. HLA-linked congenital adrenal hyperplasia results from a defective gene encoding a cytochrome P-450 specific for steroid 21-hydoxylation. *Proc Natl Acad Sci U S A* 1984;81: 7505–7509.
22. Nebert DW, Gonzalez FJ. P450 genes: structure, evolution, and regulation. *Annu Rev Biochem* 1987;56:945.
23. Strauss JF III, ed. Steroid hormones: synthesis, metabolism, and action in health and disease. *Endocrinol Metab Clin North Am* 1991;20:4.
24. Munck A, Naray-Fejes-Toth A. Glucocorticoid action. In: DeGroot LJ, ed. *Endocrinology*, 3rd ed, vol 2. Philadelphia: WB Saunders, 1995.
25. Miesfeld RL. Biochemistry of glucocorticoid action. In: DeGroot LJ, ed. *Endocrinology*, 3rd ed, vol 2. Philadelphia: WB Saunders, 1995.
26. Levine LS, Dupont B, Lorenzen F, et al. Cryptic 21-hydroxylase deficiency in families of patients with classical congenital adrenal hyperplasia. *J Clin Endocrinol Metab* 1980;51:1316.
27. Migeon CJ, Rosenwaks Z, Lee PA, et al. The attenuated form of congenital adrenal hyperplasia as an allelic form of 21-hydroxylase deficiency. *J Clin Endocrinol Metab* 1980;51:647.

28. Miller WL. Congenital adrenal hyperplasia. *Endocrinol Metab Clin North Am* 1991;721.
29. Globerman H, Amor M, New MI, et al. A nonsense mutation causing steroid 21-hydroxylase deficiency. Program and abstracts, Bat-Sheva Seminar on molecular approaches to hormone action. Tiberias, Israel, October, 1987.
30. Amor M, Parker KL, Globerman H, et al. Amino acid substitution in the CYP21B gene causing steroid 21-hydroxylase deficiency. *Proc Natl Acad Sci U S A* 1988;85:1600.
31. Speiser PW, Amor M, New MI, et al. Molecular genetic basis for nonclassical 21-hydroxylase deficiency. *N Engl J Med* 1988;319:19.
32. Rodrigues NR, Dunham I, Yu C-Y, et al. Molecular characterization of the HLA-linked steroid 21-hydroxylase B gene from an individual with congenital adrenal hyperplasia. *EMBO J* 1987;6:1653.
33. Speiser PW, Agdere L, Ueshiba H, et al. Aldosterone synthesis in patients with salt-wasting congenital adrenal hyperplasia (21-hydroxylase deficiency) and complete absence of adrenal 21-hydroxylase (P450c21). *N Engl J Med* 1991;324:145–149.
34. Pang SP, Wallace MA, Hofman L, et al. Worldwide experience in newborn screening for classical congenital adrenal hyperplasia due to 21-hydroxylase deficiency. *Pediatrics* 1988;81:866–874.
35. Speiser PW, Dupont B, Rubinstein P, et al. High frequency of nonclassical steroid 21-hydroxylase deficiency. *Am J Hum Genet* 1985;37:650–667.
36. Temeck JW, Pang S, Nelson C, et al. Genetic defects of steroidogenesis in premature pubarche. *J Clin Endocrinol Metab* 1987;64:609.
37. Kuttenn F, Couillin P, Girard F, et al. Late onset adrenal hyperplasia in hirsutism. *N Engl J Med* 1986;313:224.
38. Lobo RA, Goebelsmann U. Adult manifestation of congenital adrenal hyperplasia due to incomplete 21-hydroxylase deficiency mimicking polycystic ovarian disease. *Am J Obstet Gynecol* 1980;138:720.
39. Bonaccorsi AC, Adler I, Figueiredo JG. Male infertility due to congenital adrenal hyperplasia: testicular biopsy findings, hormonal evaluation, and therapeutic results in three patients. *Fertil Steril* 1987;47:664.
40. Levine LS, Dupont B, Lorenzen F, et al. Genetic and hormonal characterization of cryptic 21-hydroxylase deficiency. *J Clin Endocrinol Metab* 1981;53:1193.
41. Pang S, Hotchkiss J, Drash AL, et al. Microfilter paper method for 17alpha-progesterone radioimmunoassay: its application for rapid screening for congenital adrenal hyperplasia. *J Clin Endocrinol Metab* 1977;45:1003.
42. Hofman LF. Screening infants for congenital adrenal hyperplasia: the Washington experience. In: Therrll BL, ed. *Advances in neonatal screening* [Excerpta Medica Intl Congr Series, vol. 741]. Amsterdam: Elsevier, 1987:287.
43. Klingensmith GJ, Garcia SC, Jones HW, et al. Glucocorticoid treatment of girls with congenital adrenal hyperplasia: effects on height, sexual maturation, and fertility. *J Pediatr* 1977;90:996.
44. Mulaikal RM, Migeon CJ, Rock JA. Fertility rates in female patients with congenital adrenal hyperplasia due to 21-hydroxylase deficiency. *N Engl J Med* 1987;316:178.
45. Forest MG, Dorr HG. Prenatal treatment of congenital adrenal hyperplasia due to 21-hydroxylase activity [abstr 10]. *Pediatric Res* 1994;33[suppl 3]:53.
46. Laue L, Rennert OM. Congenital adrenal hyperplasia: molecular genetics and alternative approaches to treatment. *Adv Pediatr* 1995;42:113.
47. Temeck JW, Pang S, Nelson C, et al. Genetic defects of steroidogenesis in premature pubarche. *J Clin Endocrinol Metab* 1987;64:609.
48. Lucky AW, Rosenfield RI, McGuire J, et al. Adrenal androgen hyperresponsiveness to adrenocorticotropin in women with acne and/or hirsutism: adrenal enzyme defects and exaggerated adrenarche. *J Clin Endocrinol Metab* 1986;62:840.
49. Wischusen J, Baker HWG, Hudson B. Reversible male infertility due to congenital adrenal hyperplasia. *Clin Endocrinol* 1981;14:571.
50. New MI, Lorenzen F, Lerner AJ, et al. Genotyping steroid 21-hydroxylase deficiency: hormonal reference data. *J Clin Endocrinol Metab* 1983;57:320.
51. Rosler A, Leiberman E. Enzymatic defects of steroidogenesis: 11β-hydroxylase deficiency congenital adrenal hyperplasia. In: New MI, Levine LS, eds. *Adrenal diseases in childhood*. Basel: Karger, 1984:47–71.
52. Zachmann M, Tassinari D, Prader A. Clinical and biochemical variability of congenital adrenal hyperplasia due to 11β-hydroxylase deficiency. *J Clin Endocrinol Metab* 1983;56:222.
53. Zerah M, Schram P, New MI. The diagnosis and treatment of nonclassical 3β-HSD deficiency. *Endocrinologist* 1991;1(2):75.
54. Yanase T, Simpson ER, Waterman MR. 17 alpha-hydroxylase/17, 20-lyase deficiency: from clinical investigation to molecular definition. *Endocrinol Rev* 1991;12(1):91.
55. Young HH. Genital abnormalities. In: *Hermaphroditism and relation adrenal diseases*. Baltimore: Williams & Wilkins, 1937:273–276.
56. Jones HWJ, Jones GES. The gynecological aspects of adrenal hyperplasia and allied disorders. *Am J Obstet Gynecol* 1954;68:1330.
57. Gross RE, Randolph J, Crigler CF Jr. Clitoridedomy for sexual abnormalities: indications and techniques. *Surgery* 1966;59:300.
58. Masters WH, Johnson VE. *Human sexual responses*. Boston: Little, Brown, 1966.
59. Lattimer JK. Relocation and recession of the enlarged clitoris with preservation of the glans: an alternative to amputation. *J Urol* 1961;86:113.
60. Sotiropoulos A, Morishima A, Homsy Y, et al. Long-term assessment of genital reconstruction in female pseudohermaphrodites. *J Urol* 1976;115:599.
61. Ansell JS, Rajfer J. A new and simplified method for concealing the hypertrophied clitoris. *J Pediatr Surg* 1981;16:681.
62. Stefan H. Surgical reconstruction of the external genitalia in female pseudohermaphrodites. *Br J Urol* 1967;39:347.
63. Rajfer J, Ehrlich RM, Goodwin WE. Reduction clitoroplasty via a ventral approach. *J Urol* 1982;128:341.
64. Spence HM, Allen TD. Genital reconstruction in the female with adrenogenital syndrome. *Br J Urol* 1973;45:126.
65. Mininberg DT. Phalloplasty in congenital adrenal hyperplasia. *J Urol* 1982;128:355.

66. Allen LE, Hardy BE, Churchill BM. The surgical management of the enlarged clitoris. *J Urol* 1982;128:351.
67. Fay S, Brosman S. Surgical management of female congenital adrenal hyperplasia (adrenogenital syndrome). *J Urol* 1974;112:118.
68. Parrott TS, Sheffen M, Hester TR. Reduction clitoroplasty and vaginal construction in a single operation. *Urology* 1980;16:367.
69. Hendren WH, Donahue PK. Correction of congenital abnormalities of the vagina and perineum. *J Pediatr Surg* 1980;15:751.
70. Braren V. Vaginal amplification using a posterolateral Y-V plasty. *J Urol* 1981;126:645.
71. McDougal WS, Lorenz RA, Burr IM. Congenital adrenal hyperplasia. In: Scott HW, ed. *Surgery of the adrenal glands*. Philadelphia: JB Lippincott, 1990:277–286.

*Medical and Surgical Management of
Adrenal Diseases,* edited by Joseph C. Cerny.
Lippincott Williams & Wilkins, Philadelphia © 1999.

9

Neuroblastoma

Craig A. Smith and *Ricardo González

*Department of Surgery, University of Illinois at Chicago, College of Medicine at Peoria,
Peoria, Illinois 61603; *Department of Pediatric Urology, Children's Hospital of Michigan,
Wayne State University, Detroit, Michigan 48202*

Neuroblastoma, ganglioneuroblastoma, and ganglioneuroma comprise the neuroblastic tumors that develop from primordial neural crest tissue. During embryogenesis, neural crest cells migrate and eventually differentiate into the adrenal medulla, parathyroid, parafollicular cells, autonomic nervous system, and nerve sheath cells.

The variation in locations and degrees of histopathologic differentiation of neuroblastic tumors result in an array of enigmatic presentations, demonstrating diverse clinical and biologic characteristics as well as behavior. These tumors exhibit highly malignant behavior when observed in older children with regional or disseminated disease but have the propensity for demonstrating spontaneous regression as well as spontaneous and induced differentiation into benign neoplasms (1,2).

As originally described by Breslow and McCann (3), age at diagnosis remains an important predictor of the outcome. Infants, defined as 1 year of age or less, in general fare better than older children. Recent advances in neuroblastoma treatment have followed identification of biochemical and genetic variables with independent prognostic significance. The result has been an increasing ability to distinguish prognostic subsets of patients based on clinical and biologic features so as to better define the relative risk of recurring disease and, therefore, the development of risk-related therapy that is not based solely on age or stage (4).

INCIDENCE

Neuroblastoma is the third most common malignancy in childhood, the second most malignant solid tumor of childhood, and the most common malignant tumor of infancy (5). Neuroblastomas account for 6% to 10% of all childhood cancers and at least 15% of all cancer-related deaths in children (6). The prevalence is approximately 1 in 8,000 live births, with about 525 new cases of neuroblastoma per year being reported in the United States (7). Evidence indicates that the incidence is fairly uniform throughout the world, at least in the industrialized nations. The incidence is 10.5 per million per year in white children and 8.8 per million per year in black children. Neuroblastoma has a slight male predominance (1.1:1.0) (7). Because there is a propensity for spontaneous regression of neuroblastoma in situ, the actual incidence of the tumor is probably much higher than reported.

ETIOLOGY

Environmental

Environmental exposures appear to play a minimal, if any, role in the development of neuroblastoma. Reports on fetal exposure to hydantoin and alcohol suggest an increased risk of neuroblastoma, although this association has not been confirmed with certainty (8). A few studies have linked paternal occupational exposure to electromagnetic fields and maternal use of hair coloring products with the development of neuroblastoma, but they have not been confirmed by other studies (9).

Genetics

There are clear genetic influences in neuroblastoma. Knudson and Strong (10) estimate that approximately 20% of all neuroblastomas could be the result of a terminal mutation with an autosomal dominant pattern of inheritance. Their two-mutation theory of the origin of childhood cancers seems to fit when regression analysis is performed on neuroblastoma data. Concerning a hereditary predisposition to neuroblastoma, a number of reports of familial neuroblastoma, as well as bilateral and multifocal disease, have been documented (11).

PATHOGENESIS

Advances in the treatment of neuroblastoma have stemmed from a better understanding of the lesion at both the cellular and molecular levels. As a result, better methods of tumor diagnosis and subclassification have been developed and are useful for predicting clinical behavior and following disease activity.

Natural History

The concept of in situ neuroblastoma has been used to support the argument that many neuroblastomas arise and regress spontaneously. Cases of complete regression of neuroblastoma in infants have been well documented (12). Also, neuroblastic nodules are uniformly present in all fetuses studied between 17 and 20 weeks of gestation (13). These nodules completely regress by the time of birth or shortly afterward. In 1963, neuroblastic nodules were identified by Beckwith and Perrin in infants younger than 3 months of age who had died of other causes; this finding left the impression that neuroblastoma may be more common with a high rate of

spontaneous regression (14). However, the actual frequency of neuroblastomas that are detected clinically or by mass screening and that subsequently regress without treatment most likely represents only 2% to 5% of all patients with neuroblastoma (15,16). Neuroblastic nodules seen in earlier studies were most likely remnants of fetal adrenal development. However, neuroblastic cell rests may be the cells from which neuroblastomas develop, at least in the adrenal medulla (4).

DNA Index

Look and colleagues (17), as well as others, have demonstrated that determination of the DNA index (DI) of neuroblastomas from infants provides important information that can predict the response to particular chemotherapeutic regimens as well as the outcome (17). Tumors with a hyperdiploid DNA content or index (DI > 1) are most likely to have lower stages of disease and respond to cyclophosphamide and doxorubicin, whereas tumors with a diploid DNA content (DI = 1) are more likely to have advanced stages of disease and do not respond to this combination (17). Although this analysis cannot detect specific chromosome rearrangements such as deletions, translocations, or gene amplification, it is simple to perform and correlates with biologic behavior.

N-*myc* Amplification

Neuroblastomas have been characterized cytogenetically and gene amplification has been noted in some patients. The amplified region is derived from the distal short arm of chromosome 2, which contains the protooncogene N-*myc*. Brodeur and colleagues (18) have demonstrated that N-*myc* amplification occurs in about 25% to 30% of primary untreated neuroblastomas and is often associated with advanced stages of disease. Amplification is found in 5% to 10% of patients with low stages of disease and stage IV-S, and in 30% to 40% of patients with advanced disease. N-*myc* amplification, if it is going to occur, is present at the time of diagnosis, suggesting an intrinsic biologic property of a subset of very aggressive tumors (19).

Chromosome Defects

Deletions of the short arm of chromosome 1 are found in 70% to 80% of near-diploid tumors that have been karyotyped (20). The deletions of chromosome 1 are somewhat variable in their proximal breakpoints, but the region of consistent deletion has been mapped to subbands of 1p36, which revealed loss of heterogenicity (LOH) for the deleted allele (21). 1p36 may contain a suppressor gene that is important in malignant transformation or progression. There is a strong correlation between LOH from chromosome 1p and N-*myc* amplification, suggesting that these two genetic events may be related (21).

PATHOLOGY

On gross section, neuroblastomas are usually encapsulated and firm. When lesions are larger, there may be penetration of the pseudocapsule with infiltration of the surrounding tissues. Cystic areas throughout the tumor are not uncommon.

Histologically, neuroblastoma is one of the *small blue round cell* neoplasias of childhood. Other small blue round cell tumors from which neuroblastoma must be differentiated include Ewing's sarcoma, non-Hodgkin's lymphoma, primitive neural ectodermal tumors, and undifferentiated soft-tissue sarcomas (rhabdomyosarcoma). The histologic subtypes of the neuroblastic tumor appear to correlate with the normal differentiation patterns of the sympathetic nervous system. The three classic histopathologic patterns include neuroblastoma, ganglioneuroblastoma, and ganglioneuroma, which reflect a spectrum of maturation and differentiation.

The typical neuroblastoma is composed of small, uniformly sized cells containing dense hyperchromatic nuclei and scant cytoplasm. The presence of neuritic processes or neuropil is a pathognomonic feature of all but the most primitive neuroblastomas. The Homer-Wright pseudorosette is composed of neuroblasts surrounding areas of eosinophilic neuropil (Fig. 9-1). Pseudorosettes may occur in 15% to 50% of neuroblastoma cases (22). Ganglioneuroma is the solely differentiated benign counterpart of neuroblastoma. It consists primarily of mature ganglion, neuropil, and schwannian cells (Fig. 9-2). Ganglioneuroblastoma defines a heterogenous group of tumors with histopathologic features between those of neuroblastoma and ganglioneuroma. Some clinicians refer to some neuroblastomas as maturing neuroblastomas if they contain less than 50% maturing or mature ganglion cells, whereas ganglioneuroblastomas have more extensive maturation elements (Fig. 9-3). Ganglioneuroblastomas may be either focal or diffuse, with diffuse patterns being less aggressive in clinical behavior.

Prognostic classification of neuroblastoma based on histopathologic features has been attempted by several investigators. The Shimada index is the most widely acclaimed. It is based on patient age, the presence or absence of schwannian stroma, degree of differentiation, and the mitosis karyorrhexis index (23). A retrospective evaluation of the Shimada method in approximately 300 cases treated by the Children's Cancer Study Group (CCSG) identified favorable and unfavorable patient subsets. When compared with other clinical features, these histologic patterns were independently predictive of the outcome, and stage was prognostically less important than histologic grade (23).

Joshi and colleagues (24) developed a predictive measure independent of age or stage, looking specifically at the presence of calcification and a low mitotic rate (<10 mitoses per high-power fields). A grading system was therefore developed combining tumors with both features (grade II) or absence of both features (grade III). When these grades were combined with age older than or younger than 1 year, surgical pathologic staging of low- and high-risk groups emerged (24). These groups closely correlated with the Shimada favorable and unfavorable groups. The reported advan-

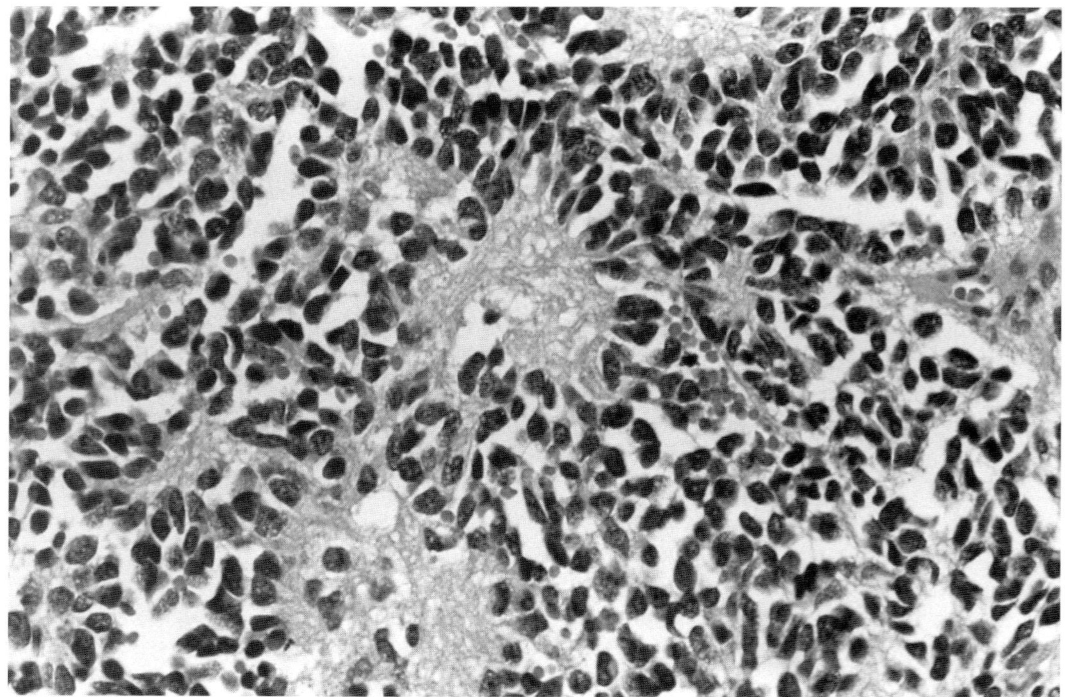

FIG. 9-1. Neuroblastoma: small round blue cell tumor with Homer-Wright pseudorosettes. (Courtesy of Raja Rabah, M.D., Department of Pathology, Children's Hospital of Michigan, Detroit, MI.)

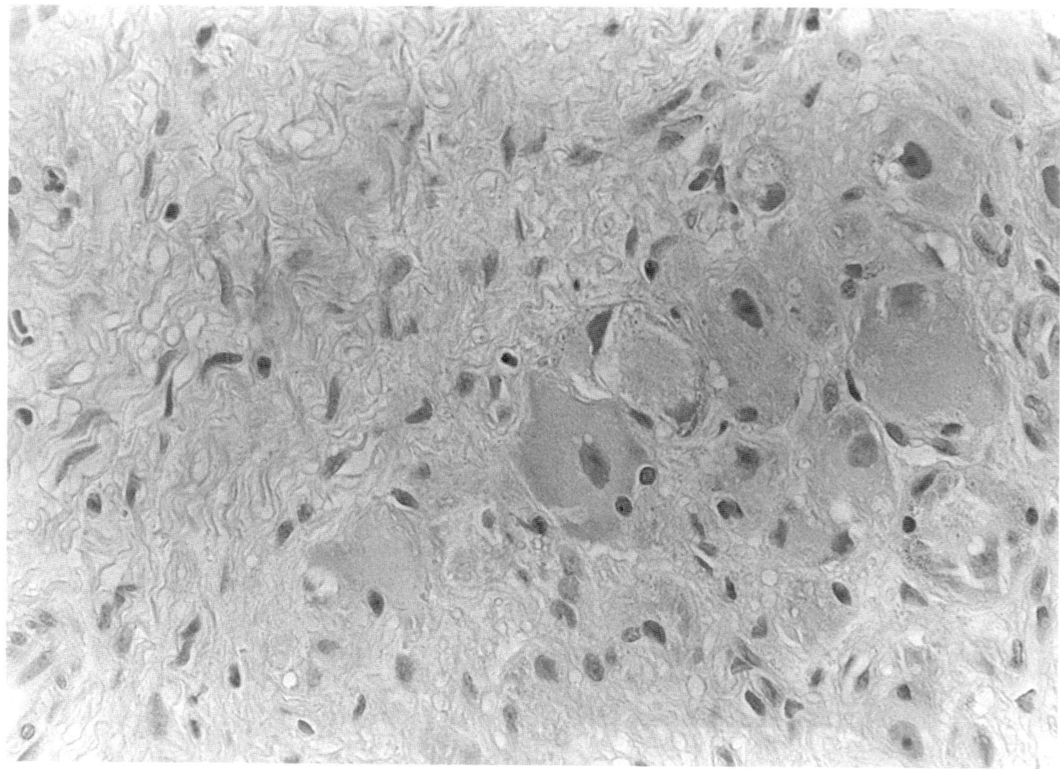

FIG. 9-2. Ganglioneuroma: schwannian stroma-rich tumor with aggregates of ganglion cells. (Courtesy of Raja Rabah, M.D., Department of Pathology, Children's Hospital of Michigan, Detroit, MI.)

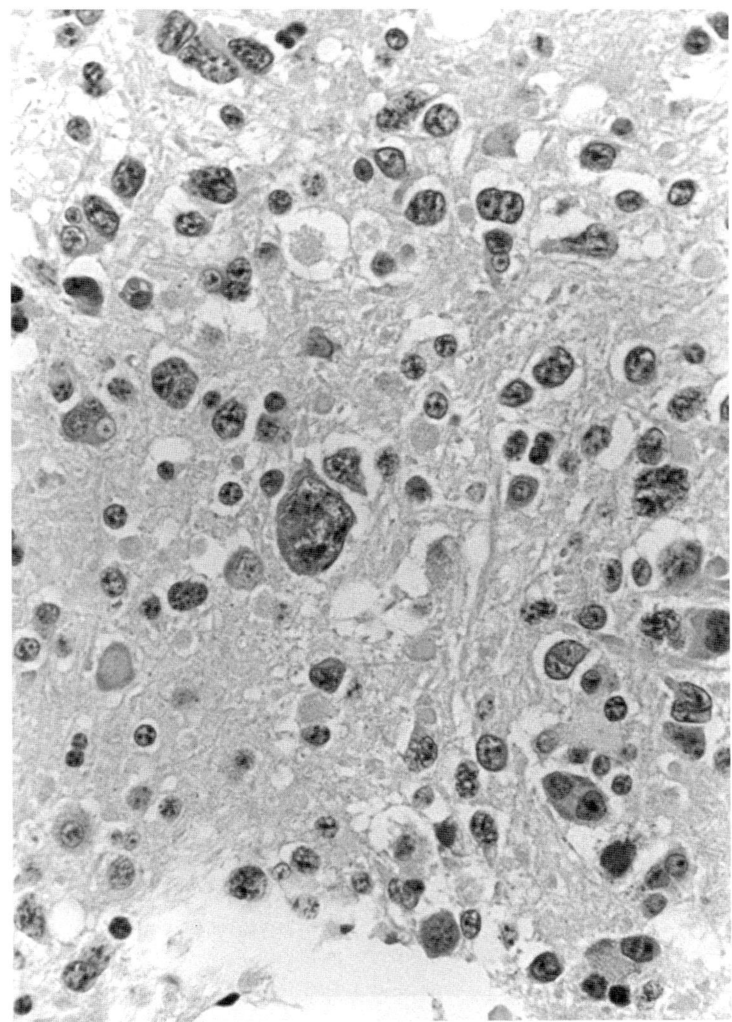

FIG. 9-3. Ganglioneuroblastoma: mixture of small round tumor cells with large, atypical cells with some ganglionic differentiation. (Courtesy of Raja Rabah, M.D., Department of Pathology, Children's Hospital of Michigan, Detroit, MI.)

tage of the Joshi method was simplicity in determining the histologic features and prognostic categories (24).

PRESENTATION

Neuroblastomas may occur anywhere in the sympathetic chain from the head to the pelvis. The presentation and differential diagnosis depend on the site of the tumor. Most primary tumors occur in the abdomen (65%), although the frequency of adrenal tumors is slightly higher in children (40%) than in infants (25%). Infants also have more thoracic and cervical primary tumors (Fig. 9-4) (4).

Neuroblastoma is the most common malignancy detected in the newborn period. Therefore, some of these tumors develop antenatally and may be detectable by maternal ultrasound. In most neuroblastomas detected prenatally, favorable clinical and biological features have been identified neonatally (25). Diagnosis of the suspected tumor was usually made between 26 and 39 weeks of gestation

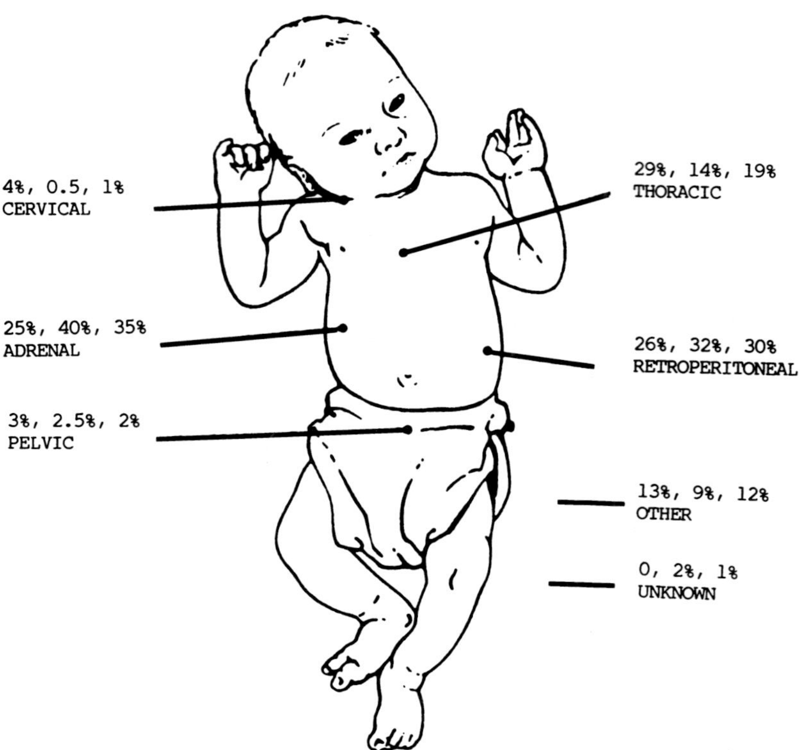

FIG. 9-4. Distribution of neuroblastoma in infants.

(26). Eleven of 11 newborns studied for N-*myc* amplification had none, and eight of ten patients were aneuploid (DI > 1) (25). Stage IV disease has been identified in three newborns with prenatally detected neuroblastoma (25,26). In these newborns who had metastatic disease, all three had fetal hydrops and their mothers had hypertension or preeclampsia. The authors concluded that staging of neuroblastoma prenatally is difficult but that mothers with no evidence of hypertension or preeclampsia appear to have minimal risk of their fetuses having widely disseminated disease (26).

In patients with apparently localized disease, the rate of regional lymph metastases may be as high as 35%. If lymph nodes are malignant outside the cavity of origin (although this is considered disseminated disease), the patient's outlook is better than if another disseminated disease is present.

Hematogenous spread occurs in the following descending order of frequency: bone marrow, bone, liver, skin. Metastases to the lung and brain are rare, usually occurring in relapsing or end-stage disease.

The proportion of patients with localized, regional, or metastatic disease is age dependent. In a recent Pediatric Oncology Group (POG) study, the incidence of localized tumors, regional lymph node spread, and disseminated disease was 39%, 18%, and 25%, respectively, in infants (18% had stage IV-S disease), compared to 19%, 13%, and 68%, respectively, in older children (4).

Abdominal disease often manifests as complaints of fullness and discomfort and rarely as gastrointestinal tract dysfunction. Massive abdominal tumors may lead to respiratory compromise or venous and lymphatic drainage compression, with eventual scrotal and lower extremity edema.

High thoracic and cervical masses can be associated with Horner's syndrome, which consists of unilateral ptosis, myosis, and anhidrosis. Large thoracic primary tumors may lead to superior vena cava syndrome, and cervical masses from primary or metastatic neuroblastoma may be confused with infectious adenopathy.

Proptosis and periorbital ecchymoses may result from retrobulbar and orbital infiltration by tumor. Skin involvement is seen almost exclusively in infants with stage IV tumors identified as bluish, nontender subcutaneous nodules. Constitutional symptoms associated with disseminating disease, including failure to thrive and fever, often help distinguish neuroblastoma clinically from Wilms' tumor, in which patients appear much healthier.

Paraneoplastic syndrome has been associated with both localized and disseminating neuroblastoma. Opsomyoclonus (myoclonic jerking and random eye movement) or cerebellar ataxia has been observed in up to 4% of patients with neuroblastoma. These symptoms often disappear with successful therapy.

DIAGNOSTIC EVALUATION

In 1988, criteria for diagnosis, staging, and response to treatment in patients with neuroblastoma were prepared by the international group of conferees and corresponding participants who represented most of the major pediatric oncology groups (27). It was concluded that the minimum criteria for diagnosis of neuroblastoma are confirmed if (a) an unequivocal pathologic diagnosis is made from tumor tissue using standard methods, including immunohistology or electron microscopy if necessary, or (b) the bone marrow contains unequivocal tumor cells (e.g., syncytia) *and* urine contains increased urinary catecholamine metabolites [vanillylmandelic acid (VMA) or homovanillic acid (HVA) is elevated more than three standard deviations above the mean per milligram of creatinine, corrected for age]. Some oncologists have used compatible radiographic or scintigraphic appearance with increased urinary catecholamine metabolites to establish the diagnosis of neuroblastoma. However, the need for tissue to assess appropriate biologic variables and establish the prognosis prevent this approach from being recommended presently.

Bone marrow aspiration is routine in suspected cases of neuroblastoma. This test may be diagnostic in that up to 70% of aspirates in children with neuroblastoma are abnormal. To standardize bone marrow sampling, as well as other diagnostic tests and studies indicated in determining the extent of disease, international conferees on neuroblastoma staging devised the minimum recommended tests in the evaluation of patients with neuroblastoma (Table 9-1) (27). Presently, neuroblastoma-

TABLE 9–1. *Minimum recommendation tests for determining extent of disease*

Tumor site	Tests
Primary	Three-dimensional measurement of tumor by CT scan, MRI, or ultrasound
Metastases	Bilateral posterior iliac bone marrow aspirates and core biopsies (4 adequate specimens necessary to exclude tumor)
	Bone radiographs and either scintigraphy by ^{99m}Tc-diphosphonate or ^{131}I– (or ^{123}I–) MIBG or both
	Abdominal and liver imaging by CT scan, MRI, or ultrasound
	Chest radiograph (anterior-posterior and lateral) and chest CT scan
Markers	Quantitative urinary catecholamine metabolites (VMA and HVA)

CT, Computed tomography; MRI, magnetic resonance imaging; MIBG, metaiodobenzylguanidine; VMA, vanillylmandelic acid; HVA, homovanillic acid.

For evaluation of bone metastases, ^{99m}Tc-diphosphonate scintigraphy is recommended for all patients and is essential if MIBG scintigraphy is negative in bone.

From ref. 27 with permission.

specific immunocytology of marrow aspirates is being used increasingly and may obviate the need for marrow biopsies.

Catecholamine Excretion

The major metabolites of catecholamine production by neuroblastoma are VMA and HVA. From 90% to 95% of neuroblastoma cases exhibit an elevation of one or both products. However, some patients occasionally have normal catecholamine excretion (28). The most common location of these nonsecreting tumors is the chest. To date, no clear-cut correlation has been identified between the pattern of catecholamine excretion and age, symptoms, or histologic pattern of the tumor.

Although neuroblastoma produces catecholamines, hypertension is an uncommon symptom. It is suggested that norepinephrine may be metabolized within the tumor itself and thus does not reach active systemic levels. An alternative theory proposed by Imashuku and colleagues (29) is that tyrosine hydroxylase, the initial enzyme in catecholamine synthesis, is subject to normal feedback inhibition by norepinephrine, dopamine, and 3, 4-dihydroxy-phenylalanine (Fig. 9-5).

Because it is cumbersome to obtain 24-hour urine collections in infants and small children to quantitate catecholamine metabolites, simpler assay methods have been developed. A filter spot test for VMA was developed by LaBrosse, with 75% positivity for neuroblastoma (30). However, although VMA and HVA screening tests are useful, the general consensus is that confir-

CATECHOLAMINE METABOLISM

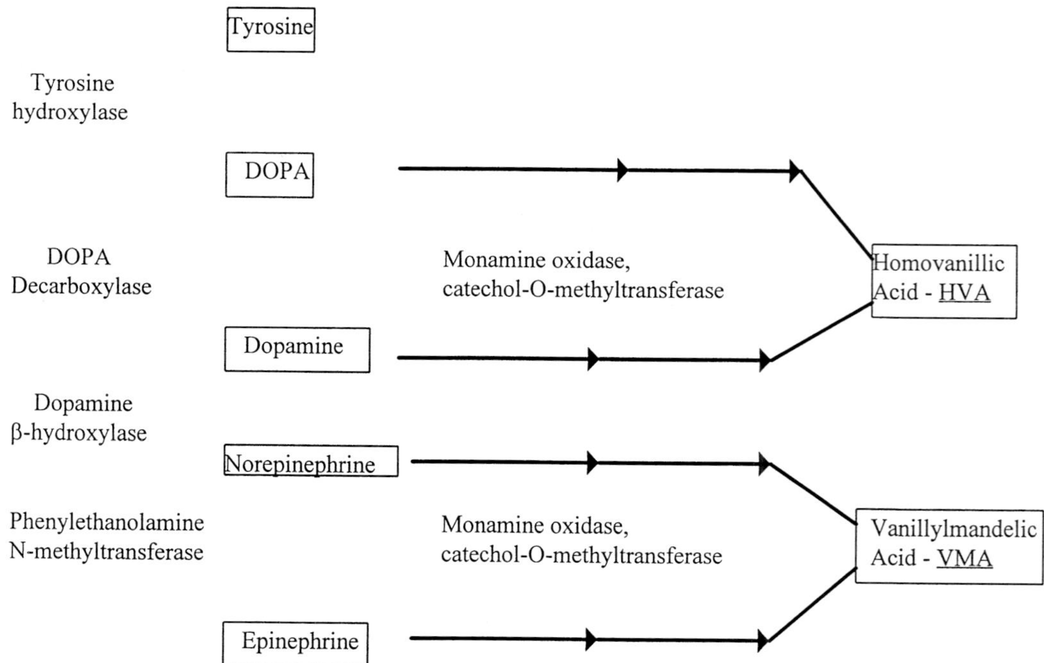

FIG. 9-5. Pathway of catecholamine metabolism. Shown is a simplified diagram of catecholamine synthesis and metabolism. Homovanillic acid and vanillylmandelic acid are the urinary catecholamine metabolites usually measured.

mation by more specific quantitative assays is usually appropriate. Concerning the catecholamine metabolism cascade, the final enzyme found in the adrenal chromaffin cells and in most pheochromocytomas is phenylethanolamine N-methyltranferase, which converts norepinephrine to epinephrine (see Fig. 9-5). Neuroblastoma cells lack this last enzyme, and therefore epinephrine is not produced.

Imaging and Laboratory Evaluation

The conventional diagnostic imaging studies include plain radiographs, bone scintigraphy, ultrasound, computed tomography (CT) scan, and magnetic resonance imaging (MRI). A chest radiograph is routinely obtained, with careful attention being paid to the posterior mediastinum and ribs for tumor extension and erosion (Fig. 9-6).

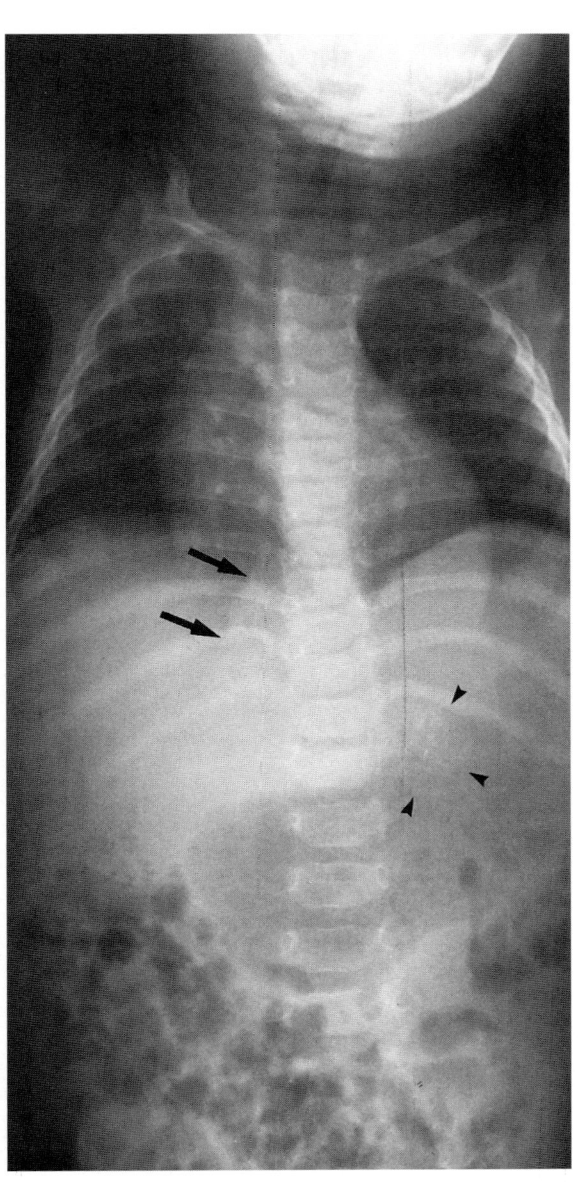

FIG. 9-6. Abnormal right paraspinal density (*arrows*) with subtle adjacent eleventh and twelfth rib erosions and speckled calcifications in the left upper quadrant (*arrowheads*) are plain film findings consistent with neuroblastoma. (Courtesy of Susan Roubal, M.D., Department of Pediatric Imaging, Children's Hospital of Michigan, Detroit, MI.)

The potential specificity and sensitivity of metaiodobenzylguanidine (MIBG) scintigraphy for evaluation of bone and soft-tissue involvement in neuroblastoma is attractive. This compound is taken up by catecholaminergic cells, which include most neuroblastomas. Radiolabeled MIBG scintigraphy thus becomes potentially a very specific and sensitive method for assessment of the primary tumor and metastatic disease. MIBG scintigraphy is becoming more readily available in the United States and has been used widely in Europe. If MIBG is not available, ^{99m}Tc-diphosphonate will remain the standard for evaluation of bone disease (Fig. 9-7), and CT and MRI scans are the standard methods for evaluation of soft-tissue disease.

When attempting to distinguish Wilms' tumor from neuroblastoma radiographically, a speckled pattern of calcification is seen in up to half of the neuroblastoma cases on a plain film and in up to 80% of cases on CT scan (Fig. 9-8). A speckled pattern seen with calcification in neuroblastomas is in contrast to the less frequent calcification seen in Wilms' tumor (approximately 10%), which tends to be curvilinear because of previous hemorrhage into the tumor. In a suprarenal neuroblastoma, the kidney is inferiorly and laterally displaced, with characteristic maintenance of a normal caliceal pattern (Fig. 9-9). Intrarenal Wilms' tumor usually causes calyceal distortion.

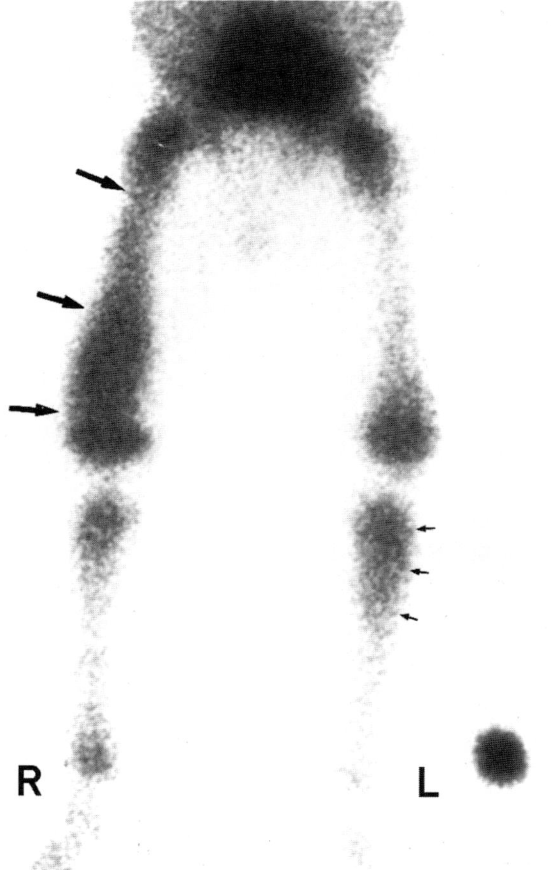

FIG. 9-7. 99m-Tc bone scan demonstrates obvious abnormally increased activity along the right femur (*large arrows*) and more subtle activity in the left proximal tibia (*small arrows*), both indicative of skeletal metastatic disease. (Courtesy of Susan Roubal, M.D., Department of Pediatric Imaging, Children's Hospital of Michigan, Detroit, MI.)

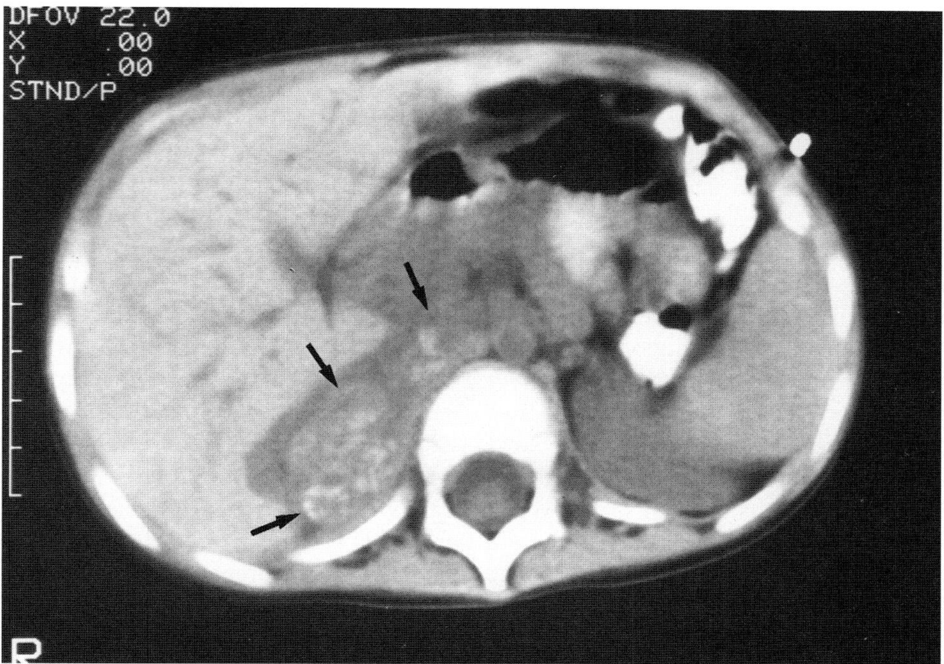

FIG. 9-8. Characteristic stippled calcifications (*arrows*) in the right adrenal and paracaval region on a noncontrast axial computed tomography scan. (Courtesy of Susan Roubal, M.D., Department of Pediatric Imaging, Children's Hospital of Michigan, Detroit, MI.)

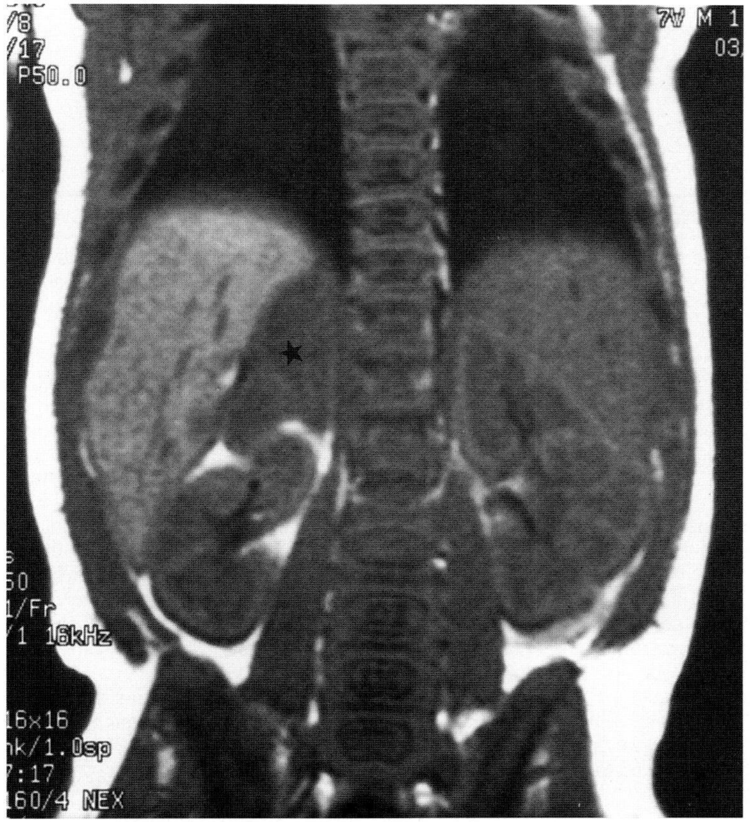

FIG. 9-9. Coronal noncontrast T1-weighted MRI demonstrates a low-signal right adrenal neuroblastoma (*asterisk*) with inferior displacement of the right kidney. (Courtesy of Susan Roubal, M.D., Department of Pediatric Imaging, Children's Hospital of Michigan, Detroit, MI.)

STAGING

The most commonly used staging system for neuroblastoma has been the CCSG staging system developed by Evans and colleagues in 1971 (31). The POG and the International Unit Against Cancer Group also proposed staging systems, and there have been various modifications of all prestaging systems used by various practicing pediatric oncologists. In general, the various staging systems give comparable results in distinguishing low-stage, good-prognosis patients from high-stage, poor-prognosis patients. However, some differences in the staging systems are substantial, in particular at the intermediate stages. Because of differences in the respective staging systems, the results of one group cannot be readily compared with those of other groups. As a result, the International Neuroblastoma Staging System (INSS) was proposed, and has led to uniformity in staging patients with neuroblastoma for clinical trials and biologic studies worldwide (Table 9-2) (27).

PROGNOSIS

Neuroblastomas demonstrate both clinical and biological heterogeneity. Clinically, the stage and age of the patient at diagnosis and the site of the primary lesion are the most important variables. As of 1992, the 5-year disease-free survival rate of patients with stage 1, 2, and 4S disease was between 70% and 90%, whereas in patients with stage 3 and 4 disease it ranged from 10% to 70% (32) (Table 9-3). Infants younger than 1 year of age with the same stage of disease do significantly better, particularly in comparison with those having advanced stages of disease. Patients with nonadrenal abdominal tumors appear to do better than those with tumors originating in the adrenal glands. Patients with mediastinal neuroblastomas, even those with positive nodes, Horner's syndrome, cord compression, or bone erosion, have improved survival rates, with a 5-year actuarial survival rate reported as high as 88% (33). Location of the primary tumor, however, does not appear

TABLE 9–2. *Staging systems for neuroblastoma*

CCSG system[a]	International (INSS)[b]
Stage I: tumor confined to the organ or structure of origin	Stage 1: localized tumor confined to the area of origin; complete gross excision, with or without microscopic residual disease; indentifiable ipsilateral and contralateral lymph nodes negative microscopically
Stage II: tumor extending in continuity beyond the organ or structure of origin, but not crossing the midline. Regional lymph nodes on the ipsilateral side may be positive	Stage 2A: unilateral tumor with incomplete gross excision and identifiable ipsilateral and contralateral lymph nodes negative microscopically
	Stage 2B: unilateral tumor with complete or incomplete gross excision, with positive ipsilateral regional lymph nodes and identifiable contralateral lymph nodes negative microscopically
Stage III: tumor extending in continuity beyond the midline. Regional lymph nodes may be involved bilaterally	Stage 3: tumor infiltrating across the midline with or without regional lymph node involvement, or unilateral tumor with contralateral regional lymph node involvement, or midline tumor with bilateral lymph node involvement
Stage IV: remote disease involving the skeleton, bone marrow, soft tissue, and distant lymph node groups (see stage IV-S)	Stage 4: dissemination of tumor to distant lymph nodes, bone, bone marrow, liver, and/or other organs (except as defined in stage 4S)
Stage IV-S: as defined in stages I or II, except for the presence of remote disease confined to the liver, skin, or marrow (without bone metastases)	Stage 4S: localized primary tumor as defined for stages 1 or 2 with dissemination limited to liver, skin, and/or bone marrow

CCSG, Children's Cancer Study Group; INSS, International Neuroblastoma Staging Systems.
[a]From ref. 31 with permission.
[b]From ref. 27 with permission.

TABLE 9–3. *Incidence and prognosis as of 1992*

Stage	Incidence	Survival at 5 yr
Stage 1	5%	≥90%
Stage 2A Stage 2B	10%	70–80%
Stage 3	25%	40–70% (depending on completeness of surgical resection)
Stage 4	60%	>60% if age at diagnosis is <1 yr; 20% if age at diagnosis is >1 yr and <2 yr; 10% if age at diagnosis is >2 yr
Stage 4S	5%	>80%

From ref. 32 with permission.

to add substantially to the prognostic variables of age and stage (4).

Biologic variables including genetic features, pathology, and serum markers appear to have predictive values with independent prognostication. The serum markers include ferritin, nonspecific enolase (NSE), a cell membrane ganglioside (G_{D2}), and lactic dehydrogenase. The genetic features currently in use as prognostic markers include tumor cell DI, N-*myc* oncogene copy number, and deletion or loss of heterozygosity (LOH) involving chromosome 1p, among others. Investigators are continuing to examine all biologic variables to determine over time, with large patient populations evaluated, which single variable or combination of variables will become most predictive of the outcome in addition to the clinical features of patient age, stage, and primary tumor location.

Genetic Features

As discussed earlier, diploid tumors (DI = 1), tumors with N-*myc* amplification, and those with loss of heterozygosity of chromosome 1p are well-established independent genetic expressions associated with a poor prognosis.

Serum Markers

Gangliosides (sialic acid–containing glycosphingolipids) are present on the membranes of neuroblastoma cells and are shed into the circulation. In more differentiated neuroblastoma, gangliosides are absent and are present in only small quantities in the serum. The most characteristic ganglioside on human neuroblastoma cell membranes is G_{D2}. G_{D2} shed by tumor cells may be increasingly evident during tumor progression and is therefore a useful marker of disease activity (34).

NSE is a cystoplasmic protein with enolase activity that is found in neural cells and is detectable in the serum. When serum NSE was analyzed in patients with neuroblastoma, a level greater than 100 ng/mL correlated significantly with a poor prognosis ($p < .01$) (35).

Serum ferritin has emerged as a most important variable. In some patients with actively growing neuroblastoma tumors, ferritin levels are increased (36). Ferritin levels are rarely elevated in patients with low-stage disease, whereas up to half of patients with advanced disease have significant elevation (≥142 ng/mL), and those with increased levels have a much lower progression-free survival ($p < .01$) (36). If serum ferritin is not elevated in stage III cases, the prognosis is improved (76% versus 23% without evidence of disease at 2-year follow-up). In stage IV disease, the difference is less dramatic (27% versus 3%) (36).

CLASSIFICATIONS

In the past 5 to 10 years, biologic variables highly predictive of clinical behavior have been used to further develop subsets of patients with neuroblastoma. There is increasing evidence for at least two or three genetic subsets of neuroblastoma that are highly predictive of clinical behavior.

A recent classification proposed by Brodeur and validated by Bourhis and colleagues takes into account abnormalities in chromosome 1p, N-*myc* copy number, and assessment of DNA content, coupled with age and stage of disease, allowing three distinct genetic subsets of neuroblastoma to be identified (37,38). The first subtype is characterized by a hyperdiploid or near-triploid karyotype with few if any cytogenic abnormalities. These patients are usually infants with localized disease and have a good prognosis, with survival rate greater than or equal to 90%. The second subtype has a near-diploid karyotype, again with no N-*myc* amplification, but usually with loss of heterogenicity at the 1p36 band. These patients are usually older than 1 year and have advanced-stage disease that progresses slowly and is often fatal, with approximately 25% to 50% survival rate. The third group has a near-diploid or tetraploid karyotype with 1p allelic loss, amplification of N-*myc*, or both. These patients are generally older, with advanced, rapidly progressive disease and a dismal prognosis, with survival rate less than or equal to 5%.

Brodeur updated his review of the three subtypes in 1995, noting nearly identical survival rates as previously published (39). In addition to the three genetic features, he added expression of TRKA, a protooncogene with independent prognostic significance. TRKA expression is usually high in subtype one, low in subtype two, and absent in subtype three (42). These genetic characteristics have allowed neuroblastomas to be categorized into three subtypes with distinct clinical features and behavior (Table 9-4).

In the past, neuroblastoma was considered to be a disease with a better outcome if diagnosed early. However, it is apparent that the tumors occurring in infants are genetically different from those in older children and that a genetically favorable subtype seldom, if ever, evolves into an unfavorable one. Brodeur has inferred that molecular pathology of the tumor may be better at predicting the outcome than patient age or disease stage alone (39).

TREATMENT

Excluding complete resection of primary tumors and infants with stable stage 4S disease, chemotherapy remains the backbone of the multimodality therapy for neuroblastomas. Chemotherapy, surgery, and radiotherapy each have a role, as determined by the natural history of individual cases, considering stage, patient age, and biologic and genetic features.

Surgery

Depending on the timing, operative procedures can have diagnostic as well as therapeutic functions. Surgery performed before any other therapy is used can establish the diagnosis, provide tissue for biologic studies, help stage the tumor, and attempt to completely excise the tumor if feasible. In delayed primary or second-look surgery, the surgeon determines the response to therapy and removes residual disease when possible. Present-day chemotherapy both consolidates and reduces the size of primary tumors as well as large lymph node metastases. Therefore, sacrifice of vital structures to achieve resection at diag-

TABLE 9–4. *Clinical/genetic aubtypes of neuroblastoma*

Feature	Type 1	Type 2	Type 3
Karyotype or ploidy	Hyperdiploid/triploid	Near diploid/near tetraploid	Near diploid/near tetraploid
N-*myc* gene	Normal	Normal	Amplified
TRKA	High	Low	Absent
Chromosome 1p	Normal	±1p LOH	±1p LOH
Age	Usually <12 mo	Usually >12 mo	Usually >12 mo
INSS stage	Usually 1, 2, 4S	Usually 3, 4	Usually 3, 4
Outcome	>90%	25–50%	5%

LOH, loss of heterogenicity.

nosis should be avoided, especially in infants, in whom the prognosis is excellent in most cases.

Gross examination of lymph nodes to exclude or define lymph node metastases is inaccurate in up to 25% of cases (40). Ideally, lymph nodes superior and inferior to the primary tumor should be sampled, with documentation made of their location. In situations in which lymph node sampling is a formidable task with a potential risk, the value of additional information regarding lymph node status may not provide a benefit over other prognostic factors and features that are presently being evaluated.

The surgical complication rate in neuroblastoma is between 5% and 25% (41). An aggressive attempt to resect abdominal tumors at diagnosis has led to the highest incidence of complications. Complications generally are lower for delayed second-look procedures after tumor shrinkage by chemotherapy (42). A recent study reviewing infants with metastatic neuroblastoma suggests that complete or greater than 95% resection of the primary tumor was associated with a statistically significant improvement in survival rate (43). This same effect has not been substantiated in children older than 1 year of age.

Advances in surgical technology have led to the introduction of ultrasonic aspiration and laparoscopy in the treatment of neuroblastoma (44,45). Ultrasonic aspiration provided nearly complete tumor resection, minimized blood loss, and did not damage adjacent organs, as reported in 12 patients from the Kaiser Permanente Medical Center in California (44). The locations of these tumors included the abdomen (five), chest (five), and neck (two). All patients underwent subsequent chemotherapy or autologous bone marrow transplantation. Recurrent local disease led to death in two patients, and one died of metastatic disease.

Laparoscopic adrenalectomy has been reported in three patients identified by mass screening in Japan who had small, localized adrenal tumors (<20 mm in diameter) (45). All three tumors were well encapsulated and completely excised. Both studies suggest that less invasive measures may be used surgically, with less potential risk in surgical control of local small as well as bulky disease.

Chemotherapy

Neuroblastoma is clearly responsive to chemotherapy and is the predominant modality of management. Cyclophosphamide, cisplatin, doxorubicin, and the epipodophyllotoxins [teniposide (VM-26) and etoposide (VP-16)] yield complete response and partial response rates ranging from 34% to 45%. They have become the cornerstone of multiagent regimens (4).

Drug combinations have evolved to take advantage of drug synergism, mechanisms of cytotoxicity, and differences in side effects. The drug pairs cyclophosphamide plus doxorubicin and cisplatin plus teniposide, used separately and in combination, take advantage of combining non–cell-dependent, cycle-specific agents (cyclophosphamide, cisplatin) followed by cell-dependent drugs (doxorubicin, teniposide) (46,47). Treatment in children with these combinations has resulted in improved response rates with a minimal increase in toxicity.

Radiation Therapy

Although neuroblastoma is considered a radiosensitive tumor, as demonstrated in vitro, on a clinical level the results have been more variable. Historically, radiation has been used in the multimodality management of residual neuroblastoma, bulky unresectable tumors, and disseminated disease. Its role continues to be refined with the improvement of multiagent chemotherapy and the increasing trend toward risk-related treatments.

Current uses include patients with INSS stage 2B and 3 disease in conjunction with chemotherapy regimens for autologous bone marrow transplants and palliative management of pain in patients with end-stage disease.

131-I-MIBG

MIBG is used for scintigraphic imaging of neuroblastoma as well as other neuroendocrine tumors. MIBG is an analogue of guanethidine, which resembles norepinephrine in molecular structure and is selectively taken up by tissues and tumors derived from the neural crest.

Initially, 131-I-MIBG was used in patients with advanced neuroblastoma who had received intensive pretreatment with chemotherapy or radiation therapy (48). The results were encouraging, which prompted the use of 131-I-MIBG at the time of diagnosis with the expectation that the tumor response might be greater than in pretreated, resistant patients. Hoefnagel and colleagues (49) evaluated 31 children with inoperable neuroblastoma (10 stage 3, 21 stage 4) with first-line 131-I-MIBG (49). A 72% to 81% objective response rate was seen, which is better than that often reported in conventional chemotherapy treatment. Nineteen patients had had complete or greater than 95% resection of the residual tumor. With combined MIBG-targeted therapy and surgery, one-third of the patients achieved a complete response. This study and others suggest that the results of MIBG therapy and surgery alone were comparable to those of multidrug chemotherapy and were less toxic.

Concerns regarding the use of MIBG have centered on the absence of good pharmacokinetic data, the accuracy of methods for determining the radiotherapy dosage, and the lack of in vitro cell kill in the absence of bulky disease (50). The results of future studies addressing these concerns, as well as increased availability of MIBG in the United States, should help clarify its role in the treatment of neuroblastoma.

Immunotherapy

Two features of neuroblastoma suggest that it may be treatable by exploiting the body's own defense system: (a) the unusual behavior of stage 4S neuroblastomas, which show spontaneous regression, and (b) the spontaneous maturation of malignant tumors in some stage 2 patients.

However, although some advanced renal cell carcinomas have responded to interleukin-2 (IL-2), the effect on neuroblastoma has been marginal at best. A 1995 phase II trial using recombinant IL-2 in nine children with refractory neuroblastomas noted an immunostimulatory effect but no measurable antitumor effects (51). The future role of immunotherapy will probably focus on the post–bone marrow transplant patient population.

Screening

The question of whether screening in infants with neuroblastoma would improve their prognosis was first addressed in Japan more than 20 years ago. Since then, more than 7 million children have been screened and more than 650 cases of neuroblastoma have been detected. Mass screening pilot studies have also been conducted throughout North America and Europe.

The likelihood of having a positive test for urinary catecholamines depends on the number of tumor cells or the size of the tumor. The detection limit appears to be approximately 5 g of tumor weight or about 5×10^9 tumor cells. Also, 25% of patients do not excrete VMA in excess and about 10% are nonexcretors of both VMA and HVA (52). Therefore, it is estimated that 21% of neuroblastoma patients in a screened population will have false-negative results and will later be proven to have neuroblastoma (52).

Currently, nationwide neuroblastoma mass screening for 6-month-old infants in Japan is detecting approximately 110 neuroblastoma cases annually, with a survival rate of 97% (53). The sensitivity of the initial screening at 6 months (positive cases/positive cases–false-negative cases) is about 75%, and the prognosis of false-negative cases is unfavorable. Because of the suboptimal sensitivity at first screening, investigators have recommended a second screening to rescue false-negative cases at 18 months.

A study by Suita and colleagues (54) noted that advanced cases of neuroblastoma detected by mass screening often have biologic variables indicating a good prognosis (54). In this study, patients with advanced neuroblastoma not detected by mass screening had a 5-year survival rate of 25%, whereas all patients whose tumors were detected by mass screening were alive after conventional therapy. The accumulating body of genetic information suggests that there are at least two or three different subsets of neuroblastoma. The more favorable group presents earlier and therefore is the predominant group detected by mass screening (54). This theory seems much more plausible than the one suggesting that all neuroblastomas begin with a more favorable genotype and phenotype and evolve into a more aggressive tumor with adverse genetic features.

Future Outlook

Clinical advances in the future will most likely be closely linked to progress made in the laboratory investigation of neuroblastomas. In the absence of new, highly active chemotherapeutic or immunotherapeutic agents, the immediate focus of research, chemotherapy, and radiotherapy concerns more effective use of the currently available therapies. This approach has improved cure rates in other malignancies, in particular leukemia.

Presently, urinary catecholamine metabolites are used to follow patients with neuroblastoma, but they are not as sensitive as α-fetoprotein or β-human chorionic gonadotropin are in following germ cell testicular tumors (4). Serum ferritin, NSE, G_{D2}, and other new markers may be used in the future to follow the response to treatment more effectively and to predict early relapse. Such markers might obviate the need for multiple diagnostic imaging studies and marrow sampling while patients are in remission.

DI, N-*myc* amplification, chromosome 1p deletion, and serum ferritin have proved to be significant prognostic variables. It remains to be determined which of these are most powerful when subjected to multivariant analysis and whether these or other variables will supersede more conventional clinical features such as age, stage, and primary tumor site. In the future, there will be a continuing effort to translate promising biologic studies into clinical application and better understanding of the mechanisms of neuroblastoma transformation and progression that can eventually be used clinically.

REFERENCES

1. Everson TC, Cole WH. Spontaneous regression of neuroblastoma. In: Everson TC, Cole WH, eds. *Spontaneous regression of cancer*. Philadelphia: WB Saunders, 1966:88.
2. Cushing H, Wolbach SB. The transformation of a malignant paravertebral sympathicoblastoma into a benign ganglioneuroma. *Am J Pathol* 1927;3:203.
3. Breslow N, McCann B. Statistical estimation of prognosis for children with neuroblastoma. *Cancer Res* 1971;31:2098.
4. Brodeur GM, Castleberry RP. Neuroblastoma. In: Pizzo PA, Poplack DG, eds. *Principles and practice of pediatric oncology*, 2nd ed. Philadelphia: JB Lippincott, 1992:739.
5. Young JL, Miller RW. Incidence of malignant tumors in U.S. children. *J Pediatr* 1975;86:254.
6. Matthay KK. Neuroblastoma: a clinical challenge and biologic puzzle. *CA: Cancer J Clin* 1995;45:179.
7. Young JL, Ries LG, Silverberg E, et al. Cancer incidence, survival, and mortality for children younger than 15 years. *Cancer* 1986;58:598.
8. Seeler RA, Israel JN, Royal JE, et al. Ganglioneuroblastoma and fetal hydantoin-alcohol syndromes. *Pediatrics* 1979;63:524.
9. Wilkins JRI, Hundley VD. Paternal occupational exposure to electromagnetic fields and neuroblastoma in offspring. *Am J Epidemiol* 1990;131:995.
10. Knudson AG, Strong LC. Mutation and cancer: neuroblastoma and pheochromocytoma. *Am J Hum Genet* 1972;24:514.
11. Kushner BH, Gilbert F, Helson L. Familial neuroblastoma: case reports, literature review, and etiologic considerations. *Cancer* 1986;57:1887.
12. Haas D, Alin AR, Miler C, et al. Congenital pathologic maturation and regression of stage IV-S neuroblastoma without treatment. *Cancer* 1988;62:818.
13. Ikeda Y, Lister J, Bouton JM, et al. Congenital neuroblastoma, neuroblastoma in situ, and the normal fetal development of the adrenal. *J Pediatr Surg* 1981;16:636.
14. Beckwith J, Perrin E. In situ neuroblastoma: a contribution to the natural history of neural crest tumors. *Am J Pathol* 1963;43:1089.
15. McWilliams NB. Stage IV-S neuroblastoma: treatment controversy revisited. *Med Pediatr Oncol* 1986;14:41.
16. Carlsen NL. How frequent is spontaneous remission of neuroblastomas? implications for screening. *Br J Cancer* 1990;61:441.

17. Look AT, Hayes FA, Nitschke R, et al. Cellular DNA content as a predictor of response to chemotherapy in infants with unresectable neuroblastoma. *N Engl J Med* 1984;311:231.

18. Brodeur GM, Seeger RC, Schwab M, et al. Amplification of *N-myc* in untreated human neuroblastoma correlates with advance disease stage. *Science* 1984;244:1121.

19. Brodeur GM, Hayes FA, Green AA, et al. Consistent N-*myc* copy number in simultaneous or consecutive neuroblastoma samples from sixty individual patients. *Cancer Res* 1987;47:4248.

20. Hayaski Y, Kanda N, Inaba T, et al. Cytogenic findings and prognosis in neuroblastoma with emphasis on marker chromosome 1. *Cancer* 1989;63:126.

21. Fong CT, Dracopoli NC, White PS, et al. Loss of heterozygosity for the short arm of chromosome 1 in human neuroblastomas: correlation with N-*myc* amplification. *Proc Natl Acad Sci U S A* 1989;86:3753.

22. Russell DS, Rubensten LJ. Tumors of peripheral neuroblasts and ganglion cells. In: *Pathology of tumors of the central nervous system*. Baltimore: Williams & Wilkins, 1989:900.

23. Shimada H, Chatten J, Newton WA Jr, et al. Histopathologic prognostic factors in neuroblastic tumors: definition of subtypes of ganglioneuroblastoma and an age-linked classification of neuroblastomas. *J Natl Cancer Inst* 1984;73:405.

24. Joshi V, Cantor A, Alschuler G, et al. Prognostic significance of histopathologic features of neuroblastoma: a grading system based on the review of 211 cases from the Pediatric Oncology Group [abstr]. *Proc Am Soc Clin Oncol* 1991;10:311.

25. Saylors RL, Cohn SL, Morgan ER, et al. Prenatal detection of neuroblastoma by fetal ultrasonography. *Am J Pediatr Hematol Oncol* 1994;16:356.

26. Jennings RW, LaQuaglia MP, Leong K. Fetal neuroblastoma: prenatal diagnosis and natural history. *J Pediatr Surg* 1993;28:1168.

27. Brodeur GM, Seeger RC, Barratt A, et al. International criteria for diagnosis, staging, and response to treatment in patients with neuroblastoma. *J Clin Oncol* 1988;6:1874.

28. Voorhees MI. Neuroblastoma with normal urinary catecholamine excretion. *J Pediatr* 1971;78:680.

29. Imashuku S, LaBrosse EH, Johnson EM Jr, et al. Tyrosine hydroxylase in neuroblastoma. *Biochem Med* 1971;5:2229.

30. Evans AE, Blore J, Hadley R, et al. The LaBrosse spot test: a practical aid in the diagnosis and management of children with neuroblastoma. *Pediatrics* 1971;47:913.

31. Evans AE, D'Angio GJ, Randolph J. A proposed staging for children with neuroblastoma: Children's Cancer Study Group A. *Cancer* 1971;27:374.

32. Philip T. Overview of current treatment of neuroblastoma. *Am J Pediatr Hematol Oncol* 1992;14:97.

33. Filler RM, Traggis DG, Jaffe N, et al. Favorable outlook for children with mediastinal neuroblastoma. *J Pediatr Surg* 1972;7:136.

34. Ladisch S, Wu Z-L. Circulating gangliosides as tumor markers. *Prog Clin Biol Res* 1985;175:277.

35. Zeltzer PM, Marangos PJ, Evans AE, et al. Serum neuron specific enolase in children with neuroblastoma: relationship to stage and disease course. *Cancer* 1986;57:1230.

36. Hann HW, Stahlhut MW, Evans AE. Serum ferritin as a prognostic indicator in neuroblastoma: biological effect of isoferritins. *Prog Clin Biol Res* 1985;175:331.

37. Brodeur GM. Neuroblastoma: clinical significance of genetic abnormalities. *Cancer Surv* 1990;9:673.

38. Bourhis J, De Vathaire F, Wilson GD, et al. Combined analysis of DNA ploidy index and N-*myc* genomic content in neuroblastoma. *Cancer Res* 1991;51:33.

39. Brodeur GM. Molecular basis for heterogeneity in human neuroblastomas. *Eur J Cancer* 1995;31A:505.

40. Wilson ER, Altshuler GI, Smith EL, et al. Gross observation does not predict regional lymph node metastasis in the surgicopathologic staging of neuroblastoma [abstr]. *Proc Am Soc Clin Oncol* 1989;8:304.

41. Azizkjan RG, Shaw A, Chandler JG. Surgical complications of neuroblastoma. *J Clin Oncol* 1991;9:789.

42. Berthold F, Utsch S, Holschneider AM. The impact of preoperative chemotherapy on resectability of primary tumor and complication rate in metastatic neuroblastoma. *Z Kinderchir* 1989;44:21.

43. DeCou JM, Bowman LC, Rao BN, et al. Infants with metastatic neuroblastoma have improved survival with resection of the primary tumor. *J Pediatr Surg* 1995;30:937.

44. Applebaum H, Feinfeld LE. Ultrasonic resection of neuroblastomas: long-term local tumor control. *Arch Surg* 1995;130:905.

45. Yamamoto H, Yoshida M, Sera Y, et al. Laparoscopic surgery for neuroblastoma identified by mass screening. *J Pediatr Surg* 1996;31:385.

46. Green AA, Hustu HO, Kumar M. Sequential cyclophosphamide and doxorubicin for induction of complete remission in children with disseminated neuroblastoma. *Cancer* 1981;48:2310.

47. Hayes FA, Green AA, Caspar J, et al. Clinical evaluation of sequentially scheduled cisplatin and VM26 in neuroblastoma: response and toxicity. *Cancer* 1981;48:1715.

48. Mastrangelo R. Editorial: the treatment of neuroblastoma with 131-I-MIBG. *Med Pediatr Oncol* 1987;15:147.

49. Hoefnagel CA, De Kraker J, Valdes Olmos RA, et al. 131-I-MIBG as a first-line treatment in high-risk neuroblastoma patients. *Nucl Med Communications* 1994;15:712.

50. O Donoghue JA, Wheldon TE, Babich JW, et al. Therapeutic implications of the uptake of radiolabeled MIBG for the treatment of neuroblastoma. In: Evans AE, D Angio GJ, Knudson AGJ, et al, eds. *Advances in neuroblastoma research*, vol 3. New York: Wiley-Liss, 1991:455.

51. Bauer M, Reaman GH, Hank JA, et al. A phase II trial of human recombinant interleukin-2 administered as a 4 day continuous infusion for children with refractory neuroblastoma, non-Hodgkin's lymphoma, sarcoma, renal cell carcinoma, and malignant melanoma: a Children's Cancer Group study. *Cancer* 1995;75:2959.

52. Nishi M, Miyake H, Takeda T, et al. Cases of neuroblastoma missed by the mass screening programs. *Pediatr Res* 1989;26:603.

53. Sawada T. Past and future of neuroblastoma screening in Japan. *Am J Pediatr Hematol Oncol* 1992;14:320.

54. Suita S, Zaizen Y, Yano H, et al. How to deal with advanced cases of neuroblastoma detected by mass screening: a report from the Pediatric Oncology Study Group of the Kyushu area of Japan. *J Pediatr Surg* 1994;29:559.

Medical and Surgical Management of
Adrenal Diseases, edited by Joseph C. Cerny.
Lippincott Williams & Wilkins, Philadelphia © 1999.

10

Anesthesia for Adrenal Surgery

H. Michael Marsh and *J. G. Kim

Department of Anesthesiology, Wayne State University School of Medicine, Detroit, Michigan 48201;
**Department of Anesthesiology, Henry Ford Hospital, Detroit, Michigan 48202*

Adrenal surgery is performed for resection of cortical or medullary adrenal tumors or of hyperplastic adrenal glands. The major risk for the patient undergoing adrenalectomy stems from inadequate preoperative preparation of the patient, or from inadequate treatment for, or misdiagnosis of perioperative complications from the anesthesia and surgery. In adrenal disease, the highest perioperative risks are from undiagnosed pheochromocytoma, with an incidental need for surgical treatment, or from unrecognized adrenal hypofunction and acute circulatory failure.

This chapter outlines, from the anesthesiologist's viewpoint, the perioperative management of the patient undergoing adrenal surgery. Many excellent reviews are available (1–3). Herein, we emphasize those basic principles that we believe are essential to good care for these patients.

PREOPERATIVE PREPARATION

The three major groups of medical conditions in patients with adrenal disease that necessitate preoperative preparation are listed in Table 10-1. The major surgical complications are listed in Table 10-2. Preoperative preparation should anticipate or correct these conditions, thus preventing disastrous complications.

Adrenocortical Hyperfunction

Cushing's Syndrome

Exposure to excessive circulating glucocorticoid for a prolonged period causes Cushing's syndrome (Fig. 10-1) (4). However, only 10% to 25% of these patients require adrenal surgery, because transsphenoidal microadrenectomy or hemihypophysectomy is the preferred treatment for Cushing's disease, which accounts for 75% of patients with the syndrome, and extirpation of the primary tumor is preferred for the ectopic adrenocorticotropic hormone (ACTH) syndromes, which account for a further 10% to 15% of patients with Cushing's syndrome. The annual incidence of Cushing's syndrome is estimated at 6 per 1 million population.

Conn's Syndrome

Primary hyperaldosteronism is more rare than Cushing's syndrome, with an estimated annual incidence of 0.2 to 0.4 per 1 million

TABLE 10–1. *Major adrenal-associated conditions*

Adrenocortical hyperfunction
Adrenocortical hypofunction
Pheochromocytoma
Major surgical complications from adrenalectomy
Emergencies

TABLE 10–2. *Major surgical complications*

Blood loss
Stress
Tumor emboli
Pneumothorax
Third spacing
Hypertensive crisis
Perioperative myocardial infarction
Hypotensive crisis
Nelson's syndrome
Cardiac dysrhythmias
Hypoglycemia-stroke

population (5–7). The hypertension and hypokalemia are indistinguishable from those seen in Cushing's syndrome, but the other features of that syndrome are missing in these patients. Most cases of Conn's syndrome are caused by adrenal tumors (55%–60%) or hyperplasia (35%–40%), although extraadrenal sites of aldosterone production, including ovarian arrhenoblastoma and renal tumors, are also described (8). Adrenal surgery is often indicated for patients with Conn's syndrome.

Preoperative Preparation

Preoperative preparation is similar for patients with Cushing's and Conn's syndromes, addressing primarily the hypertension and electrolyte disturbances. Differences in preparatory regimens are engendered by individual differences among the patients based on the extent of disease progression and symptoms, other features that may be seen, and the site of the lesion. Only minor differences are engendered by the differing potential for intraoperative and postoperative complications inherent in the different surgical approaches that might be planned.

The anesthesiologist should first make sure that the diagnosis of the cause for Cushing's or Conn's syndrome is firmly established, through review of the history and test results and from the written consultation notes. The site of the lesion and the nature of the planned surgical procedure should also be clear. Although lack of a specific preparatory regimen appears to pose no proven problem for these patients, when adequate steroid supplementation is pro-

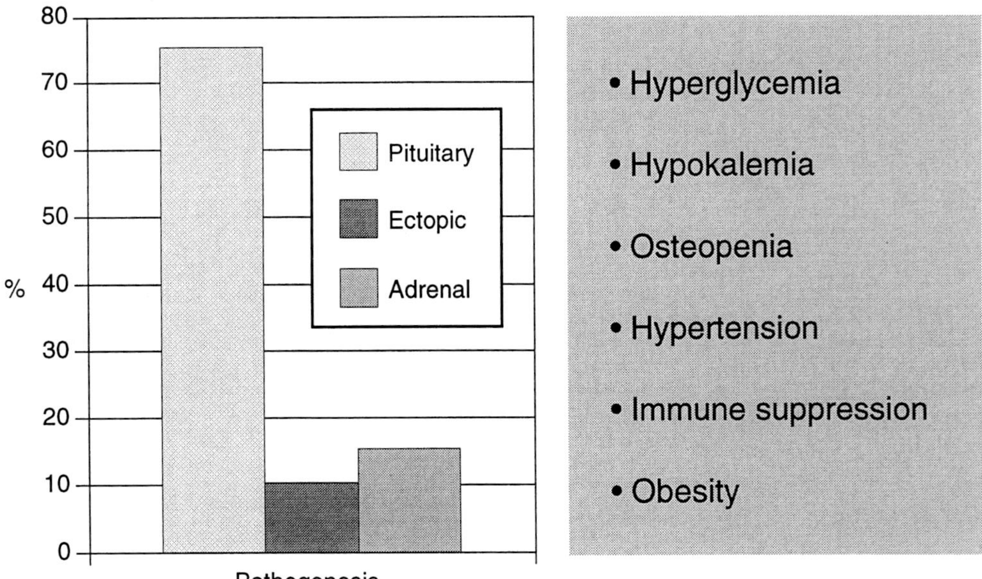

FIG. 10-1. The pathogenesis of adrenocortical Cushing's syndrome include primary pituitary and ectopic ACTH producing tumors, and adrenal tumors occurring with the frequency shown in the figure. The primary features of the syndrome are listed to the right.

vided perioperatively, the prudent anesthesiologist will attempt to optimize the patient's state before surgery with regard to three symptoms: hypertension, hypokalemia, and, for the patient with Cushing's syndrome, hyperglycemia. Furthermore, there would be some attempt to establish coronary risk, partly because patients with Cushing's syndrome of long duration are believed to have accelerated coronary atherosclerosis and partly because cardiomegaly or heart failure may develop in patients with long-standing, severe hypertension.

Carney's syndrome, a rare familial syndrome characterized by primary adrenocortical nodular disease, cardiac myxoma, pigmentation, mammary fibroadenoma, testicular tumor, and gigantism and acromegaly, has also been described (9,10). These patients have cardiac manifestations as well as Cushing's syndrome.

The risks from changed body habitus with obesity and from osteopenia associated with Cushing's syndrome also need to be considered, but as with the immune suppression inherent in the elevated glucocorticoid levels, no specific preparation is recommended.

Hyperglycemia is seen in about 66% of patients with Cushing's syndrome. It is usually mild, but 10% to 15% of patients with the syndrome become diabetic and require insulin treatment. Close observation of the blood glucose level is recommended, particularly in the postresection period when hypoglycemia may develop.

Hypertension and hypokalemia in Cushing's syndrome (11) are caused by a combination of factors, including mineralocorticoid effects of cortisol, induction of excess renin substrate resulting from hypercortisolism, increased sensitivity to beta-agonists because of cortisol, and, finally, production of other steroids from the cortex such as 18-hydroxycorticosterone and aldosterone. Hypomagnesemia may develop in both of these syndromes. It may contribute to dysrhythmia and possibly exacerbate hypertension if not corrected. In Conn's syndrome, the hypertension is primarily related to increased plasma volume and is mild to moderate in severity. In non-iatrogenic Cushing's syndrome of long-standing, by contrast, hypertension may be severe, lead to sequelae, and contribute to death. In one series of patients dying with active Cushing's syndrome, hypertension or atherosclerosis caused 40% of the deaths (12). Preoperative preparation should include attempts to control the hypertension and to replenish potassium stores. Potassium-sparing diuretics, either spironolactone or amiloride, with potassium supplements should be used.

Changed body habitus with obesity and a "buffalo hump" may occasionally pose an airway difficulty. The usual algorithms [American Society of Anesthesiologists (ASA) difficult airway algorithm] will suffice. Osteopenia, capillary fragility, skin and subcutaneous tissue friability, and poor wound healing necessitate extra care in positioning and protecting these patients perioperatively. There is a close relation between the cytokines and the hypothalamic-pituitary-adrenal axis (HPA) in the response to stimuli for the immune–inflammatory reaction in both humans and animals (13). In Cushing's syndrome, suppression of the immune response poses special difficulties in both prevention and management of infections. Care in protecting these patients from exposure to cross-infection is necessary. The relation between the cytokines and the HPA may also explain some of the symptoms from acute withdrawal of steroids and adrenal insufficiency, a potential problem for the adrenalectomized patient in the postoperative period (14).

Finally, all these patients should receive steroid supplementation for the perioperative period of stress and to prevent the withdrawal syndrome after resection of the gland (15). Several suitable regimens are in use. The equivalent of 200 to 300 mg cortisol per day is recommended for the high-stress period of 24 to 72 hours, barring prolonged stress from complications, in which case steroids may need to be continued. An appropriate tapering regimen then follows.

Adrenocortical Hypofunction

Occasionally, exploration of the adrenal must be undertaken in situations in which adrenal suppression or destruction has occurred (Table 10-3). Adrenal insufficiency arising from too little glucocorticoid or mineralocorticoid production may be present, predisposing the patient to the possibility of an adrenal crisis in response to stress. Usually, this is a postoperative complication following removal of the adrenals with inadequate or too rapid withdrawal of steroid therapy. Acute adrenal insufficiency may also arise spontaneously in association with sudden destruction of the adrenal cortex, or it may follow drug therapy with one of the inhibitors of biosynthesis of the steroids (aminoglutethimide suppressing c20-hydroxylation of cholesterol; ketoconazole inhibiting P450 side chain cleavage of hydroxylated cholesterol; trilostane inhibiting 3-β-hydroxylation of the steroid precursors; and metyrapone inhibiting 11-β-hydroxylation, with accumulation of deoxycorticosterone and 11-deoxycortisol) or with the adrenal cortical cell cytotoxic agent mitotane (15).

Adrenal suppression should be suspected in any patient receiving high-dose steroid therapy for at least 1 week during the previous 12 months. Adrenal insufficiency manifests with fever, myalgia, arthralgia, and malaise, and stress may induce a crisis with acute cardiovascular collapse (16). Classic features of Addison's disease—pigmentation, lymphocytosis, and eosinophilia with hypovolemia and hyponatremia—need not be present (17). The patient should still receive prophylactic steroid coverage for stress episodes.

Pheochromocytoma

The incidence of pheochromocytoma in the population is estimated at about four times that of primary hyperaldosteronism, a rate of 0.8 to 1.6 per 1 million population annually, or about 0.04% of all hypertensive patients, according to one survey from the Mayo Clinic (18). Patients referred to the Cleveland Clinic showed the reverse pattern, with primary hyperaldosteronism being more prevalent than pheochromocytoma (19). However, this was a selected population with a 6% rate of surgically correctable secondary hypertension. All secondary causes of hypertension cases account for about 1% of all hypertensives patients in the United States, according to many other data sources (20). Because both conditions are rare, this incidence rate remains somewhat controversial (Table 10-4).

The clinical manifestations of pheochromocytoma arise from excessive secretion of catecholamines from chromaffin tissue tumors; 10% are extraadrenal, 10% occur in children, 10% are multiple or bilateral, 10% recur after surgery, 10% are malignant, and 10% are familial. The familial types include multiple endocrine neoplasia (MEN) types 2A (Sipple's syndrome) and 2B (21); neuroectodermal dysplasias including neurofibromatosis, von Recklinghausen's disease, tuberous sclerosis, Sturge-Weber syndrome, and von Hippel-Lindau disease. Other hormones, including vasoactiveintestinal polypeptide (VIP), opioids, calcitonin, and ACTH, are also secreted by these tumors, in addition to the catecholamines (22).

Early diagnosis and localization of pheochromocytoma is important to prevent progression of the disease and early death. The

---

TABLE 10–3. *Adrenal hypofunction*

Addison's disease
Suppression
Panhypopituitarism
Hypovolemia
Hyponatremia
Addisonian crisis (hypotension, stress response)

TABLE 10–4. *Pheochromocytoma*

Adrenal, 90%
Malignant, 5%–10%
MEN 2A and B
Multiple hormones [catecholamines, VIP
    (vasoactive intestinal polypeptide), opioids,
    Calcitonin, ACTH]
Hypertension
Hypovolemia
Hyperglycemia
Hypermetabolism
MEN 2 (hypercalcemia)
Myocarditis

ACTH, adrenocorticotropic hormone; MEN, multiple endocrine neoplasia.

stepwise evaluation of patients in whom the diagnosis is suspected should proceed, based on the sensitivity and specificity of the available tests, from measurement of urinary metabolites (metanephrines and vanillylmandelic acid) and plasma catecholamines, which have moderate to low sensitivity but high specificity if positive, to either a provocative challenge with glucagon if the blood pressure is not elevated or measurement of plasma catecholamines after clonidine suppression in the face of persistent hypertension. Computed tomography, magnetic resonance imaging, or I-131-metaiodobenzylguanidine (MIBG) scanning may be used to provide anatomic localization of the tumor (23).

Emphasis on preoperative preparation is aimed at controlling hypertension and its associated hypovolemia (Table 10-5). Evaluation for myocarditis should also be carried out and may delay surgery while some recovery is allowed. Autopsy series of patients who died of active pheochromocytomas reveal that about 50% of such patients had an active myocarditis at the time of death, often with left ventricular failure and pulmonary edema (24). These changes are usually reversible with control of the hypertension. Delay of 10 to 14 days after hypertension is controlled is recommended for myocardial recovery. This regimen is untested for efficacy.

Evaluation for hypercalcemia arising from hyperparathyroid overactivity or hyperplasia, and for associated medullary thyroid carcinoma, is also necessary in patients who may have pheochromocytoma as part of the MEN syndromes. Patients from known MEN kindreds may be seen, in the future, having had prophylactic thyroidectomy in childhood (25). Screening for the RET protooncogene in these families is providing a tool for prediction of the development of medullary thyroid carcinoma in these patients (26). Hypermetabolism, weight loss, and stress-induced hyperglycemia may also be present in any patient with pheochromocytoma. These features also resolve with control of the catecholamine effects. For unknown reasons, patients with pheochromocytoma are also susceptible to development of gallstones: a 30% incidence has been reported (27). These may become a problem in the postoperative period if prolonged supportive care is needed or a critical complication develops.

Traditionally, it is held that death during surgery for pheochromocytoma is reduced by a preparatory regimen. Alpha-blockade, with later introduction of beta-blockade for persistent tachycardia, should be started about 10 to 14 days preoperatively to allow volume readjustment from the contracted state associated with the active disease and possibly for recovery from associated myocarditis. The following criteria for adequate preparation have been suggested: blood pressure (BP) less than 160/90 on two measurements in the 36 hours preceding surgery, with systolic BP decreasing more than 15% on going from the supine to the standing position but without decreasing below 80/45 after standing for 2 minutes. In addition, there should be no ST or T-wave abnormalities for the 24-hour period before surgery and premature ventricular contractions should be infrequent. Drug therapy may include (a) phenoxybenzamine alone, or with prazosin, terazosin, or doxazosin for alpha-blockade, (b) labetalol, for its combined alpha- and beta-blocking properties, as the first choice when adding a beta-blocker, although others may also be used, and (c) α-methyltyrosine to reduce the production of catecholamines by the tumor. Because of their shorter period of action and titratability, nipride (vasodilator) or phentolamine (alphablocker) may be used to control acute hypertensive crises that occur either before or during surgery. Esmolol (a short-acting beta-blocker) may be used to control ventricular dysrhythmia (28). Maintenance of serum

TABLE 10–5. *Emergencies associated with pheochromocytoma*

Hypertensive crisis
Hypotensive crisis
Cardiac dysrhythmias
Cardiac failure (myocarditis with or without acute myocardial infarction)
Hypoglycemia

magnesium in the range 2-4 mmol/L with infusions of magnesium sulfate has also been shown to reduce the dysrhythmic potential and to lower BP in patients with pheochromocytoma (29).

At the Cleveland Clinic, a more recent preparatory regimen consists of alpha-adrenergic blockade and calcium channel blockers for patients with persistent hypertension, about 50% of those with pheochromocytoma (30). These authors believe that this regimen provides equally safe conditions for their patients and that there are advantages for surgery on the nonblocked patient (31). This conclusion remains somewhat controversial.

INTRAOPERATIVE MANAGEMENT

Standard anesthetic management can be tolerated well by the properly prepared patient with any of the diseases necessitating adrenal surgery. General anesthesia and endotracheal intubation is usually preferred for all approaches to the adrenal gland. Regional and local anesthesia for obstetric or lower abdominal or extremity surgery in patients with these diseases is also very well tolerated and may be preferred for the less well prepared patient.

Monitoring

Pulse oximetry, electrocardiography, a precordial (later becoming an esophageal) stethoscope, temperature probe, and noninvasive BP monitoring should be started as the patient is placed on the operating table. End-tidal CO_2 and inspired oxygen measurement is commenced as intubation takes place. When pheochromocytoma is suspected or known to be present, invasive arterial BP monitoring should have begun before induction, because this stress may be sufficient to trigger significant hemodynamic change even in the prepared patient. Vasodilatory (nipride) and short-acting beta-blocker (esmolol) drips should be available if needed anytime the affected gland is manipulated during surgery. They must also be available when vascular

cannulation is performed by the anesthesia team.

Central venous pressure (CVP) or pulmonary artery (PA) catheter placement can occur after induction, but prior placement is preferred. Baseline hemodynamic measurements made well before induction allow evaluation of the adequacy of volume replacement and of the alpha-blocking regimen used before surgery. Magnesium sulfate administration can commence at this time, if used. CVP is recommended for any patient undergoing adrenal surgery because of the potential for massive blood loss.

We have also found it useful to have a rapid infusion system available and to use cell saver technology for these patients in the unlikely (but not unknown) eventuality of sudden, unexpected massive blood loss. During right-sided adrenalectomy, there is a heightened risk of caval or portal venous injury, which may necessitate partial or complete caval occlusion for surgical repair. To prevent severe hypotension with this intervention, rapid infusion through an upper limb or superior caval line at rates of up to 300 to 500 mL/min may be needed for 10 to 15 minutes. This infusion counteracts the decrease in venous return caused by the caval occlusion or replaces suddenly lost blood. After completion of the venous repair, phlebotomy may be needed if blood loss did not occur. Asking the surgeon to briefly occlude the aorta may also be necessary to reduce pooling in the lower extremities and splanchnic bed if the situation becomes complicated.

Transesophageal echocardiography, if available, may also be useful during surgery for pheochromocytoma to assess cardiac function and to aid in the differential diagnosis if there is hemodynamic collapse or severe instability. Air embolus, tumor embolus, and thromboembolus have been described during such procedures.

Fluids and Blood

In the anticipation of massive blood loss and third spacing, large-bore intravenous lines with access to the superior vena cava are necessary. Infusion of drugs should also be anticipated, and nipride, phentolamine, esmolol, phenylephrine, and dopamine should be at hand. Fluids should be adequately warmed. In addition, means for surface warming of the patient and a head cover should be used to conserve the patient's body heat. Acid-base balance should be maintained and blood gas analyses performed as indicated.

Induction and Maintenance

In the patient with pheochromocytoma, one should avoid using any agent that might cause histamine release or directly trigger activation of the tumor. Many combinations of drugs have been used, and there are several safe choices (32). Combined epidural and general anesthesia can be safely tailored to the needs of these patients. This combination has also been used to provide pain relief in the postoperative period, with infusion of narcotics or local anesthetics through the catheter after emergence from general anesthesia (33). One should anticipate swings in BP (34), dysrhythmia, and the usual surgical complications, and prepare to deal with them if they should arise.

POSTOPERATIVE CARE

Emergence and Postoperative Care

If the patient has shown hemodynamic instability, is hypothermic (temperature less than 34°C), or continues to have a large third-space fluid replacement requirement in the postoperative period, intensive care unit (ICU) admission and management should be considered. Because the incidence of pneumothorax has been reported to be as high as 20%, a chest radiograph is recommended on return to the recovery area or the ICU, even in the absence of signs or symptoms. Blood glucose levels should be carefully monitored throughout the operative and postoperative periods. Action should be taken as indicated

by these values, noting that either increased or decreased values many be seen at various stages of the procedure (35).

Complications

Surgical mortality rate with adrenal resection is on the order of 1% to 3% for unilateral adrenalectomy in the prepared patient with pheochromocytoma. With Cushing's syndrome necessitating bilateral adrenalectomy, a 5% to 10% mortality rate has been reported, with a high incidence of perioperative complications, and the majority of deaths occurring in the postoperative period. A 10% or higher rate of mortality has been noted for the unprepared patient with unsuspected pheochromocytoma (36).

Roizen and colleagues (37) report a 100% incidence of salvos of ventricular tachycardia in a series of 22 patients undergoing pheochromocytoma resection and a high incidence of other ventricular dysrhythmia. About 50% of these patient had high levels of catecholamine for 1 to 3 days after surgery, with persistent hypertension. James (29) noted that none of the patients in his series of 16 patients with sustained elevations of magnesium demonstrated dysrhythmias. This demands prospective testing.

Hemodynamic instability is most common in patients with pheochromocytoma. Profound hypotension, necessitating the use of fluids and vasopressors, frequently occurs intraoperatively, particularly following adrenalectomy. Massive blood loss is seen in only a few patients undergoing adrenal resection. Air embolus and tumor embolus have also been reported.

Long-term survival varies with the natural history of the underlying disease. However, the prognosis for cure and for control of BP in patients undergoing resection of an adrenal tumor producing either aldosterone or catecholamine is very good. Patients with malignant pheochromocytoma had a 44% 5-year survival rate in one series from the Mayo Clinic (36). Survival rates of more than 95% for 5 years, with recurrence rates less than

10% have been reported for benign pheochromocytoma. A recent report of survival after surgical management of extraadrenal pheochromocytoma of the heart from two centers, noted a 24% mortality rate from reconstruction of the native heart after curative resection of the tumor (38). These authors suggest that cardiac transplantation may be an option for these patients, and they report one case with a good outcome.

About 95% of patients who have resection of an aldosterone-producing adenoma become normotensive and normokalemic 3 to 6 months after surgery. However, hypertension redevelops in 20% to 25% over the ensuing 2 to 3 years. Bilateral adrenal hyperplasia carries a less satisfactory prognosis for correction of the hypertension after resection. Only 15% of patients become normotensive after bilateral adrenalectomy for hyperplasia. Surgery for idiopathic hyperaldosteronism with bilateral hyperplasia is therefore performed only to treat symptomatic hypokalemia that does not respond to medical therapy.

Recent introduction of laparoscopic techniques to adrenal surgery allows removal of adrenal tissue with less postoperative pain and more rapid recovery (39). The published series since 1992 currently exceeds 162 cases and includes pheochromocytomas. Intraoperative fluctuations in BP during removal of pheochromocytoma are reported to be similar whether the laparoscopic or surgical technique is used.

A major risk exists for the pregnant patient with an unsuspected pheochromocytoma, because, in this population, the diagnosis is frequently missed. The hypertension responds to all the standard treatments for preeclampsia, including magnesium, but the stress of delivery may cause a crisis. There is a risk of both maternal and fetal mortality. As Weiss reports (40), Schenker and others reviewed outcomes from pheochromocytoma detected during pregnancy first in 1971, and again in 1982 after the introduction of alpha- and beta-blockers to therapy. Maternal mortality rate decreased from 18% to 10.6%, but fetal

mortality rate remained high, 50% and 46%, respectively, before and after these new therapies were in use. This population deserves close attention.

SUMMARY POINTS

1. The safety of the patient undergoing adrenal surgery depends on adequate diagnosis and preparation for the endocrine dysfunction, with anticipation of the possible surgical complications that may occur.
2. The major risk is undiagnosed pheochromocytoma, particularly in the pregnant patient; in these cases, fetal mortality rate is still close to 50% and maternal mortality rate is close to 10%.
3. The anesthesiologist is responsible and accountable as a team member for pharmacologic management of endocrine dysfunction in the perioperative period, and for detecting and treating complications as they occur. This demands full knowledge of the pathogenesis and pathophysiology of the endocrinopathies, as well as knowledge of the complete range of perioperative management skills. One must anticipate the risk of venous injury, of diaphragmatic involvement or injury during adrenal surgery, in addition to the usual range of hemodynamic and other risks in these patients.

REFERENCES

1. Christopherson R. Anesthesia for endocrine surgery. In: Rogers MC, Tinker JH, Covino BG, et al, eds. *Principles and practice of anesthesiology.* St. Louis: Mosby-Year Book, 1993:2035.
2. Sieber FE. Evaluation of the patient with endocrine disease and diabetic mellitus. In: Rogers MC, Tinker JH, Covino BG, et al, eds. *Principles and practice of anesthesiology.* St. Louis: Mosby-Year Book, 1993:278.
3. Roizen MF. Diseases of the endocrine system. In: Katz J, Benumof JL, Kadis LB, eds: *Anesthesia and uncommon diseases,* 3rd ed. Philadelphia: WB Saunders, 1990:245.
4. Cushing HW. The basophil adenomas of the pituitary body and their manifestations (pituitary basophilism). *Bull Johns Hopkins Hosp* 1932;50:137–195.
5. Conn JW. Primary aldosteronism: a new clinical syndrome. *J Lab Clin Med* 1955;45:3–17.

6. Conn JW. Aldosteronism and hypertension. *Arch Intern Med* 1961;107:813.

7. Conn JW. Aldosteronism in man. *JAMA* 1963;183:775.

8. Abdelhamid S, Müller-Lobeck H, Phal S, et al. Prevalence of adrenal and extraadrenal Conn syndrome in hypertensive patients. *Arch Intern Med* 1996;156:1190–1195.

9. Carney JA, Gordon H, Carpenter PC, et al. The complex of myxomas, spotty pigmentation, and endocrine overactivity. *Medicine (Balt)* 1985;64:270–283.

10. Danoff A, Jormak S, Lorber P, et al. Adrenocortical micronodular dysplasia cardiac myxomas, lentigenes, and spindle cell tumors: reports of a kindred. *Arch Intern Med* 1987;147:443–448.

11. Abboud CF, Giuliani ER. Endocrines and the heart. In: Giuliani ER, Fuster V, Gersh BJ, et al, eds. *Cardiology: fundamentals and practice*, 2nd ed. St. Louis: Mosby, 1991:2087.

12. Plotz CM, Knowlton AI, Ragan C. The natural history of Cushing's syndrome. *Am J Med* 1952;13:597–614.

13. Chrousos GP. Hypothalamic-pituitary-adrenal axis and immune-mediated inflammation. *N Engl J Med* 1995;332:1351–1362.

14. Papanicolaou DA, Tsigos C, Oldfield EH, et al. Acute glucocorticoid deficiency is associated with plasma elevations of interleukin 6: does the latter participate in the symptomatology of the steroid withdrawal syndrome and adrenal insufficiency? *J Clin Endocrinol Metab* 1996;81:2303–2306.

15. Schimmer BP, Parker KL. Adrenocorticotrophic hormone; adrenocortical steroids and their synthetic analogs; inhibitors of the synthesis and actions of adrenocortical hormones. In: Hardman JG, Limbird LE, eds. *The pharmacological basis of therapeutics,* 9th ed. New York: McGraw-Hill, 1996;1459.

16. Engquist A, Backer OG, Jarnum S. Incidence of postoperative complications in patients subjected to surgery under steroid cover. *Acta Chir Scand* 1974;140:343–346.

17. Guttman PH. Addison's disease. *Arch Pathol* 1930;10:742.

18. Tucker RM, Labartue DR. Frequency of surgical treatment for hypertension in adults at the Mayo Clinic from 1973 through 1975. *Mayo Clin Proc* 1977;52:549–555.

19. Gifford RW. Evaluation of the hypertensive patient with emphasis on detecting curable causes. *Milbank Mem Fund Q* 1969;37:170–186.

20. Zachariah PK, Osmundson PJ. Cardiovascular manifestations of hypertension. In: Giuliani ER, Fuster V, Gersh BJ, et al, eds: *Cardiology: fundamentals and practice*, 2nd ed. St. Louis: Mosby, 1991:2003.

21. Sipple JH. The association of pheochromocytoma with carcinoma of the thyroid gland. *Am J Med* 1961;31:163.

22. Benowitz NL. Pheochromocytoma. *Adv Intern Med* 1990;35:195–219.

23. Bravo EL, Gifford RW. Current concepts—pheochromocytoma: diagnosis, localization, and management. *N Engl J Med* 1984;311:1298–1303.

24. Sjoerdsma A, Englemann K, Waldmann TA, et al. Pheochromocytoma: current concepts of diagnosis and treatment, combined clinical staff conferences at the NIH. *Ann Intern Med* 1966;65:1302–1326.

25. Wells SA, Chi DD, Toshima K, et al. Predictive DNA testing and prophylactic thyroidectomy in patients at risk for multiple endocrine neoplasia type 2A. *Ann Surg* 1994;220:237–250.

26. Wohlk N, Cote GJ, Evans DB, et al. Application of genetic screening information to the management of medullary thyroid carcinoma and multiple endocrine neoplasia type 2. *Endocrinol Metab Clin North Am* 1996;25:1–25.

27. Gifford RW, Kvale WF, Maher FT, et al. Clinical features, diagnosis and treatment of pheochromocytoma: a review of 76 cases. *Mayo Clin Proc* 1964;39:281.

28. Nicholas E, Deutschman CS, Allo M, et al. Use of esmolol in the intraoperative management of pheochromocytoma. *Anesth Analg* 1988;67:1114–1117.

29. James MFM. Use of magnesium sulphate in the anaesthetic management of phaeochromocytoma: a review of 17 anaesthetics. *Br J Anaesth* 1989;62:616–623.

30. Boutros AR, Bravo EL, Zanettin G, et al. Perioperative management of 63 patients with pheochromocytoma. *Cleve Clin J Med* 1990;57:613–617.

31. Gifford RW, Manger WM, Bravo EL. Pheochromocytoma. *Endocrinol Metab Clin North Am* 1994;23:387–404.

32. Berman ML. Anesthetic management of pheochromocytoma. In: Scott: *Surgery of the adrenal gland.* Philadelphia: Lippincott, 1989:233–240.

33. Cousins MJ, Rubin RB. The intraoperative management of pheochromocytoma with total epidural sympathetic blockade. *Br J Anaesth* 1974;46:78–81.

34. Roizen MF, Hunt TK, Beaupre PN, et al. The effect of alpha-adrenergic blockade on cardiac performance and tissue oxygen delivery during excision of pheochromocytoma. *Surgery* 1983;94:941–945.

35. Chambers S, Espiner EA, Donald RA, et al. Hypoglycemia following removal of pheochromocytoma: case report and review of the literature. *Postgrad Med J* 1982;58:503–506.

36. Van Heerden JA, Sheps SG, Hamberger B, et al. Pheochromocytoma: current status and changing trends. *Surgery* 1982; 91:367–373.

37. Roizen MF, Horrigan R, Koike M, et al. A prospective randomized trial of four anesthetic techniques for resection of pheochromocytoma. *Anesthesiology* 1982;57:A43.

38. Jeevanandam V, Oz MC, Shapiro B, et al. Surgical management of cardiac pheochromocytoma: resection versus transplantation. *Ann Surg* 1995;221:415–419.

39. Weisnagel SJ, Gagner M, Breton G, et al. Laparoscopic adrenalectomy. *Endocrinologist* 1996;6:169–178.

40. Weiss JA. Nongynecologic surgery during pregnancy. In: Norris MC, ed. *Obstetric anesthesia.* Philadelphia: JB Lippincott, 1993:201.

*Medical and Surgical Management of
Adrenal Diseases,* edited by Joseph C. Cerny.
Lippincott Williams & Wilkins, Philadelphia © 1999.

11

Pheochromocytoma

Robert A. Bonzani and *Norman W. Thompson

Department of Urology, Henry Ford Hospital, Detroit, Michigan 48202;
**Department of Endocrine Surgery, University of Michigan Medical Center, Ann Arbor, Michigan 48109*

Pheochromocytoma is a clinical entity that continues to fascinate the medical and surgical community. It is a rare endocrine neoplasm, which, if untreated, is most often fatal, but, if diagnosed, can be safely excised in 90% of cases (1).

Pheochromocytomas are catecholamine-producing tumors arising from cells within the sympathetic nervous system; they are predominantly located within the adrenal gland, although they may appear anywhere along the sympathetic chain, from the base of the skull to the urinary bladder.

Pheochromocytoma can occur at any age, from infancy to old age, being quite uncommon after age 60. They account for only 0.1% to 0.2% of all cases of diastolic hypertension (2), and they have an incidence of 0.005% to 0.1% in the general, unscreened population (3). The etiology of pheochromocytoma is unknown, although chromosomal deletions and point mutations have been identified in both the sporadic and familial forms of the disease (4).

EMBRYOLOGY

Pheochromocytomas arise from chromaffin cells, which are of neuroectodermal origin. At about the fourth week of gestation, this neuroectodermal tissue separates away from the adjacent, newly formed neural tube. It eventually becomes positioned between this neural tube and the true ectoderm. This tissue is then neural crest, and cells from this crest begin migrating throughout the developing embryo, ultimately differentiating into the peripheral sympathetic nervous system, paraganglionic system, and adrenal medulla.

These embryologic relationships help one better understand the coexistence of other diseases, such as von Hippel-Lindau disease, with pheochromocytoma; affected tissues in these disorders are derived from adjacent neuroectodermal areas.

PATHOPHYSIOLOGY

Synthesis of norepinephrine begins in the cytoplasm of the cells (Fig. 11-1).This metabolic pathway continues until the compound dopamine forms and is then taken up by intracellular granules and converted to norepinephrine by the enzyme dopamine β-hydroxylase. Granular concentration of norepinephrine establishes an equilibrium with free norepinephrine that freely diffuses into the cytoplasm of the cell; free norepinephrine can be converted into epinephrine via the action of phenylethanolamine n-methyl transferase. This newly formed epinephrine can be readily stored in separate intracellular granules within the cell.

Epinephrine constitutes 85% of the catecholamine component of the adrenal medulla, and, in adults, represents the sole source of epinephrine in the body. This has important clinical significance: an epinephrine-producing tumor, in adults, is invariably localized within the adrenal medulla (5). Ep-

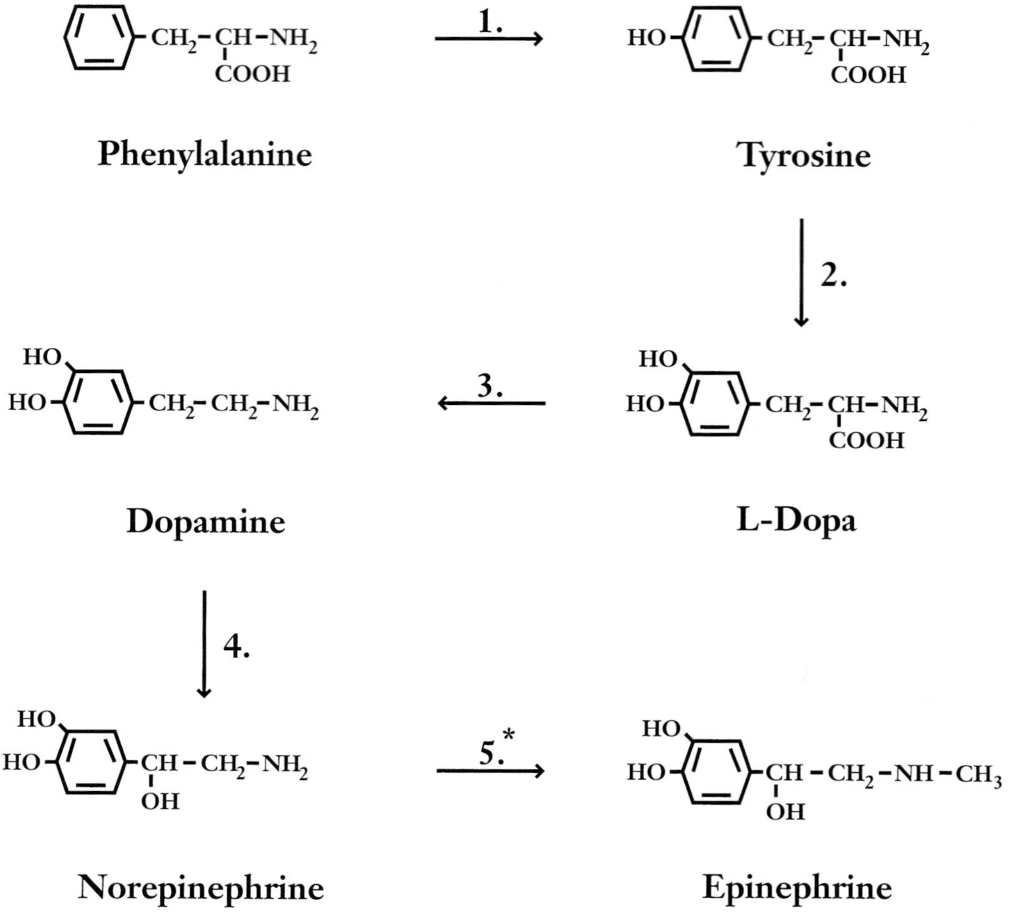

Phenylalanine   1. →   **Tyrosine**

2.

Dopamine   ← 3.   **L-Dopa**

4.

Norepinephrine   5.* →   **Epinephrine**

1. Phenylalanine hydroxylase
2. Tyrosine hydroxylase
3. Dopa decarboxylase
4. Dopamine β-hydroxlase
5. Phenylethanolamine n-methyl transferase
*** this enzymatic reaction occurs exclusively in the adrenal medulla**

FIG. 11-1. Major steps in the synthesis of the catecholamines norephinephrine and epinephrine. Enzymes are numbered and identified. (Modified from Coupland RE. *The Natural History of the Chromaffin Cell.* London: Longman S. Green, 1965;192–194.)

inephrine, four to six times more potent than norepinephrine, displays alpha activity, through the action of peripheral vasoconstriction, and beta activity, via vasodilation (to a lesser degree than vasoconstriction) (5).

In addition, tachycardia and inotropism occur as a result of the beta-receptor status of the heart.

Norepinephrine has predominantly alpha-agonist activity, promoting marked peripheral vasoconstriction and reflex bradycardia as its chief effects.

Pheochromocytoma may secrete norepinephrine, epinephrine, or both. They may be secreted continuously, resulting in sustained hypertension, or they may be released intermittently, yielding paroxysmal hypertensive episodes. The reason for these variations is not clear. They have also been well documented to secrete a variety of other substances, including calcitonin, vasoactive intestinal peptide (VIP), neuropeptide Y, dopamine, serotonin, parathyroid-like hormone, and adrenocorticotropic hormone (ACTH) (6,7).

Twenty-one cases of ACTH-secreting pheochromocytomas are reported in the world literature, 20 of which were benign (8).

Grossly, pheochromocytomas vary in size from microscopic foci to 30 cm in diameter, averaging approximately 5 cm in length. Macroscopic tumor can weigh as little as 2 g or as much as 4 kg, with 70% weighing less than 70 g. Smaller tumors (<5 g) tend to store catecholamines poorly, releasing large amounts of biologically active norepinephrine and epinephrine into the plasma. Because of this, smaller tumors tend to exhibit more severe signs and symptoms, and are diagnosed earlier than larger tumors, which bind and store catecholamine well. Norepinephrine and epinephrine are metabolized and broken down within larger tumors; thus, in contrast to smaller pheochromocytomas, they yield lower plasma and urinary catecholamine metabolites, and they present later because of their less severe symptoms (5).

On gross appearance, pheochromocytoma appears lobulated because trabeculated fibrous tissue projects inward from its capsule. Cut section reveals a gray to pink-tan color, with areas of hemorrhage and necrosis frequently present in larger tumors. Cystic areas may be on the capsular surface.

Microscopically, tumor cells closely resemble normal adrenal medulla. They are arranged in alveolar-shaped clusters, separated by endothelial-lined spaces. Numerous vessels are present, reflecting the abundant vascularity of these tumors. Tumor cell cytoplasm may be granular, basophilic, or eosinophilic. Nuclei are round or oval, with prominent nucleoli. Mitotic figures are scarce. Nuclear gigantism and hyperchromatasia are seen but are not indicators of malignancy. As a rule, histologic appearance alone cannot distinguish between benign and malignant tumors (9). Additionally, capsular or vascular invasion does not imply malignancy; these findings have been seen in benign pheochromocytomas (10). Currently, the only definitive criterion for malignancy is the spread of the tumor to distant sites: lymph nodes, bone, lung, liver, brain, and the central nervous system are the most common sites.

Because histologic examination cannot diagnose malignancy, some investigators have tried to identify any prognostic factors that may imply a malignant course. Tumor size and local tumor extension at the time of surgical exploration have been suggested, as has DNA ploidy. In a study of 184 pheochromocytoma patients by Nativ and colleagues, 84% of those with vascular endothelial invasion and 100% of patients with regional or distant metastases had either aneuploid or tetraploid DNA content. All 12 patients dying of their disease had abnormal DNA ploidy, whereas no patient with diploid DNA died (11).

Even though this strongly suggests that DNA ploidy testing can be an important prognostic variable in delineating benign from malignant pheochromocytoma, other recent studies cast some doubt on the reproducibility of these findings (12).

INCIDENCE AND CHARACTERISTICS

Pheochromocytomas occur at a rate of about 1 in 1,000,000 to 1 in 50,000 persons per year and about 1 in 1,000 hypertensive individuals (3). Peak incidence of pheochromocytomas occur during the fourth and fifth decades of life, although age ranges from 5 months to 82 years. One review cites a slight female predilection (13); others show no difference in incidence (5). Additionally, another study has shown a slightly more common incidence in the right adrenal gland (14), whereas others cite equal incidence rates (15,16).

TABLE 11–1. *Pheochromocytoma characteristics and distribution*

	Adrenal location (%)	Extraadrenal location (%)	Multiple tumors (%)	Malignant tumors (%)	Bilateral tumors (%)
Stenström et al. (24)	78	22	—	—	—
Hartley et al. (25)	89	11	11	7	—
St. John Sutton et al. (26)	91	9	19	11	10
Gifford et al. (27)	90	10	—	—	—
Samaan et al. (21)	85–95	5–15	—	—	—
Stein et al. (23)	85–95	5–15	—	—	10
Neuman et al. (28)	84	16	8	11	—
Proye et al. (29)	86.5	13.5	—	15.5	9.4
Chong et al. (20)	—	9.8	7	13.4	4.4
Whalen et al. (31)	—	18	—	—	—

Traditionally, pheochromocytomas have been described by the rule of tens: 10% bilateral, 10% extraadrenal, 10% familial, 10% metastatic, 10% malignant, and 10% pediatric. This description has held up fairly well over time. Numerous studies have found that sporadic pheochromocytoma occurs in the adrenal medulla 78% to 95% of the time (Table 11-1) (14,16–22). Multifocality is seen in 7% to 19% of these pheochromocytomas (13,17,18,21), whereas the incidence of bilaterality ranges from 4.4% to 9.4% (13,16, 19,22,23). The percentage of malignant pheochromocytomas varies from 7% to 15.5% (13,18,19,21,22).

EXTRAADRENAL PHEOCHROMOCYTOMA

Traditionally, 10% of all pheochromocytomas were believed to lie outside the adrenal medulla. A recent review by Whalen and colleagues summarized the literature to date and reported the incidence to be 18% (24). Eighty-five percent of extraadrenal pheochromocytomas are infradiaphragmatic; 98% of all pheochromocytomas lie below the diaphragm, with 1% residing in the cervical region and the remaining 1% being located intrathoracically (24). To better delineate the nature and location of these extraadrenal tumors, the term *paraganglion system* was developed as a replacement for the term *pheochromocytoma*. It is defined as a widely dispersed collection of specialized neural crest cells, arising in association with the segmental or collateral autonomic ganglia, that migrate to one of three final destinations:

1. Adjacent to arterial vessels and cranial nerves of the head and neck
2. Alongside the sympathetic plexus and chains, extending from the neck to the pelvis
3. Adrenal medulla

Thus, these extraadrenal tumors can occur anywhere along the sympathetic nervous system (Fig. 11-2). Certain variants are specifically named. A *chemodectoma* arises from paraganglia of the carotid body. A *glomus jugulare* tumor has its origins in paraganglia of the intracranial branches of the ninth and tenth cranial nerves. *Ganglioneuromas* arise from postganglionic sympathetic neurons. All extraadrenal chromaffin tissues behave similarly to those within the adrenal medulla. Even though trends are emerging to support use of these anatomic descriptions, the label of "pheochromocytoma" is still very much ingrained into the medical literature, and because of its universal recognition, it is used here to apply to all variants of these neural crest tumors.

Unlike adrenal pheochromocytomas, extraadrenal tumors usually present in the second and third decades of life. They are usually less than 5 cm in diameter and weigh 20 to 40 g (2). They are further characterized by an

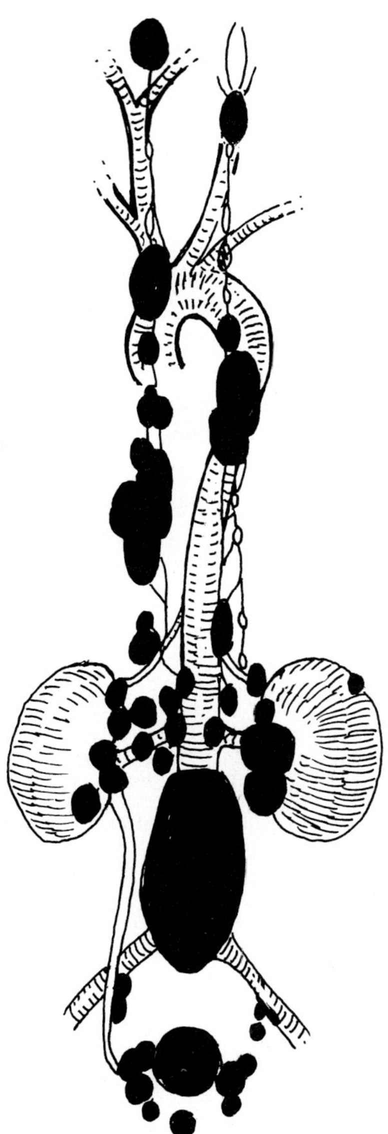

FIG. 11-2. Distribution of extraadrenal pheochromocytoma along the sympathetic axis. Approximately 1% are in the cervical region; 1% lie intrathoracically.

aberrant, large blood supply. They are also two to three times more likely to be malignant than adrenal pheochromocytomas (13,23). Certain extraadrenal variants warrant special mention.

The most common location for an extraadrenal pheochromocytoma is in the organ of Zuckerkandl. This structure consists of small collections of paraganglionic tissue adjacent to the aorta between the root of the inferior mesenteric artery and the aortic bifurcation. Tumors in children arising from the organ of Zuckerkandl may secrete epinephrine, the only instance of an extraadrenal site producing epinephrine (5). They may become large enough to compress adjacent vascular and genitourinary structures, making subsequent resection difficult.

Two other sites where extraadrenal pheochromocytomas are most frequently located are the perihilar renal regions and in the groove between the aorta and inferior vena cava, at the level of the left renal vein.

Pheochromocytoma of the urinary bladder can produce severe hypertensive paroxysms, both during and after micturition (25). Changes in bladder wall tension during filling and voiding are responsible for these attacks. Painless hematuria is present in half of cases, and 80% can be visualized on cystoscopy (but only after appropriate alpha-adrenergic blockade (24).

SIGNS AND SYMPTOMS

The clinical presentation of pheochromocytoma is attributable to the physiologic effects of its circulating catecholamines. The predominant sign is hypertension. Half of cases yield sustained hypertension, whereas approximately 45% of patients experience paroxysms of high blood pressure. The remaining 5% are normotensive. It is highly unusual to correctly diagnose pheochromocytoma in the absence of hypertension, except in multiple endocrine neoplasia II (MEN II) family members at known risk, who have biochemical screening performed. Hypotension can occur, and some patients may even alternate between hypertensive and hypotensive episodes.

Another important diagnostic clue in the evaluation for pheochromocytoma is postural hypotension. When seen in a hypertensive patient *not* on hypertensive medication, it raises strong clinical suspicion for the presence of pheochromocytoma. Probable mechanisms for this include autonomic insensitivity, resulting from excessive circulating catecholamines, and hypovolemia. Postural hypotension is more common in sustained hypertension.

The classic pheochromocytoma paroxysmal "spell" yields the most striking constellation of symptoms. The typical triad consists of headache, excessive sweating or diaphoresis, and palpitations (Table 11-2) (2,26,27). Headache is by far the most common symptom in pheochromocytoma, occurring in 92% of paroxysmal patients and 72% of those with stable hypertension (2). The headache is usually characterized as severe, throbbing, and bilateral, lasting minutes to days. It may resemble tension headache. Diaphoresis can be present even in the absence of paroxysmal blood pressure elevations, and the palpitations experienced may coexist with tachycardia.

The frequency of these attacks varies from every few minutes to every few months, occurring weekly in 75% of patients. The tendency is for the episodes to increase in frequency as time progresses. Attacks last several seconds to several hours. A paroxysm can result in a blood pressure as high as 300/200 mm Hg, and be associated with fatigue and exhaustion as the attack subsides—80% resolve within 1 hour.

Many other signs and symptoms exist with pheochromocytoma and are cited in Table 11-2. Hyperglycemia is seen commonly. In patients with preexisting diabetes mellitus, impaired glucoregulation develops, sometimes presenting with diabetic ketoacidosis. This impaired glucose metabolism may be due to beta-adrenergic receptor desensitization as a modulator of insulin resistance (28). Hypoglycemia frequently develops in the immediate postoperative period, requiring intravenous glucose infusion for the initial 12 to 24 hours.

Hypercalcemia is noted, even in the absence of the MEN syndromes, which resolves after surgical resection of the tumor. In most cases, this is apparently related to the secretion of parathyroid-related peptide, which does not cross-react with any of the parathyroid hormone (PTH) assays currently used. Thus, PTH levels will be suppressed if measured.

Nausea and vomiting may occur, especially in conjunction with severe headache. Weakness and weight loss are present, despite a normal or increased appetite. Chest or abdominal pain may mimic coronary artery disease or an acute abdomen. Excessive catecholamines decrease intestinal mobility and

TABLE 11–2. *Symptom frequency in pheochromocytoma (%)*

	Manger			
	Paroxysmal	Persistent	Thomas	Hume
Headache	92	72	80	80
Excessive sweating	65	69	71	70
Palpitations	73	51	64	60
Anxiety, nervousness, and panic	60	28	22	60
Tremulousness	51	26	31	40
Nausea	43	26	42	30
Pallor	—	—	42	40
Weakness	38	15	28	25
Weight Loss	14	15	—	15
Dyspnea	11	18	19	—
Heat intolerance and flushing	13	15	18	—
Visual disturbances	3	21	11	—
Dizziness	11	3	8	—
Constipation	0	13	—	—
Paresthesias	11	0	11	—
Bradycardia	8	3	3	—
Grand mal seizures	5	3	5	—

From refs. 2, 34, and 35 with permission.

result in severe constipation, whereas the rare VIP-secreting tumor predisposes the patient to diarrhea.

These paroxysmal "spells" are elicited by multiple stimuli, including pain, tumor manipulation (such as an abdominal examination), exercise, anxiety, bladder distention or voiding (in the case of bladder pheochromocytomas), constipation, trauma, sexual intercourse, diagnostic procedures, radiographic contrast media, surgery, and anesthesia.

Additionally, certain foods, for example, tyramine-containing cheeses, beer, and wine, as well as medications, such as phenothiazines, tricyclic antidepressants, ACTH, histamine, glucagon, beta-blockers, metoclopramide, nicotine, angiotensin II analogues, and epinephrine, can all promote an attack.

Despite the striking presentation that a pheochromocytoma may elicit, the lag period between onset of symptoms and definitive diagnosis averages 4.5 years (29). This may be partially explained by the fact that clinical features may diminish in intensity over time, as adrenoreceptors downregulate in response to overstimulation by catecholamines, but it is also due to a low index of suspicion. Because of the rarity of the disease, it often is not entertained on a list of differential diagnoses, which typically includes essential hypertension, hyperthyroidism, psychosomatic illness, brain tumors, angina, migraine headaches, and diabetes mellitus. As a result, the tumor may ultimately manifest itself via an acute abdomen or cardiovascular collapse as the tumor begins to hemorrhage. Morbid events that may occur from unabated, undiagnosed catecholamine secretion include myocardial infarction, congestive heart failure, cerebrovascular accident, aortic dissection, or even death. To avoid these devastating sequelae, a high degree of suspicion must exist. The following conditions should prompt the physician to screen for the presence of pheochromocytoma:

1. Resistance to hypertensive therapy
2. Young individuals with new-onset hypertension

3. Paradoxical blood pressure elevations during beta-blocker guanethidine or ganglionic blocker treatment
4. Hypertension and new or worsening diabetes mellitus
5. Hypertensive crisis after anesthesia, surgery, or medication administration
6. Hypertension developing during pregnancy
7. Patient has family member with pheochromocytoma or MEN syndrome

Children

Ten to twenty percent of all patients with pheochromocytomas are children. These tumors display some different characteristics than those of adults. Roughly two-thirds of the pediatric pheochromocytoma population are prepubertal boys; the tumors have a much higher likelihood of being multiple (32%), bilateral (24%), and extraadrenal (15%–31%) than in adults (30). Malignancy is less common and, when present, more likely to be in an extraadrenal location.

Hypertension is much more likely to be sustained (31). Paroxysmal hypertension accounts for less than 10% of pediatric cases (2). Symptoms in children are also different. The classic triad in children includes headache, diaphoresis, and nausea rather than palpitations. Half of the children have visual complaints, with eyeground changes seen in 70%. Polyuria and polydipsia are often present as well. Twenty-five percent of children display convulsive seizures, and puffy, red, or cyanotic hands develop in up to 11% (2).

ASSOCIATED SYNDROMES

Up to 10% of pheochromocytomas are familial, inherited by itself, as part of a MEN syndrome, or in association with a neuroectodermal dysplasia (1). Familial transmission is thought to be autosomal dominant, with varying degrees of penetrance (32).

Simple familial pheochromocytomas usually present by age 20 years, are more likely to be benign than sporadic tumors, and have a much higher incidence of bilaterality—50% (16,19).

MEN syndromes were first described in 1961, when Sipple characterized a syndrome of concomitant pheochromocytoma and medullary carcinoma of the thyroid (33). This was later renamed as multiple endocrine neoplasia (MEN) type IIA, with the addition of parathyroid adenoma. In 100% of patients in families with the MEN IIA allele, medullary carcinoma of the thyroid develops; in 33%, pheochromocytoma is diagnosed (bilaterally in the majority), and 34% become hyperparathyroid (34).

MEN IIB includes pheochromocytoma, medullary carcinoma of the thyroid, and an additional complex of multiple mucosal neuromas centered around the lips, tongue, and buccal mucosa; neuromas located submucosally in the autonomic plexus of the bowel; thickened corneal nerves; and a marfanoid body habitus. Two large epidemiologic studies of MEN II families revealed the incidence of bilaterality to be 51% to 68%, and the risk of malignancy to be 3% to 4% (35,36). Extraadrenal sites were present in 4% (35), and 64% of deaths in these families were directly attributable to the pheochromocytoma (36). The diagnosis of medullary carcinoma of the thyroid usually precedes that of pheochromocytoma (29).

Other studies of MEN II families have shown genetic abnormalities. Eight of 10 MEN II kindreds were shown to have a point mutation of the RET protooncogene in chromosome 10, near its centromere, whereas the remaining two families were found to have mutations in the von Hippel-Lindau gene, present on chromosome 3 (37).

These MEN II–associated pheochromocytomas tend to secrete substantially more epinephrine than norepinephrine. Thus, with the current management of screening MEN II family members at risk after undergoing mutational analysis, an elevated urinary epinephrine level may be the only abnormality suggesting the tumor in an asymptomatic patient.

The neuroectodermal dysplasias are also associated with pheochromocytoma. Von Recklinghausen's disease, or neurofibromatosis, has one of the strongest relationships. The disease is characterized by multiple neurofibromas of peripheral nerves, presenting as subcutaneous or intradermal nodules. Other features include vascular and hairy nevi, cutaneous polyps, and café au lait spots. The prevalence of pheochromocytoma in patients with von Recklinghausen's disease is 1% to 2%. Conversely, 5% of pheochromocytoma patients have neurofibromatosis.

Von Hippel-Lindau disease consists of angiomatous malformations of the retina, cystic cerebellar hemangioblastomas, and, less commonly, spinal cord hemangioblastomas. Although classically less frequently associated with pheochromocytoma than neurofibromatosis, one series screened for pheochromocytoma and found 19% of patients to have von Hippel-Lindau disease (38).

Other neuroectodermal dysplasia linked to pheochromocytoma include Sturge-Weber syndrome, consisting of familial hemangiomas, angiomatous brain malformations, and seizures, and tuberous sclerosis, a triad of mental deficiency, epileptiform seizures, and multiple adenoma sebaceum.

LABORATORY DIAGNOSIS

Biochemical confirmation of pheochromocytoma is crucial before proceeding to definitive treatment, and the cornerstone of diagnosis remains the measurement of 24-hour urinary catecholamine levels.

Major substances that are currently used for pheochromocytoma detection include plasma catecholamine, urinary free catecholamine, urinary metanephrine, and normetanephrine, as well as urinary vanillylmandelic acid (VMA) levels. Metanephrine and VMA represent two of the main metabolites of norepinephrine and epinephrine (Fig. 11-3). Newer substance assays (chromogranin A, neuron-specific enolase, platelet catecholamines, neuropeptide Y) are still in the experimental stages; older assays for HMMA (4-hydroxy-3-methoxy-mandelic acid) have

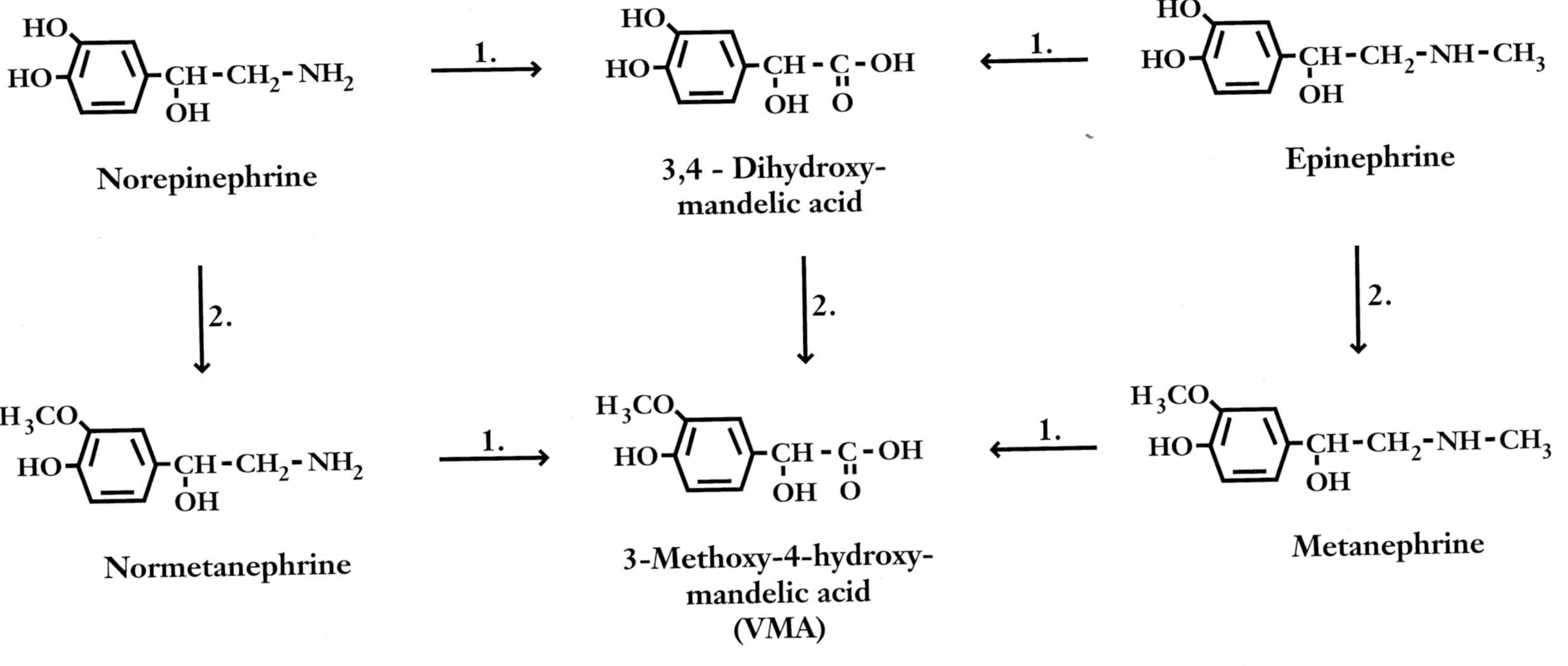

FIG. 11-3. Catecholamine degradation and metabolite formation. Enzymes are numbered and identified.

poor sensitivity and should be abandoned (39). Additionally, the measurement of plasma metanephrines has been advocated, although this test has not been widely adopted (40).

The usefulness of these assays arises from the fact that 95% to 99% of patients with pheochromocytoma have elevated levels of catecholamines in their blood or urine (41). Which assay is performed depends on availability and personal preference, although several recent studies have clearly demonstrated the superiority of urinary metanephrine levels (Table 11-3) (42,43). Peplinski and Norton report a sensitivity of 100%, and positive and negative predictive values of 83% and 100%, respectively (42). Plasma catecholamine levels serve as a very good adjunctive test. However, false-negative findings can be seen in up to 30% of patients. Probable explanations for this are that this assay is a "spot" measurement and not averaged over a 24-hour period, like a urine assay, and plasma levels are highly sensitive to stress, physical activity, and even the stimulus of phlebotomy. VMA levels are the least specific assay, with false-positive results seen with the ingestion of coffee, tea, raw fruits, and certain drugs.

Measurement of urinary catecholamines and their metabolites, despite their diagnostic accuracy, have several limitations. The collection needs to be acidified and chilled, and obtained during a paroxysm (if the patient does not have sustained hypertension), preferably while the patient is off all medications. The patient should also be at rest, something that can be difficult to achieve over a 24-hour period. For this reason, overnight urine collections have been performed to avoid the daily effects of stress and exercise. Sensitivity and specificity rates are reported to be 100% and 98%, respectively (44). We routinely obtain two 12-hour urinary collections from 8 p.m. to 8 a.m., and measure both fractionated catecholamines and metabolites, including VMA.

Many medications can interfere with these assays, yielding falsely elevated levels: Levodopa, methyldopa, ethanol, monoamine oxidase inhibitors, benzodiazepines, labetolol, and tricyclic antidepressants are the major offending agents—ethanol can also falsely decrease VMA levels (45).

A finding of elevated urinary catecholamines does not eliminate other diseases. The differential diagnosis of increased urinary catecholamines includes intracranial lesions, carcinoid syndrome, acute porphyria, factitious hypertension, clonidine withdrawal, and hypoglycemia.

Provocative and suppressive testing may be used for the minority of patients with equivocal findings, although their role in the diagnosis of pheochromocytoma has diminished sharply.

Provocative testing involves the administration of an adrenolytic agent to stimulate catecholamine production. The standard agent used is glucagon, 1 to 2 mg given intravenously in a closely monitored setting. A

TABLE 11–3. *Sensitivities and specificities of the various biochemical assays used in the detection of pheochromocytoma*

	Reference values	Sensitivity (%)	Specificity (%)	PPV (%)	NPV (%)
Plasma catecholamines	<600 pg/ml	75	20	43	50
Urinary catecholamines	<100 ng/24°	50	83	75	63
Norepinephrine	<75 ng/24°	67	83	80	71
Epinephrine[a]	<25 ng/24°	50–75	84–98	—	—
Urinary metanephrines	<1.8 mg/24°	100	80	83	100
Urinary VMA[b]	<11.0 mg/24°	80	80	80	80

PPV, Positive predictive value; NPV, negative predictive value; VMA, vanillymandelic acid.

[a]Werbel SS, Ober KP. Pheochromocytoma: Update on Diagnosis, Localization, and Management. *Med Clin North Am* 1995;79:137.

[b]Peplinski GR, Norton JA: The Predictive Value of Diagnostic Tests for Pheochromocytoma. *Surgery* 1994:116:1101–1110.

threefold or higher increase in plasma catecholamine levels, or an absolute level above 2,000 pg/mL, is diagnostic of pheochromocytoma. This test has largely been abandoned because of the obvious risk of inducing a paroxysmal attack.

The clonidine suppression test may be infrequently useful for distinguishing between pheochromocytomas and centrally mediated essential hypertension in patients with borderline catecholamine levels (46). Clonidine, a centrally acting alpha-2-agonist that inhibits neurally mediated catecholamine release, is administered as a 0.3-mg oral dose. Plasma catecholamine levels are obtained at baseline and at 3 hours after administration. A level decreasing to less than 500 pg/mL excludes the diagnosis of pheochromocytoma.

RADIOLOGIC TESTS

Following biochemical confirmation of pheochromocytoma, radiologic localization of the tumor is necessary to plan definitive surgical therapy. Not only does imaging delineate location, but it also aids in defining singularity, bilaterality, and possible multicentricity. Unsuspected metastatic lesions in bone, liver, or the lymph nodes may also be visualized. The three major modalities currently in use are computed tomography (CT) scans, magnetic resonance imaging (MRI), and 131-I-metaiodobenzlguanidine labeled nuclear scanning (MIBG). Additionally, imaging with positron emission tomography scans using isotope-labeled glucose or ephedrine, and scintiscans, with indium-labeled octreotide, are being evaluated in a number of endocrine centers.

A CT scan is the most commonly used imaging test for pheochromocytoma (Fig. 11-4). A CT scan can identify approximately 95% of all pheochromocytomas—it has the capacity to detect 1-cm tumors within the adrenal gland and 2-cm extraadrenal lesions. Sensitivity of the CT scan is 98%, with speci-

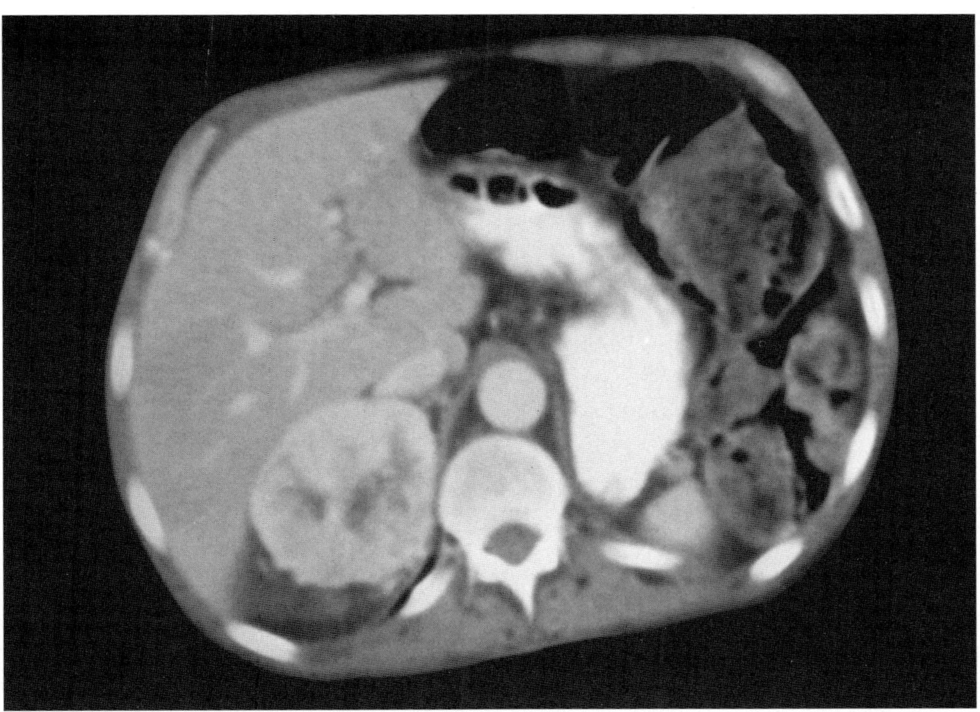

FIG. 11-4. Computed tomography scan of a right 6-cm pheochromocytoma in a 56-year-old black man with sustained hypertension, weight loss, anorexia, and weakness.

ficity of approximately 70% (47). Its easy accessibility and excellent resolution make it the initial test of choice.

Several disadvantages to the CT scan have prompted some centers to adopt MRI as their first imaging modality. The CT scan entails radiation exposure, and it does require intravenous contrast material, with its risk of inducing a paroxysm. Furthermore, a CT scan cannot distinguish pheochromocytoma from other adrenal lesions, such as cortical adenomas or metastatic deposits (48). MRI imaging, with its sensitivity and specificity of 100% and 67%, respectively, can detect 95% of all pheochromocytomas, and can usually distinguish them from other adrenal lesions by the characteristically high-signal intensity given off by the tumor on T_2-weighted images (the "light bulb" sign). MRI avoids the risks of contrast media and radiation exposure, and it enables the radiologist to image the lesion in multiple planes. It may also have better res-

olution in the detection of extraadrenal pheochromocytomas.

The 131-I-MIBG nuclear imaging scan incorporates radioactively labeled iodine into the molecular compound metaiodobenzylguanidine, a guanethidine analogue similar in structure to norepinephrine, that concentrates itself into catecholamine storage vesicles of chromaffin tissue (Fig. 11-5). The radioactive material is excreted unchanged in the urine.

MIBG scanning has reported sensitivities of 77% to 88% and specificities of 88% to 100% (43); it is thought to accurately detect 85% of all pheochromocytomas (1). The advantage of MIBG scanning is its superior ability to detect extraadrenal tumors. Small amounts of functioning chromaffin tissue are easily detected anywhere in the body. For this reason, MIBG scan is also excellent for follow-up imaging, looking for possible tumor recurrences. The disadvantages of this imaging tool are its radi-

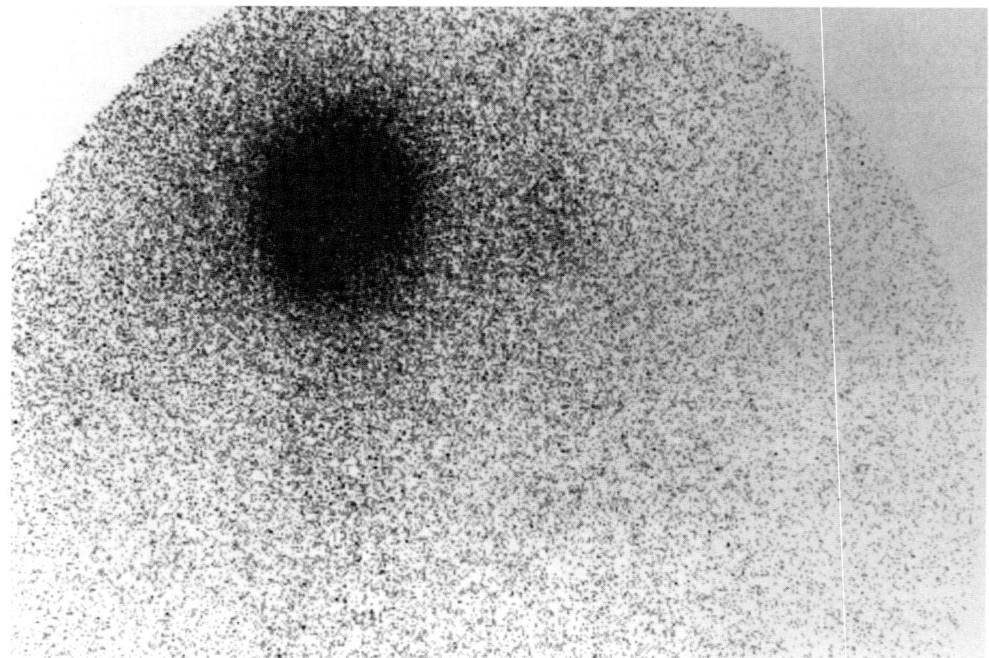

FIG. 11-5. Metaiodobenzylguanidine scan in a 19-year-old black man with hypertension. The large accumulation of radioactive tracer delineates a left-sided pheochromocytoma, but less clearly seen is uptake over the right adrenal gland. This patient was found to have bilateral pheochromocytomas.

ation exposure, its relatively high cost, and limited accessibility. False-positive results occur with neuroblastoma, carcinoid tumors, and medullary carcinoma of the thyroid. The medications that interfere with the biochemical assays for catecholamines can affect the results of MIBG scanning by pharmacologically increasing or decreasing catecholamine stores. They therefore should be discontinued for 1 week before scintigraphy.

Even though MIBG scanning is not the initial test at most centers, current indications for MIBG scanning include instances when CT (or MRI) results are negative in the scenario of classic clinical and biochemical evidence of pheochromocytoma, when follow-up imaging of recurrent or metastatic pheochromocytoma is needed, and to better delineate the functional characteristics of a tumor located on CT or MRI. We use 123-I-MIBG scans in all patients preoperatively, to confirm the CT or MRI finding, and to rule out concomitant extraadrenal pheochromocytomas (2% to 3%) or occult metastases. 123-I-MIBG can be given in a larger dose because of less radiation, increasing the sensitivity in detecting small pheochromocytomas.

PREOPERATIVE MANAGEMENT

Once the diagnosis of pheochromocytoma is firmly established, the patient must be prepared for surgical resection. Optimization of the patient requires adequate blood pressure control and correction of intravascular fluid deficits. Sometimes this is not feasible; conditions mandating emergent surgical removal include malignant hypertension, acute cardiovascular complications (sporadic ventricular arrhythmias, impending heart failure), and abdominal morbidity (tumor hemorrhage). In most cases, however, preoperative management can be instituted.

The mainstay of preoperative treatment is alpha-adrenergic blockade. Instituted 1 to 3 weeks before surgery, this normalizes blood pressure, controls paroxysms, and allows for intravascular volume expansion. Phenoxybenzamine (Dibenzyline) is the drug of choice,

because of its irreversible binding and its 100-fold greater potency at the alpha-1, rather that the alpha-2, receptor. A noncompetitive receptor antagonist, phenoxybenzamine is given initially as 10 mg orally four times daily, and may be increased 20 to 40 mg/day up to a total dose of 200 mg or more. Most patients require 40 to 80 mg/day. Endpoints of therapy include normalized blood pressure and the onset of postural hypotension.

Phentolamine (Regitine) is a competitive norepinephrine antagonist that also may be used preoperatively. It is usually given at a dosage of 50 mg every 4 hours. This agent is less effective than phenoxybenzamine, as its effects are transient (requiring more frequent dosing intervals). Side effects are prominent and include nausea, vomiting, nasal congestion, and ejaculatory dysfunction, all to a greater degree than that of the other alpha-blockers. For these reasons, phentolamine is essentially reserved for intraoperative hypertensive crises.

Prazosin is another alpha blocker once considered useful in preoperative blockade. A postsynaptic alpha-1-receptor antagonist, it is administered orally in dosages ranging from 1 to 2 mg every 6 hours. Because prazosin is a competitive inhibitor, it has the potential to be displaced off its binding sites by surges of catecholamines, such as during periods of increased stress (49). For this reason, prazosin is seldom used.

Other agents in addition to alpha-blockers have been tried in an attempt to control blood pressure and paroxysms. Captopril, an angiotensin-converting enzyme inhibitor, had initial success, but drug resistance soon developed (50). Calcium channel blockers have met with success and are reasonable alternatives for those patients refractory to alpha-blocker therapy.

Although alpha-adrenergic blockade is accepted as standard preoperative management of pheochromocytoma patients, Boutros and colleagues reported the Cleveland Clinic experience, citing successful surgical resection *without* preoperative alpha-blockade in 63 patients (51). They cite that alpha-adrenergic blockade may make surgical location of the tumor difficult, by masking the characteristic hypertensive response to intraoperative tumor manipulation. Although this study is intriguing, most endocrinologists and endocrine surgeons maintain that, in the era of such sensitive radiologic modalities, the tumor is virtually always localized preoperatively. Preoperative alpha-blockade, in conjunction with aggressive fluid intake and institution of a high-salt diet, minimizes intraoperative risk by decreasing the frequency of volatile blood pressure shifts during resection, and eliminates the profound hypotension that often occurred in unprepared patients in the past.

Other pharmacologic management centers around beta-adrenergic blockade. Treatment with beta-blockade is indicated for the appearance of tachycardia (greater than 140 beats per minute) and arrhythmias while on alpha-blocker therapy, as well as for purely epinephrine-secreting tumors. The standard agent is propranolol, a competitive beta-receptor blocker, given in dosages ranging from 10 to 40 mg two to three times daily. Beta-blockade is to be instituted only after alpha-blockade has been achieved. Unopposed beta-blockade can cause worsening hypertension by blocking the vasodilatory effects of epinephrine, resulting in enhanced pressor response to norepinephrine. More cardioselective beta-blockers such as metoprolol and atenolol may decrease this risk.

Beta-blockers must be used with caution in elderly patients and those with proven or suspected heart disease, because it may promote profound bradycardia, myocardial depression, and congestive heart failure. When used, they have been commonly instituted 3 to 7 days before surgery. We have obtained good results after only 1 day's treatment in most cases. Alpha- and beta-blockade may be continued up to the day of surgery, and the usual dose of both drugs is given orally with a sip of water on the morning of the operation. For most patients this is 10 or 20 mg of phenoxybenzamine and 10 to 20 mg of propranolol.

When beta-blockers are contraindicated, such as in myocarditis or congestive heart fail-

ure, metyrosine has been used. Metyrosine, or alpha-methylparatyrosine, is a competitive tyrosine hydroxylase inhibitor that blocks the conversion of tyrosine to L-dopa, effectively inhibiting catecholamine synthesis. Given in dosages ranging from 0.5 to 1 g orally three to four times daily, it can reduce circulating catecholamine levels by 50% to 80% (52). Side effects include crystalluria, extrapyramidal signs, sedation, diarrhea, and marked anxiety.

Anesthetic Considerations

It is crucial for the surgeon and anesthesiologist to keep in constant communication throughout the operative period, because hypertensive or hypotensive crises may quickly develop and become fatal if not recognized and treated immediately.

Critical moments during the operative period include the induction of anesthesia, intubation, and tumor manipulation. These actions make the patient most susceptible to hypertensive reactions and cardiac arrhythmias. Additionally, simple maneuvers such as transferring the patient onto the operating room table may incite a paroxysm. To be prepared for these situations, the anesthesiologist has several medications on hand.

Phentolamine and sodium nitroprusside are the two major intravenous agents used for intraoperative hypertensive crises. Phentolamine, given in a 5-mg bolus, may be repeated every 2 minutes until effective. Its onset of action is within 30 seconds, with a peak effect within 5 minutes; duration of action is 30 to 60 minutes. Sodium nitroprusside is the more physiologic antihypertensive medication, but it must be used with caution if used for prolonged periods or in patients with impaired renal function because of the risks of thiocyanate toxicity and nephrotoxicity, respectively. Either drug may be given as a continuous drip of 0.2 mg/mL to achieve normalization of blood pressure.

Anesthetic agents lower the arrhythmogenic threshold of the heart. In a pheochromocytoma patient with a preexisting tendency to development of life-threatening arrhythmias, the anesthesiologist must be prepared for these events. The drug of choice for supraventricular arrhythmias such as atrial fibrillation or flutter is intravenous esmolol, a rapid and short-acting cardioselective beta-blocker. Ventricular arrhythmias are best treated by lidocaine, given in intravenous boluses of 50 to 100 mg.

Once the tumor is removed, the source of hypertension is removed. Blood pressure decreases, and hypotension, occasionally profound, is seen. Aggressive fluid administration is mandatory; vasopressors, when required (rarely), are given on a short-term basis and imply inadequate preoperative adrenergic blockade. Blood pressure that does not decrease after tumor removal should raise the strong possibility that another tumor is present.

Hypoglycemia may become a significant problem for the first 12 to 24 hours after surgical removal of the tumor. For this reason, 10% glucose is routinely administered during this time, with frequent chemstick monitoring.

SURGICAL APPROACHES

All patients undergoing resection of pheochromocytoma need rigorous intraoperative and postoperative monitoring. Continuous arterial blood pressure measurement is necessary. A central venous pressure line, or a Swan-Ganz catheter for hemodynamic monitoring, is often necessary. Most patients do not need to be placed in the intensive care unit postoperatively unless there are severe concurrent illnesses or if labile hemodynamic pa-

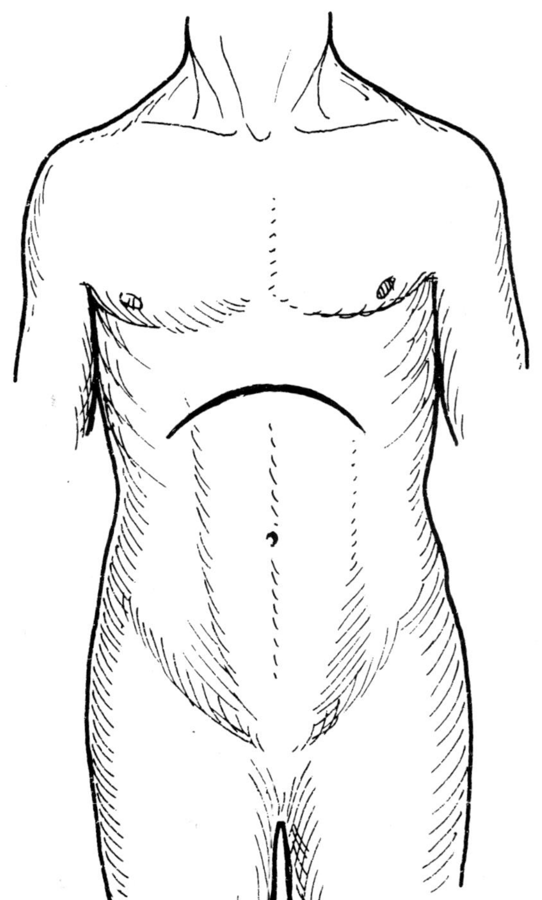

FIG. 11-6. Modified chevron, or bucket-handle, incision used most often in surgery for pheochromocytoma. (Modified from Hinman F. *Atlas of Urologic Surgery.* Philadelphia: WB Saunders, 1989:875.)

rameters are present. In most patients, blood pressure normalizes within 24 hours.

Traditionally, most surgeons used an anterior transabdominal approach. This allows inspection of both adrenal glands and the entire paraspinal axis, from diaphragm to bladder, to search for any possible additional tumors. This approach remains the standard for surgical resection of pheochromocytoma.

Two possible incisions may be made with this approach: (a) the midline vertical or (b) the bilateral subcostal, or chevron, incision. Advocates of the chevron incision cite the advantage of minimizing incisional length on the contralateral (nontumor) side and still achieving adequate abdominal exposure. Although some surgeons state that the chevron incision limits the ability of the surgeon to obtain lower abdominal and pelvic exposure, it remains the preferred incision for most endocrine surgeons resecting pheochromocytomas (Fig. 11-6).

For lesions in the left adrenal gland, exposure is facilitated by mobilizing the descending colon, spleen, and tail of the pancreas. This is achieved by laterally incising the peritoneum and dividing the splenocolic and splenorenal ligaments, allowing medial retraction of these structures (Fig. 11-7).

The left adrenal gland is best visualized by exposing the renal hilum, following the left

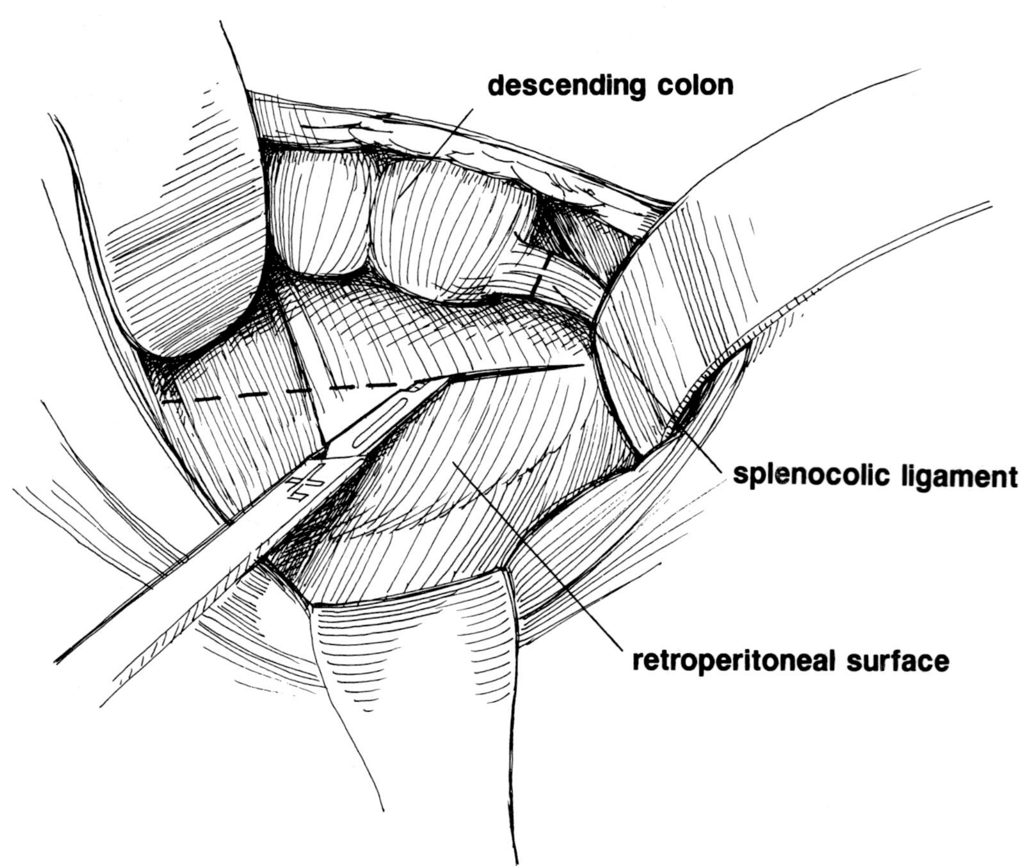

FIG. 11-7. Surgical excision of left pheochromocytoma. To obtain access into the retroperitoneal space, the peritoneum is incised lateral to the descending colon, and extended to take down the splenocolic ligament. (Modified from Hinman F. *Atlas of Urologic Surgery*. Philadelphia: WB Saunders, 1989:849.)

renal vein to its junction with the adrenal vein. The surgeon should look for posteriorly located lumbar veins draining into the adrenal vein. Another approach is through the lesser space after reflecting the omentum from the transverse colon, and then incising the retroperitoneum along the caudal border of the pancreas from superior mesenteric vein to the tail. This allows direct exposure of the renal vein near the central adrenal vein.

One of the unique aspects of pheochromocytoma surgery is that the adrenal vein is controlled *before* the arterial supply to stop further catecholamine release during tumor resection. When the vein is ready to be ligated (Fig. 11-8),

the anesthesiologist must be informed so that he or she can prepare for the decrease in blood pressure that often occurs, unless there is a large inferior phrenic vein still draining the adrenal.

Once the central adrenal vein has been divided, attention is turned toward the identification of any accessory adrenal veins. Next, the adrenal arteries are secured. Superiorly, the inferior phrenic artery is identified and ligated, followed by the aortic adrenal artery medially, and then the renal arterial supply inferiorly. The gland is then circumferentially released from its connective tissue attachments with clips or ties and removed (Fig. 11-9).

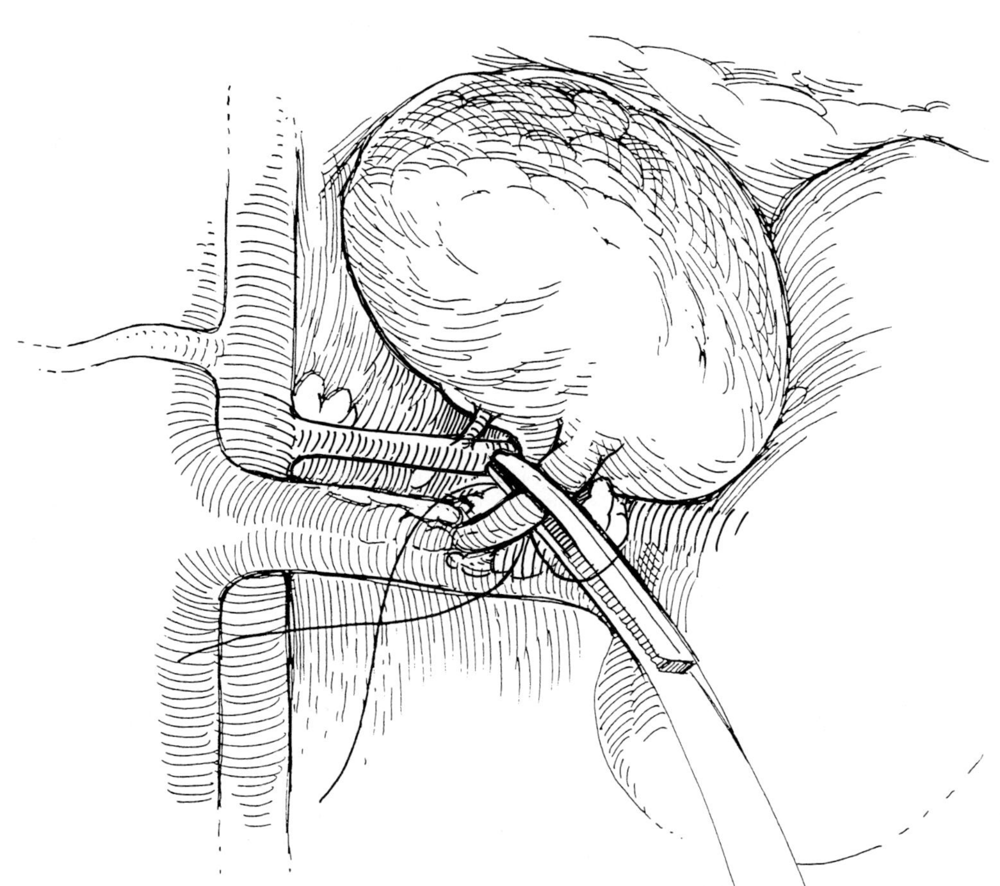

FIG. 11-8. Surgical excision of left pheochromocytoma. With minimal tumor manipulation, the adrenal vein is ligated and cut before the adrenal arterial supply. (Modified from Hinman F. *Atlas of Urologic Surgery*. Philadelphia: WB Saunders, 1989:850.)

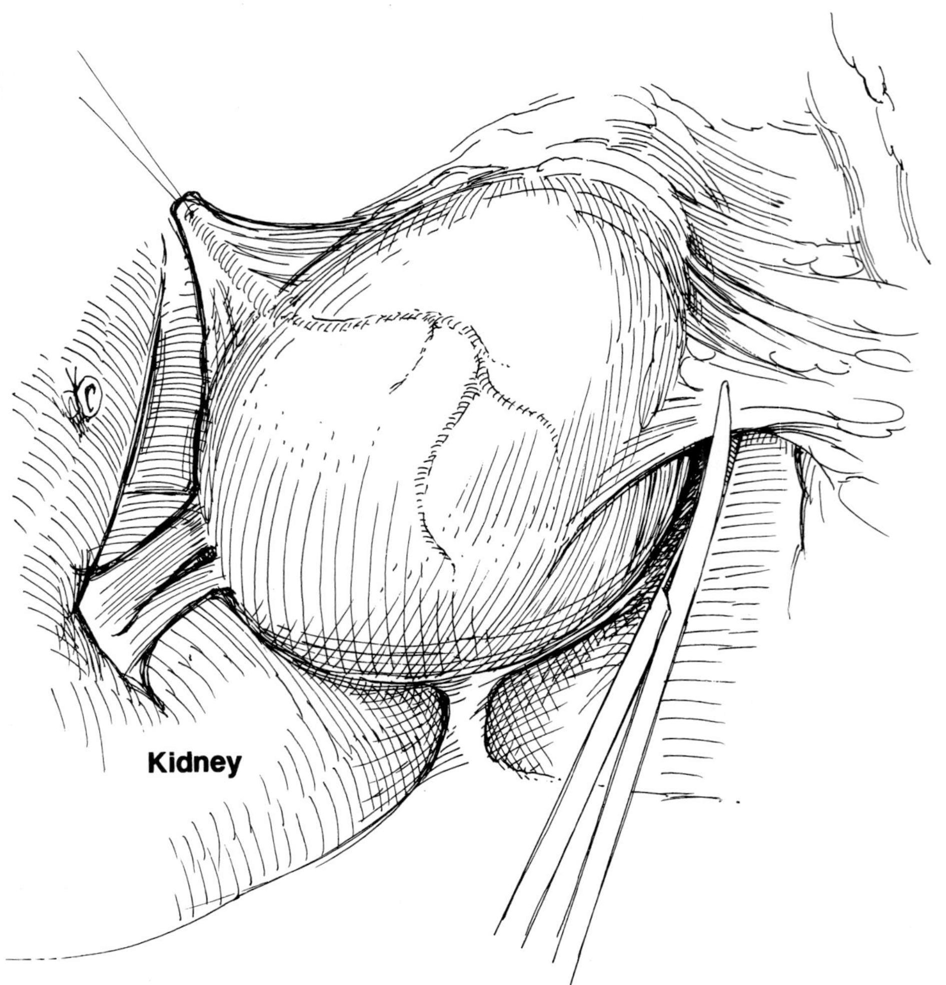

FIG. 11-9. Surgical excision of left pheochromocytoma. Once the blood supply is controlled, the connective tissue attachments can be taken down with a series of surgical clips or ties. (Modified from Hinman F. *Atlas of Urologic Surgery*. Philadelphia: WB Saunders, 1989:851.)

For right adrenal lesions, after the abdomen is entered, exposure of the adrenal gland involves freeing and retracting the surrounding viscera. The peritoneum lateral to the duodenum is sharply incised, and a Kocher maneuver is performed to retract the duodenum medially (Fig. 11-10). The hepatocolic and gastrohepatic ligaments are divided, allowing cephalad retraction of the right lobe of the liver. These actions result in easy visualization of Gerota's fascia, which is then incised. At this point, the suprarenal vena cava, right adrenal gland, and upper pole of the kidney should be seen. The kidney is reflected inferiorly, and dissection should ensue between the inferior vena cava and the tumor to isolate the short right adrenal vein. This vein inserts posteriorly and high under the liver. In some cases, cephalic retraction of the liver is facilitated by clipping and dividing one or more small hepatic veins from the caudate lobe. For very large tumors, the entire right lobe can be mobilized to allow good exposure of the central vein. In 1% to 2% of cases, the central vein drains directly into the right hepatic vein and can be torn if this anomaly is not recognized.

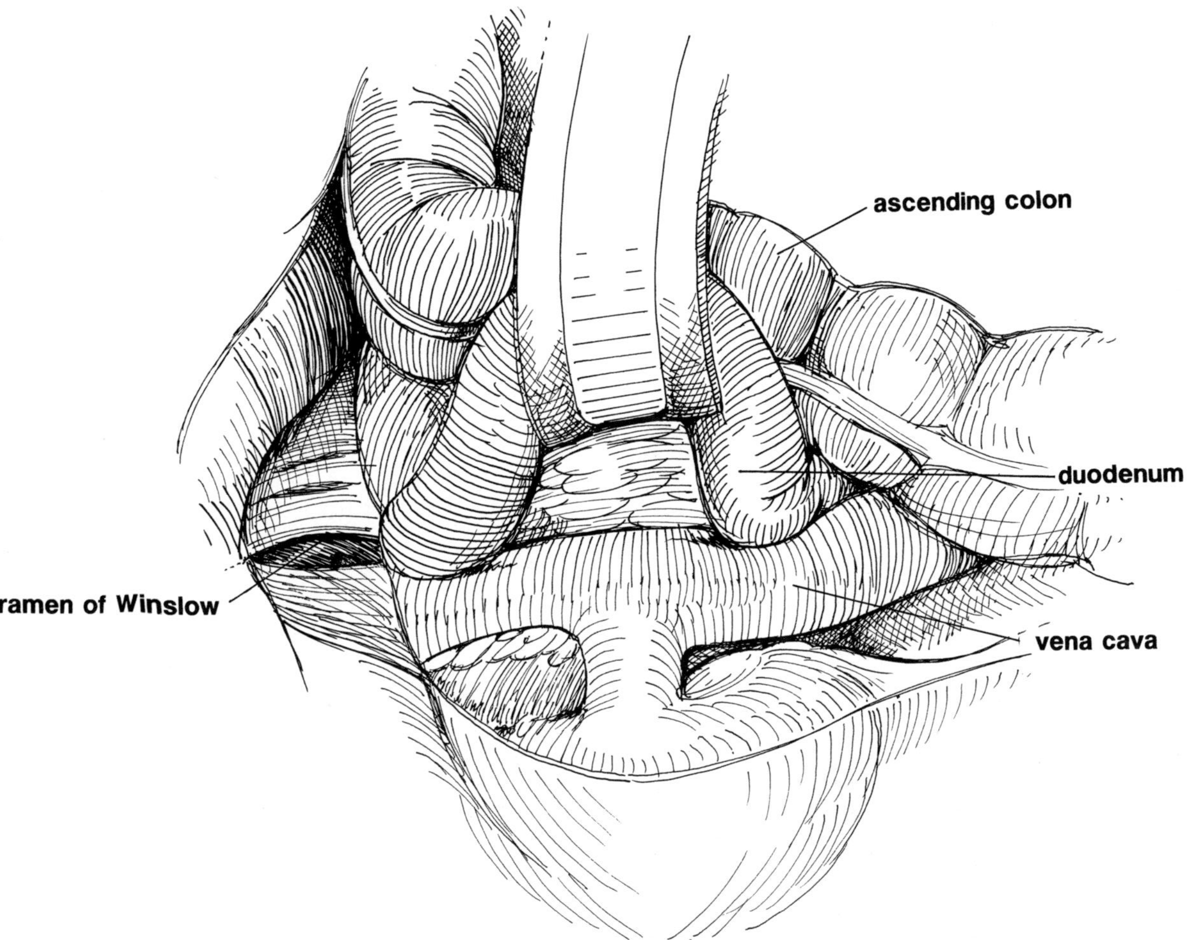

FIG. 11-10. Surgical excision of right pheochromocytoma. Retroperitoneal access is achieved by performing a standard Kocher maneuver. (Modified from Hinman F. *Atlas of Urologic Surgery.* Philadelphia: WB Saunders, 1989:852.)

Once the tumor is removed, a systematic search for contralateral and extraadrenal lesions should be sought. An absence of a blood pressure decrease should alert the surgeon to the possibility that an additional tumor remains. Invasion into adjacent tissues should be aggressively resected if possible, to maximally remove as much chromaffin tissue as possible.

Even though this transabdominal approach remains the traditional standard, some surgeons have argued that, in the era of superior radiologic imaging, tumor localization is so accurate that a less morbid retroperitoneal flank or posterior incision may be performed in cases of unilateral adrenal tumors (53). Patients with a high incidence of bilaterality (familial, pediatric, and those associated with MEN syndromes or neuroectodermal dysplasias) should still be approached transperitoneally.

A thoracoabdominal approach is generally reserved for large pheochromocytomas; it affords exposure and palpation of the entire retroperitoneal and abdominal contents. It also allows for tumors that have extended into the inferior vena cava. In these cases, the abdominal incision is complemented by a midline sternal split. Posterior approaches are usually contraindicated because they afford minimal exposure. Laparoscopic adrenalectomy for pheochromocytoma offers resection with minimal tumor manipulation, but at least one large series reported a much higher incidence of intraoperative and postoperative complications as compared to laparoscopy for other adrenal lesions (54). Nevertheless, an ever increasing number of pheochromocytomas, particularly those that are small and considered likely to be benign, are being excised laparoscopically.

For pheochromocytoma patients at high risk for tumor bilaterality (i.e., MEN syndromes) and a macroscopically normal contralateral adrenal gland, the surgeon is faced with the decision whether to perform bilateral adrenalectomy. Lairmore and colleagues reported that, in MEN II patients undergoing unilateral adrenalectomy, contralateral tumor

formation was high (52%). These recurrences were found during routine follow-up, and no patient experienced signs or symptoms from their recurrence; morbidity and mortality rates (excluding any that may have been derived from a second resection) were zero. Conversely, 23% of patients who did undergo prophylactic bilateral adrenalectomy experienced at least one episode of acute adrenal insufficiency, and one patient died of influenza (15). These authors conclude that unilateral adrenalectomy and close follow-up are indicated in this subset of patients. The great majority of our MEN II patients, however, have had grossly apparent bilateral tumors and have thus had bilateral adrenalectomies.

PHEOCHROMOCYTOMA IN PREGNANCY

Special considerations exist for the patient diagnosed with pheochromocytoma during pregnancy. Although catecholamines minimally cross the placenta, the tumor is still a significant source of fetal, as well as maternal, morbidity and mortality. Difficulty exists in differentiating pheochromocytoma from hypertension of pregnancy (preeclampsia). Hendee found only 13% of patients were correctly given the diagnosis of pheochromocytoma during their pregnancy (55).

The signs and symptoms of pheochromocytoma in pregnancy are similar to those in the nonpregnant patient, but in those patients without paroxysms, several diagnostic features aid in distinguishing between these two conditions. There is a lack of proteinuria in pheochromocytoma, as opposed to that seen in toxemia, there is generally no anuria or oliguria in pheochromocytoma, and thrombocytopenia may be present in pheochromocytoma. Also, hypertension worsens when the patient with pheochromocytoma lies supine, secondary to pressure on the tumor from the gravid uterus.

In those patients with strong evidence of pheochromocytoma, especially those women with severe and intermittent hypertension, biochemical diagnosis should be sought immediately, because a fatal hypertensive crisis can be provoked by anesthesia, vaginal delivery, or even fetal movements. Because the pregnant state does not alter the catecholamine metabolism, the diagnostic accuracy of these assays should not be altered (56).

Radiologic testing of the pregnant patient is best achieved by MRI, avoiding the exposure to ionizing radiation.

Treatment of the pregnant patient with pheochromocytoma is essentially identical to that for the nonpregnant patient. Phenoxybenzamine is administered to achieve alpha-adrenergic blockade, which has been well established to be safe throughout pregnancy; prazosin and labetolol have also been used without untoward effects in the fetus (56).

If the diagnosis is made before 23 weeks' gestation, the tumor should be resected after alpha-blockade is established; after 23 weeks, the gravid uterus usually makes abdominal exploration much more difficult and hazardous. Surgical resection should be delayed until fetal maturity, at which time simultaneous cesarean section and tumor resection should be performed (56).

Maternal and fetal mortality rates, since the introduction of adrenergic blockers, have decreased sharply over the past 30 years. Maternal mortality rate has decreased from 48% before 1969 to 17%, and fetal mortality rate has decreased from 50% to 30% (57,58). As with nonpregnant patients, a strong index of suspicion is crucial in expediting diagnosis and treatment of these tumors.

PROGNOSIS

Benign Tumors

Overall operative mortality rate for surgical resection of pheochromocytoma is less than 2%. Seventy-five percent to 80% of patients become normotensive postoperatively, whereas 20% to 25% remain hypertensive. This is probably due to underlying essential hypertension.

For benign tumors, 5-year survival rates are 96% (29). Recommended follow-up consists of repeated biochemical assays at approximately 1 week postoperatively and again at 3 to 6 months. Thereafter, annual testing is performed for at least the next 5 years. Blood pressure is also monitored at monthly intervals for the first year, then semiannually for life. Any abnormalities found should be further worked up and treated in a similar way to the initial tumor.

Malignant Tumors

Malignant pheochromocytoma carries a 5-year survival rate ranging from 36% to 60% (29,59). The incidence of malignant lesions ranges from 10% to 15%. Recurrences, when they occur, usually develop within 5 to 10 years, but they can appear as long as 20 years after surgical resection. One study by Beierwaltes, using follow-up MIBG scanning to detect metastatic recurrences, found that metastatic disease develops in 46% of all patients undergoing pheochromocytoma resection at a mean duration of 4.2 years after surgery (60).

In general, the definition of malignancy centers on the finding of tumor spread into local or distant sites. Treatment of malignant pheochromocytoma begins with surgical debulking of as much tissue as possible. Following this, several treatment modalities are available to treat residual disease. All have met with minimal success.

131-I-MIBG irradiation, using dosages that interfere with catecholamine metabolism, has been studied and been found to cause tumor regression and decreased catecholamine secretion in 25% of patients. However, all patients relapsed within 2 years (61). Another high-dose MIBG trial resulted in a 0% complete tumor response rate, with 35% partially responding (61).

Chemotherapy regimens have been used that were initially developed for neuroblastoma. Cyclophosphamide, vincristine, and dacarbazine are administered. Results of one study showed a 14% complete tumor response rate, with 43% partial responders, 21% minimal responders, and 21% nonresponders.

cytoma in children: report of nine cases and review of the first 100 published cases with follow-up studies. *J Pediatr* 1963;63:315.

31. Caty MG, Coran AG, Geagen M, et al. Current diagnosis and treatment of pheochromocytoma in children. *Arch Surg* 1990;125:978–981.

32. Cushman P. Familial endocrine tumors. *Am J Med* 1962;32:352.

33. Sipple JH. The association of pheochromocytoma with carcinoma of the thyroid gland. *Am J Med* 1961;31:163.

34. Cance WG, Wells SA Jr. Multiple endocrine neoplasia type IIA. *Curr Probl Surg* 1985;22:1.

35. Modigliani E, Vasen HM, Raue K, et al. Pheochromocytoma in multiple endocrine neoplasia type 2: European study. *J Intern Med* 1995;238:363–367.

36. Casanova S, Rosenberg-Bourgin M, Farkas D, et al. Pheochromocytoma in multiple endocrine neoplasia type 2A: survey of 100 cases. *Clin Endocrinol* 1993;38:531–537.

37. Neumann HPH, Eng C, Mulligan LM, et al. Consequences of direct genetic testing for germline mutations in the clinical management of families with multiple endocrine neoplasia, type II. *JAMA* 1995;274:1149–1151.

38. Neumann HPH, Berger DP, Sigmund G, et al. Pheochromocytomas, multiple endocrine neoplasia type 2, and von Hippel-Lindau disease. *N Engl J Med* 1993;329:1531–1538.

39. Preston RT, Lai LC. Biochemical detection of pheochromocytoma: should we still be measuring urinary HMMA? *J Clin Pathol* 1993;46:734–737.

40. Lenders JWM, Keiser HR, Goldstein DS, et al. Plasma metanephrines in the diagnosis of pheochromocytoma. *Ann Intern Med* 1995;123:101–109.

41. Sjoerdsma A, Waldeman TA, Cooperman TA, et al. Pheochromocytoma: current concepts of diagnosis and treatment. *Ann Intern Med* 1966;65:1302.

42. Peplinski GR, Norton JA. The predictive value of diagnostic tests for pheochromocytoma. *Surgery* 1994;116:1101–1110.

43. Werbel SS, Ober KP. Pheochromocytoma: update on diagnosis, localization, and management. *Med Clin North Am* 1995;79:131–153.

44. Peaston RT, Lennard TWJ, Lai LC. Overnight excretion of urinary catecholamines and metabolites in the detection of pheochromocytoma. *J Clin Endocrinol Metab* 1996;81:1378–1384.

45. Manger WM, Gifford RW Jr. Pheochromocytoma. In: Laragh JH, Brenner BM, eds. *Hypertension: pathophysiology, diagnosis, and management.* New York: Raven Press, 1990.

46. Sjoberg RJ, Simcic KJ, Kidd, GS. The clonidine suppression test for pheochromocytoma: a review of its utility and pitfalls. *Arch Intern Med* 1992;152:1193–1197.

47. Bravo EL. Pheochromocytoma: new concepts and future trends. *Kidney Int* 1991;40:544.

48. Velchik MG, Alavi A, Kressel HY, et al. Localization of pheochromocytoma: MIBG, CT, and MRI correlation. *J Nucl Med* 1989;30:328.

49. Nicholson JP Jr, Vaughn ED Jr, Pickering TG, et al. Pheochromocytoma and prazosin. *Ann Intern Med* 1983;99:477–479.

50. Israeli A, Gottehrer N, Garish D, et al. Recent developments in the diagnosis and treatment of pheochromocytomas. *Mayo Clin Proc* 1990;65:88.

51. Boutros AR, Bravo EL, Zanettin GG, et al. Perioperative management of 63 patients with pheochromocytoma. *Clev Clin J Med* 1990;57:613–617.

52. Engelman K, Horowitz D, Jequier E, et al. Biochemical and pharmacologic effects of alpha-methylparatyrosine in man. *J Clin Invest* 1968;47:577.

53. Obara T, Kanbe M, Okamoto T, et al. Surgical strategy for pheochromocytoma: emphasis on the pledge of flank extraperitoneal approach in selected patients. *Surgery* 1995;118:1083–1089.

54. Gagner M, Breton G, Pharand D, et al. Is laparoscopic adrenalectomy indicated for pheochromocytomas? *Surgery* 1996;120:1076–1080.

55. Hendee AE, Martin RP, Waters WC. Hypertension in pregnancy: toxemia or pheochromocytoma? *Am J Obstet Gynecol* 1969;105:64–70.

56. Hadden DR. Adrenal disorders of pregnancy. *Endocrinol Metab North Am* 1995;24:144–146.

57. Schenker JG, Granat M. Pheochromocytoma and pregnancy: an updated appraisal. *Aust N Z J Obstet Gynaecol* 1982;22:1.

58. Burgess GE. Alpha blockade and surgical intervention of pheochromocytoma in pregnancy. *Obstet Gynecol* 1979;53:266–270.

59. Van Heerden JA, Sheps SG, Hamberger B, et al. Pheochromocytoma: current status and changing trends. *Surgery* 1982;91:367.

60. Beierwaltes WH. Update on basic research and clinical experience with metaiodobenzylguanidine. *Med Pediatr Oncol* 1987;15:163–169.

61. Krempf M, Lumbroso J, Mornex R, et al. Use of ^{131}I-metaiodobenzylguanidine in the treatment of malignant pheochromocytoma. *J Clin Endocrinol Metab* 1991;72:455.

62. Averbuch SD, Steakley CS, Young RC, et al. Malignant pheochromocytoma: effective treatment with a combination of cyclophosphamide, vincristine, and dacarbazine. *Ann Intern Med* 1988;109:267.

Medical and Surgical Management of
Adrenal Diseases, edited by Joseph C. Cerny.
Lippincott Williams & Wilkins, Philadelphia © 1999.

12

Laparoscopic Adrenalectomy

B. Todd Heniford, *David A. Iannitti, and †Michel Gagner

Department of Surgery, Carolinas Medical Center, Charlotte, North Carolina 28232;
**Department of Surgery, Brown University School of Medicine, Providence, Rhode Island 02905;*
†Department of Surgery, The Mount Sinai Medical Center, New York, New York 10029

The fervor surrounding laparoscopic cholecystectomy, which began in the late 1980s, has rapidly expanded into many other fields of surgery. Helping to spur this enthusiasm has been the advent of less cumbersome and complex instrumentation and techniques, improved video imaging, and greater familiarity with endoscopic equipment by the operating room staff. Laparoscopic adrenalectomy was first reported in 1992. Since that time, it has moved from an acceptable option for removal of adrenal pathology to a first-line method preferred over the conventional open techniques (1–6). The development of an adequate animal model (7) and the availability of many instructional courses have promoted the popularity of laparoscopic adrenalectomy. As with the conventional methods, several techniques are available to remove the adrenal laparoscopically, with the techniques being varied according to pathology, diameter of the adrenal mass, location of the lesion, and patient morphology. Knowledge of anatomy, meticulous hemostasis, and delicate tissue handling are essential in making adrenal surgery successful (8,9). Thorough workup, including localization of the pathology and confirmation of the diagnosis by an inclusive endocrine evaluation, is also necessary.

LAPAROSCOPIC ADRENALECTOMY

The patient is placed in the lateral decubitus position with the left side up. The surgeon and assistant stand facing the abdomen (Fig. 12-1). The table is flexed, and a flank pillow is positioned under the patient's right side. The left side should be hyperextended so that the space between the costal margin and the iliac crest is exposed maximally to the point where the flank musculature begins to feel slightly tight (Fig. 12-2). The left arm is extended and suspended. The area from the umbilicus to the vertebral column and from the nipple to the mid-iliac crest should be prepared and draped. A skin incision approximately 1.2 to 1.4 cm in length is made 2 cm below and parallel to the costal margin, just medial to the anterior axillary line (Fig. 12-3).Using a muscle-splitting technique, which requires a scalpel and S-shaped retractors, the incision is extended down to the peritoneum. At this point, in patients who have not had previous surgery in this area, a Veress needle is inserted into the abdominal cavity. A saline test is performed to ensure that no abdominal organs have been injured; then CO_2 is insufflated up to 15 mm Hg. In patients who have had previous surgery in the flank region, the peritoneum is opened and a 10-mm Hassen trocar is inserted under direct vision.

A 30-degree, 10-mm laparoscope, which is used throughout the operation, is placed in the abdomen via this first port, and diagnostic laparoscopy is performed. The distal transverse, descending, and sigmoid colons are inspected, as are the inguinal area for possible hernias and the left adnexal structures in women. The spleen, superior pole of the left kidney, left lateral portion of the liver (segments II and

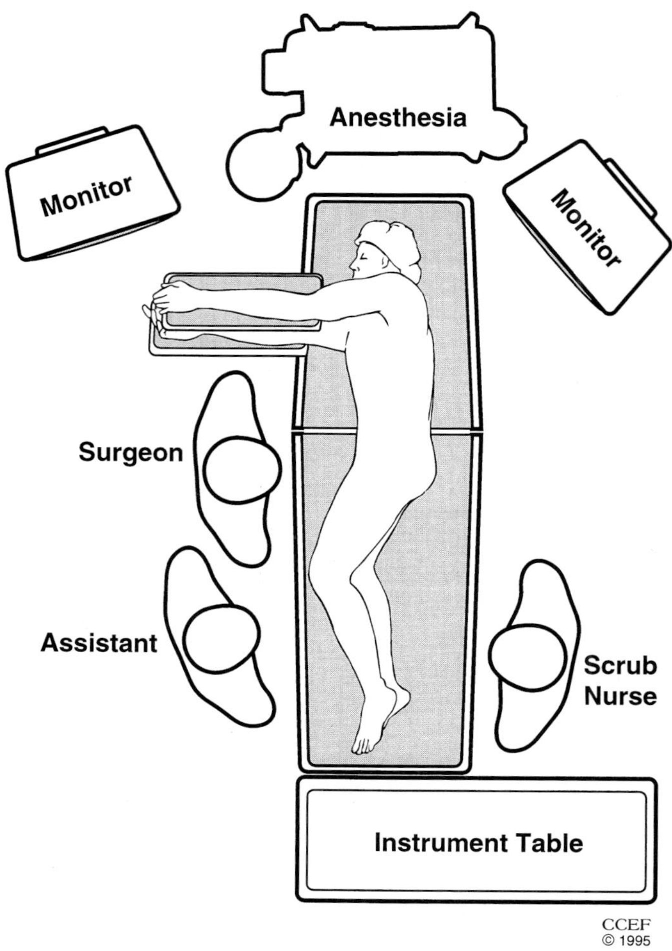

FIG. 12-1. Organization of the operating room for laparoscopic adrenalectomy. © Cleveland Clinic Education Foundation.

III), diaphragm, and greater curvature of the stomach should be closely examined. If the inspection is satisfactory, two more 10-mm trocars are inserted in the flank under laparoscopic visualization. One is placed inferior and slightly medial to the eleventh rib, and the other is inserted more anterior and medial to the initial trocar (see Fig. 12-3). All trocars should be at least 5 cm apart and, at best, 8 to 10 cm apart. It is important to keep the trocars close to the costal margin and no further posterior than 2 to 3 cm behind the level of the anterior superior spine of the iliac crest. This positioning ensures that the instruments will reach the superior-lateral aspects of the spleen and not bump the iliac crest while the surgeon is working.

The laparoscope is then placed through the most anterior trocar, and the surgeon, operating with two hands, uses the lateral two ports. A laparoscopic curved dissector (left hand) and a scissors with cautery (right hand) are used for the dissection. Minimal mobilization of the colonic flexure is necessary to uncover the retroperitoneal space and move the colon from the inferior pole of the adrenal gland. Reflecting the colon medially and inferiorly allows the instruments to be inserted more easily, avoiding inadvertent trauma to the colon. The next plane of dissection is along the lateral bor-

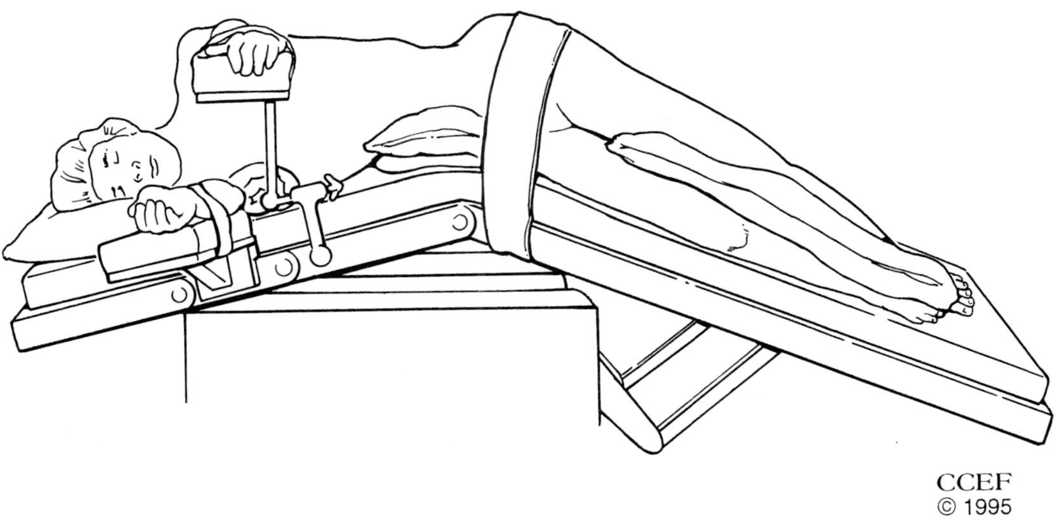

FIG. 12-2. Patient and table position for left laparoscopic adrenalectomy. © Cleveland Clinic Education Foundation.

der of the spleen at the splenorenal ligament; a short segment of the peritoneal covering 1 cm lateral to the spleen should be incised (Fig. 12-4).With a grasper in the left hand, the 1-cm peritoneal cuff created adjacent to the spleen is held and retracted to facilitate dissection in the space between the spleen and kidney. Using the peritoneum as a handle helps to avoid injuring the capsule of the spleen. This plane is carried up to the diaphragm, very close to the greater

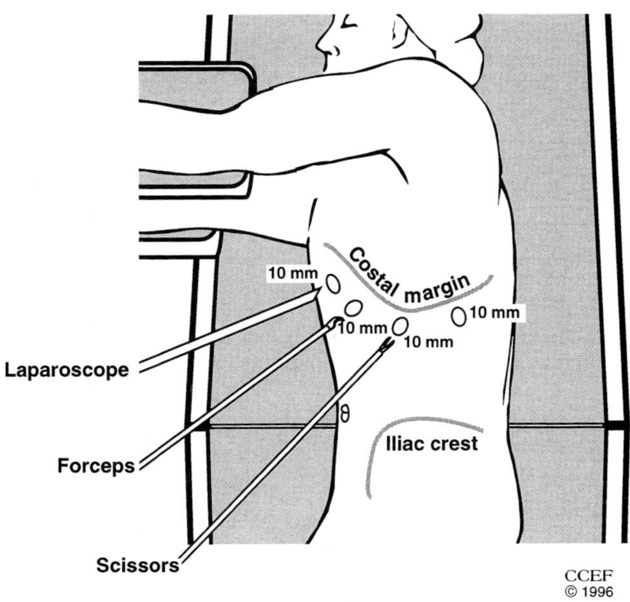

FIG. 12-3. Trocar sites for left adrenalectomy. © Cleveland Clinic Education Foundation.

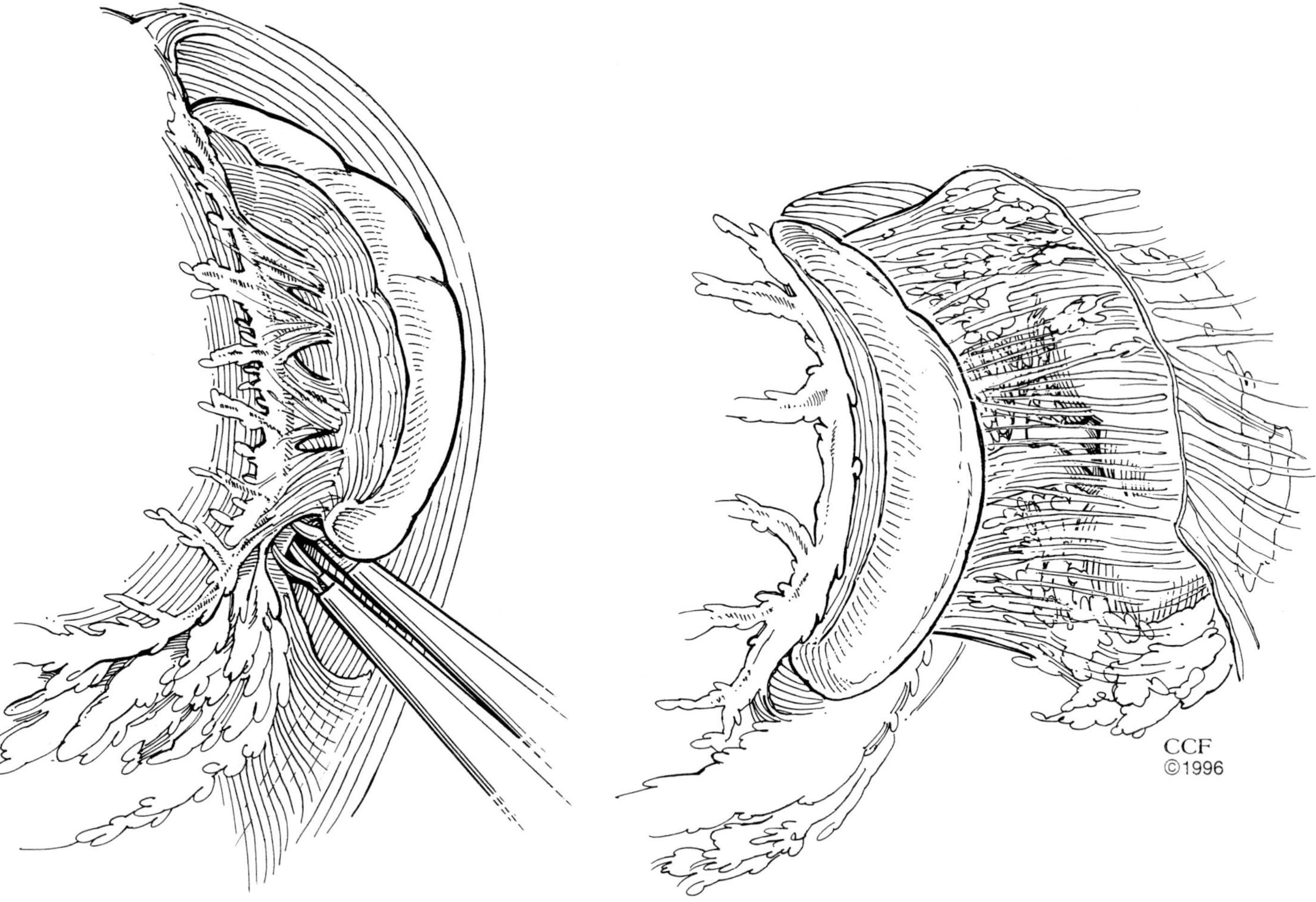

FIG. 12-4. A: Dissection of the inferior portion of the splenorenal ligament. **B:** Completed dissection of the splenorenal ligament. © Cleveland Clinic Education Foundation.

curvature of the stomach. When the short gastric vessels are identified, the dissection is stopped. Once the spleen is fully mobilized, it falls medially and the space opens in a book-like fashion. The lateral and anterior portions of the adrenal gland become visible in the perinephric fat, according to the type of perinephric fat that is present. Of the two types of fat that may be encountered, the soft, nonadherent areolar fat is easily removed using the laparoscopic scissors and cautery. The other type of fat found is dense, adherent, and contains multiple small vessels originating in the retroperitoneum. The hook cautery is used to dissect the adrenal gland from surrounding tissue. This form of dissection is more tedious and requires patience to avoid bleeding or rupture of the adrenal capsule.

Once the lateral portion of the adrenal gland has been exposed, the table is tilted to a head-up position, permitting further downward displacement of the surrounding organs. This position also allows any saline irrigation, bleeding, or oozing in that area to flow caudally. The operation is usually performed through three trocars. Occasionally, however, a fourth trocar may be necessary to further retract the spleen, kidney, or surrounding fat for better exposure of the inferior pole and lateral edge of the adrenal gland. If this additional trocar is needed, it is inserted 5 to 8 cm posterior to the most lateral port (see Fig. 12-3). This port should always be inserted after the splenorenal ligament has been divided, allowing this trocar to pass over the lateral and superior borders of the kidney. If this ligament is not taken down, the trocar may inadvertently penetrate the renal parenchyma. A fan-shaped retractor is the instrument most often used through this additional port.

The dissection can be continued inferiorly, dividing the left adrenal vein early in the operation, or superiorly, clipping the adrenal vein at the end. The direction depends on the exposure gained after the spleen has been dissected, the type of pathology, and the size of the adrenal mass. If a large adrenal mass (5 to 10 cm) must be dissected, the left adrenal vein may be more difficult to visualize. In such cases, dissecting the lateral and superior adrenal poles first allows better mobilization and easier control of the adrenal vein. In tumors 5 cm or less in diameter, dissecting and dividing the adrenal vein first is feasible. Most left adrenal veins are about 5 to 10 mm in diameter and can be controlled with medium-large titanium clips placed with a single or multifire clip applier (Ethicon Endosurgery, Johnson & Johnson, Cincinnati, OH). The adrenal vein is dissected from the gland with a right-angled instrument for a distance of approximately 1.5 to 2 cm. It is not necessary to identify its junction with the renal vein. The adrenal vein is then clipped approximately 1 cm from the gland, with one or two clips placed adjacent to the adrenal and two or three positioned distally (Fig. 12-5). Following the division of the vein, adrenal mobilization becomes much easier. It is manipulated by grasping the adherent perinephric fat to avoid rupturing the capsule. The adrenal is then pushed cranially, permitting access to its medial and superior portions. This dissection is done with the hook cautery. Anything that offers resistance should be examined and then cauterized or clipped. The adrenal branches of the inferior phrenic vessels are often quite large and should be ligated as the dissection approaches the superior-medial pole of the left adrenal gland.

Once the adrenal gland is free, hemostasis is verified by irrigation and aspiration. The gland is extracted after it has been placed in a sterile plastic bag (Fig. 12-6); bags in a variety of sizes should be available to accommodate variously sized lesions. This bag should be fairly transparent and strong so that it is easy to manipulate and will not rupture during extraction. Rupture could lead to adrenal cell seeding of the incision or abdominal cavity. The bag is removed via the original trocar site by spreading the abdominal wall musculature using a Kelly clamp. The incision may need to be enlarged to facilitate removal of the lesion if it is larger than 4 cm. Usually the wound size must be one-third to one-half the original diameter of the lesion. Drainage is seldom necessary, and this practice has

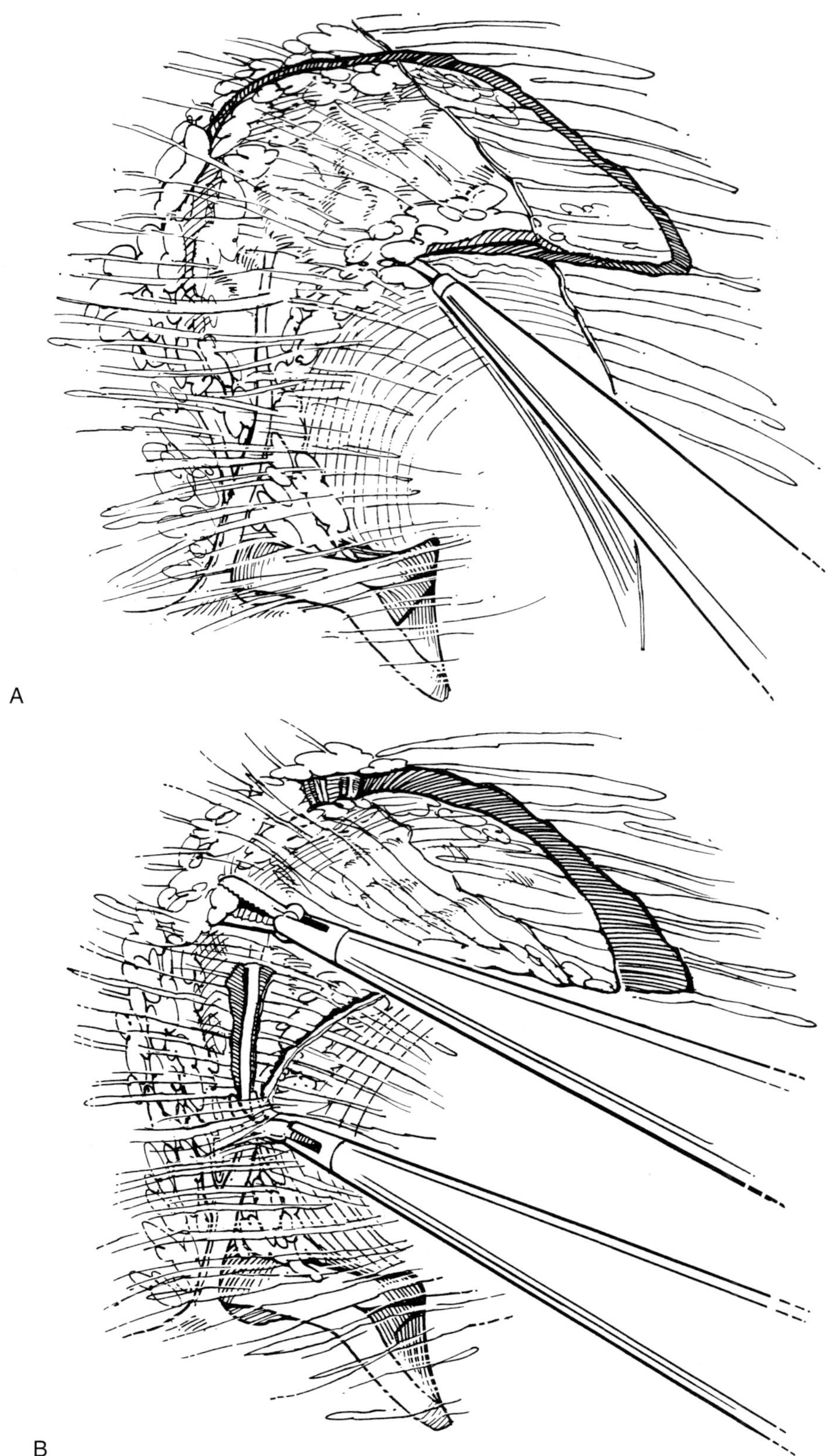

A

B

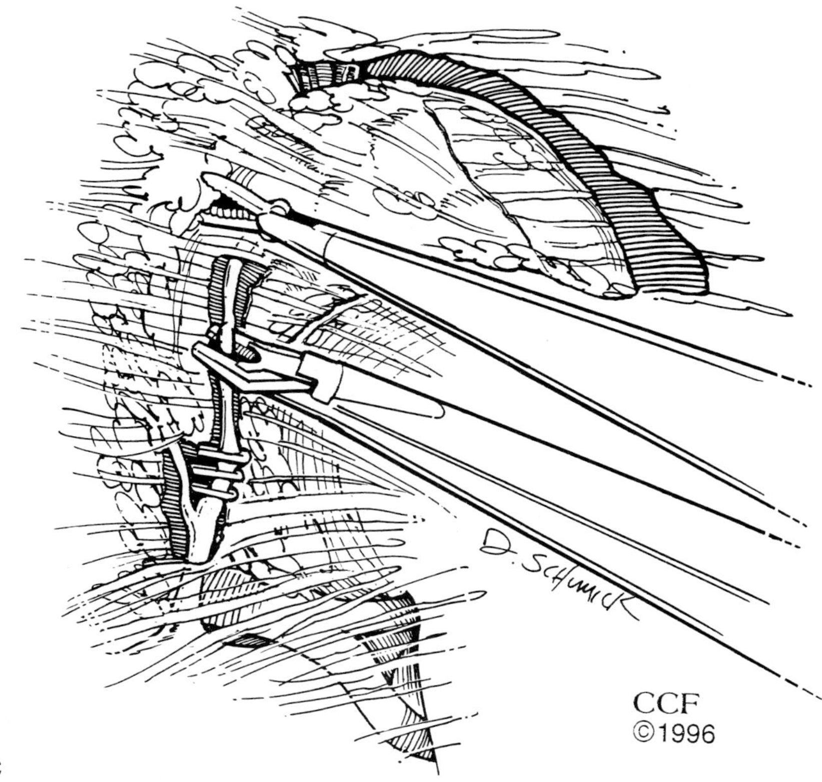

FIG. 12-5. Exposure of the left adrenal vein, with control obtained with several clips. © Cleveland Clinic Education Foundation.

been abandoned in our most recent cases. Early in the postoperative period, patients in a supine position will occasionally have leakage from their most posterior trocar site. This has not been a problem. If one uses a minimal amount of irrigation, this seepage and the need for a drain are avoided altogether. The fascial and skin incisions are closed with absorbable suture, sizes 0 and 4-0, respectively.

LAPAROSCOPIC RIGHT ADRENALECTOMY

The patient is placed in the lateral decubitus position (right side up), with the surgeons facing the patient's abdomen. Pneumoperitoneum is established in the same manner as described for a left adrenalectomy, using a partially open technique with the Veress needle or the open method in patients who have had surgery involving the right upper quadrant. Needle insertion must be done carefully to prevent injury to the liver parenchyma and resultant bleeding or to prevent gas emboli if CO_2 insufflation is initiated in the liver parenchyma. Therefore, the peritoneum is not penetrated with the needle until the liver edge is palpated. Pneumoperitoneum is maintained at 15 mm Hg during the procedure.

The initial incision is made approximately 1.2 to 1.4 cm in length, 2 cm below the costal margin, and in the anterior axillary line. A 10-mm port is placed at this location, followed by the introduction of the 10-mm, 30-degree laparoscope. A diagnostic laparoscopy from this position yields an excellent view of the right hepatic lobe, triangular ligament, diaphragm,

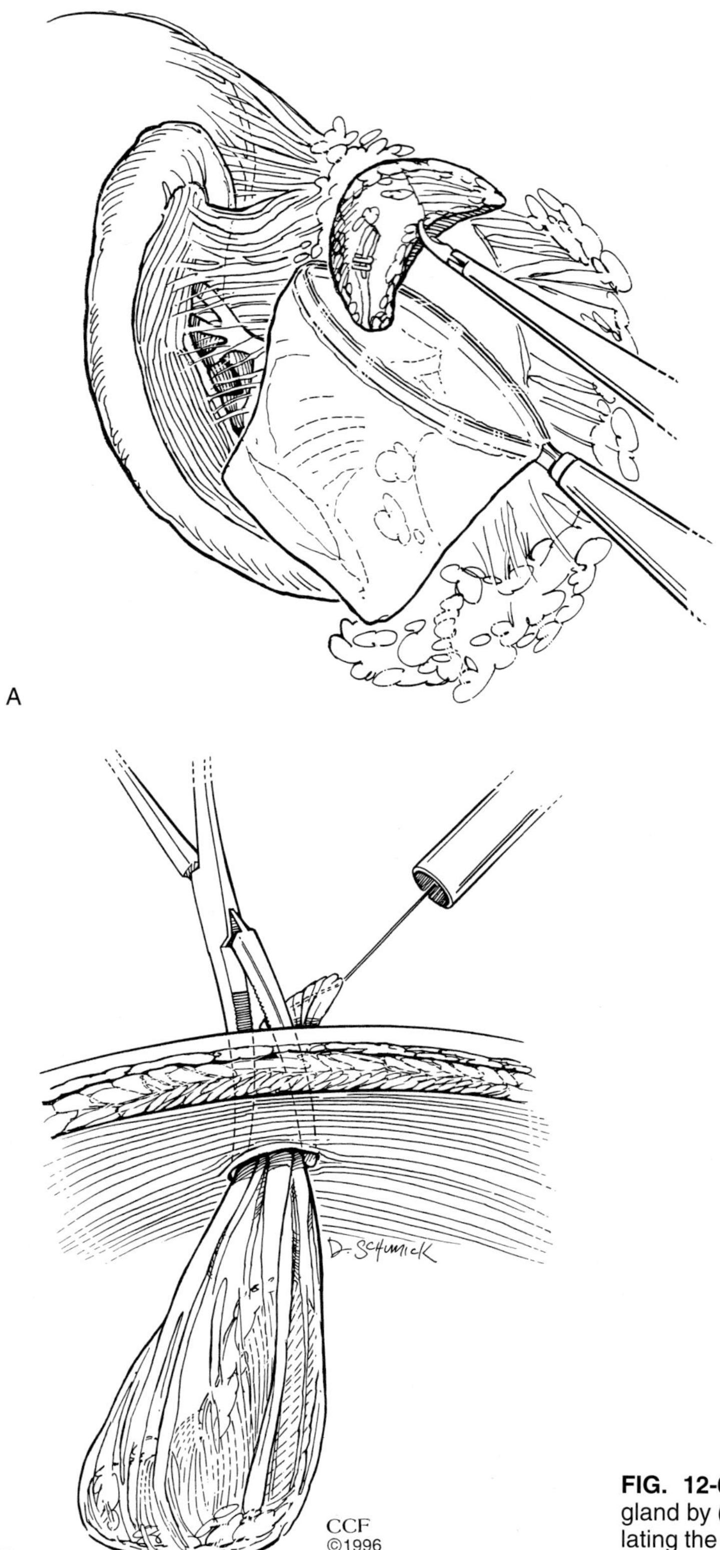

A

B

FIG. 12-6. Extraction of the left adrenal gland by **(A)** placing it into a bag and **(B)** dilating the abdominal wall. © Cleveland Clinic Education Foundation.

and ascending and proximal transverse colons. In women, the right adnexal structures may be inspected for possible pathology, and, in both sexes, the inguinal area is examined for the presence of a hernia.

Following inspection of the abdomen, three additional 10-mm trocars (four total) are placed to perform the operation. Under laparoscopic visualization, the second trocar is inserted into the right flank inferior and slightly posterior to the tip of the eleventh rib; it enters above the hepatic flexure of the colon. This portion of the colon rarely requires any mobilization. The third and fourth trocars are placed more anteriorly, approximately 2 cm from the costal margin, with the most medial port lying along the lateral border of the rectus abdominis muscle. The trocars should be at least 5 cm apart to minimize interference. As our experience with adrenal surgery has expanded, we have moved the trocar positions slightly more anterior compared to what was done in the past (10).

Four trocars are necessary because the right lobe of the liver must be retracted to expose the most medial aspect of the right adrenal gland and the inferior vena cava (Fig. 12-7). Therefore, a fan-type liver retractor is inserted in the most anterior trocar to gently reflect the right hepatic lobe medially. Special attention should be paid to this retractor during the operation to avoid inadvertent hepatic laceration. The procedure is begun with the laparoscope in the second trocar and the surgeon working through the two most lateral ports. The camera can be repositioned dorsally to obtain a better view of the superior aspect of the field of dissection; in this situation, the surgeon works via the middle two trocars.

The liver must be mobilized to obtain the best possible exposure of the junction between the adrenal gland and the inferior vena cava (Fig. 12-8). We prefer to create a right-angled plane between the anterior aspect of the right kidney and the lateral portion of the liver. This plane provides enough room to see

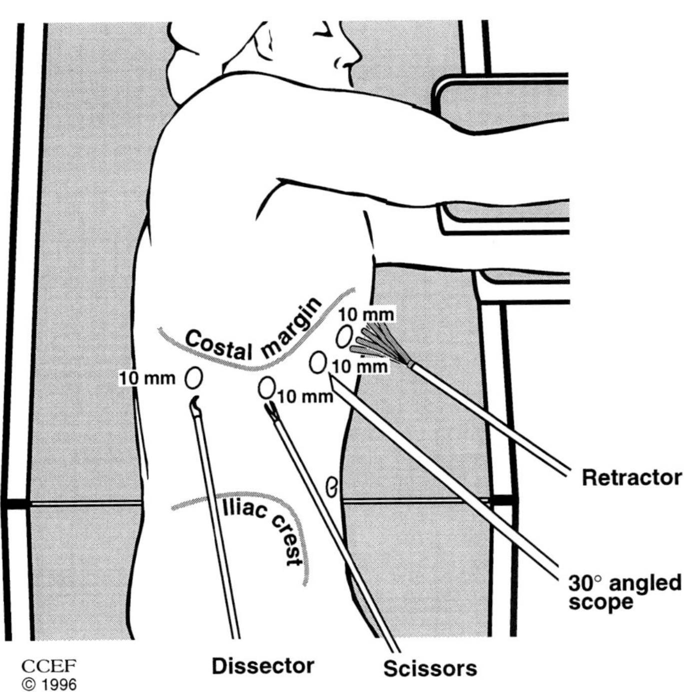

FIG. 12-7. Trocar sites for right laparoscopic adrenalectomy. © Cleveland Clinic Education Foundation.

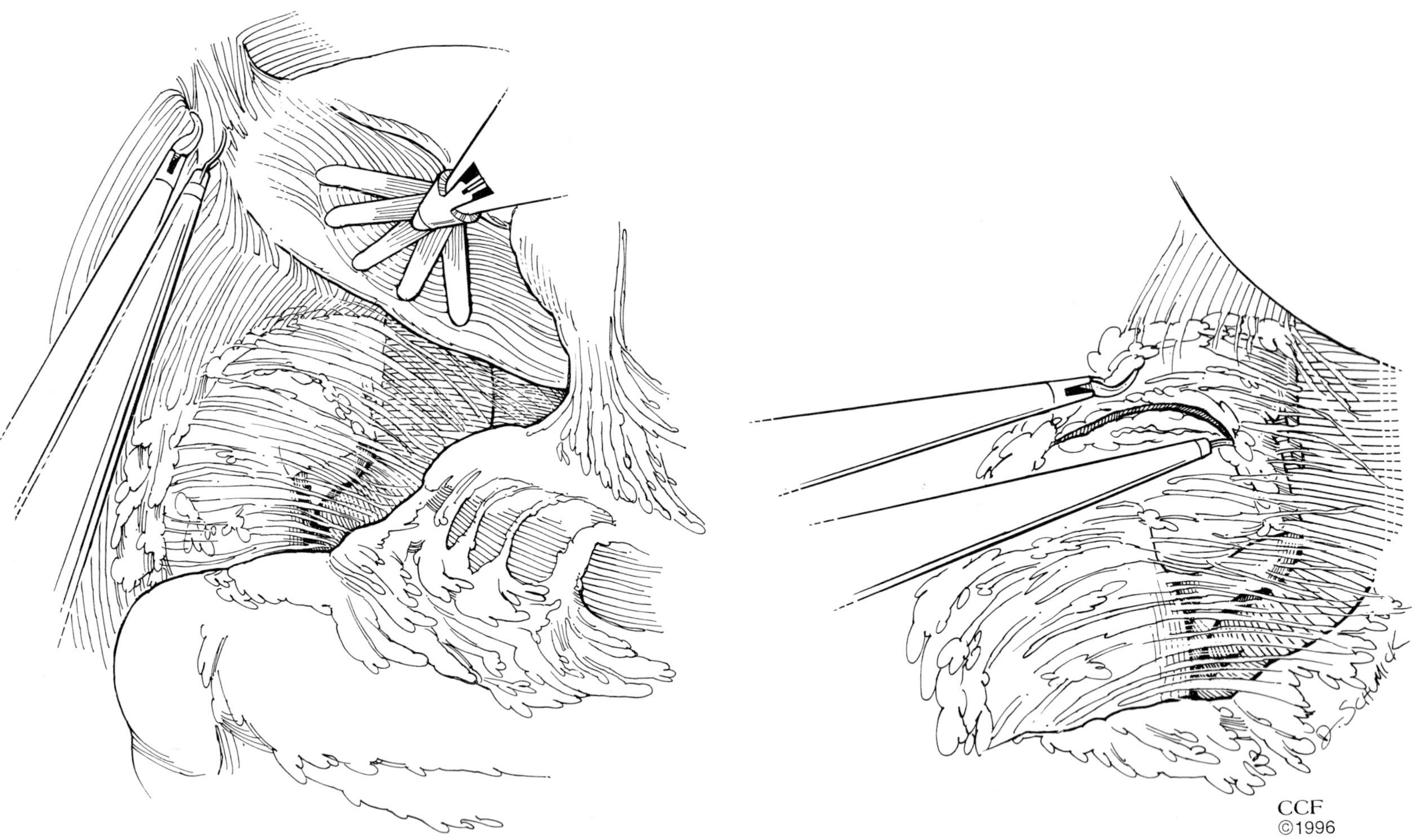

FIG. 12-8. A: Mobilization of the right hepatic attachments. **B:** Incising over the upper pole of the adrenal gland. © Cleveland Clinic Education Foundation.

and work. Therefore, the right lateral hepatic attachments and the triangular ligament are transected using laparoscopic scissors. This dissection is typically carried up to the diaphragm and permits more effective medial retraction of the liver.

The right adrenal gland is dissected next. If the mass is less than 4 cm in diameter, access to the right adrenal vein early in the operation is possible. This permits easier mobilization of the rest of the adrenal gland. The inferior portion is mobilized using the hook cautery or the

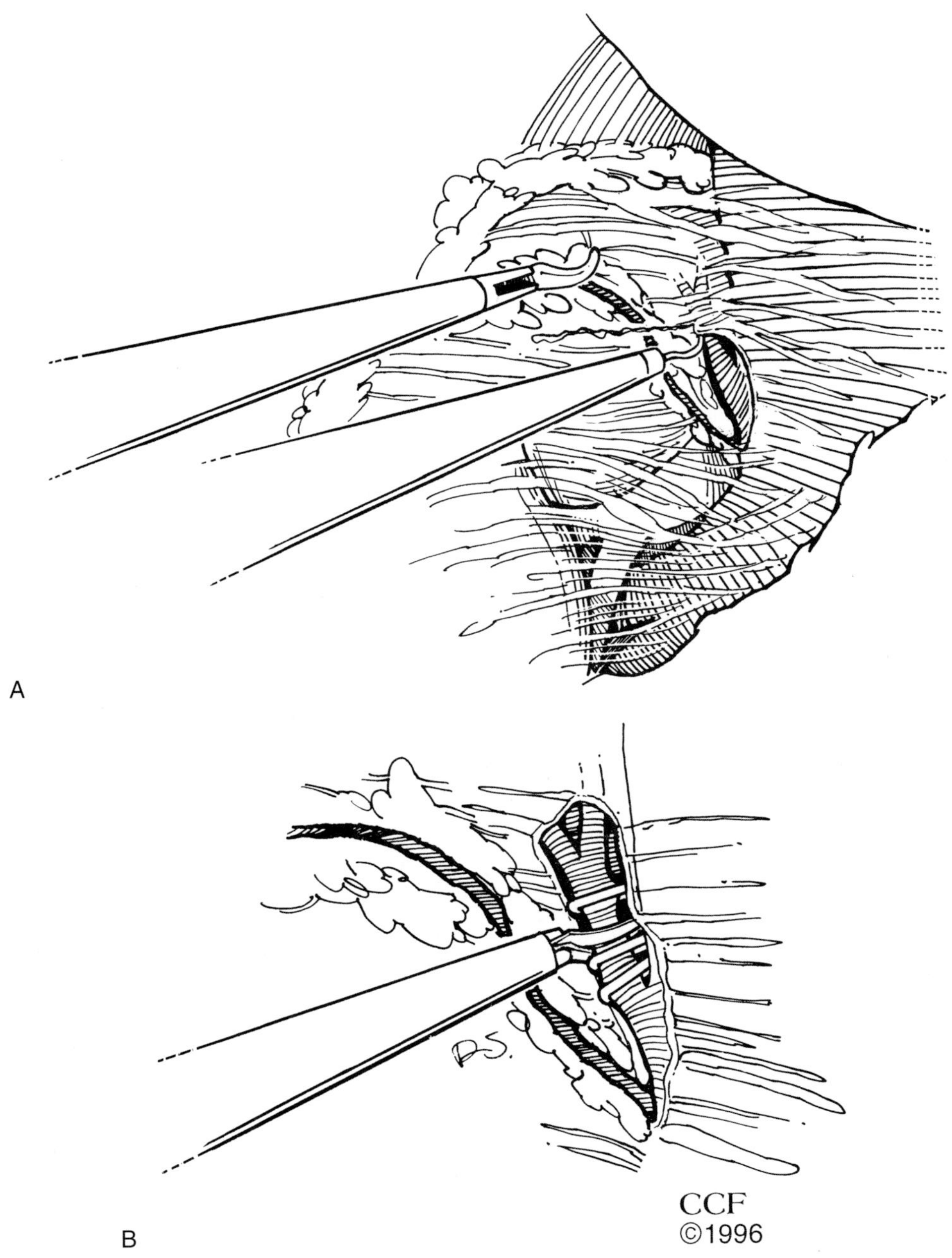

FIG. 12-9. A: Exposure of the right adrenal vein, with **(B)** subsequent clip application and transection of the vessel. © Cleveland Clinic Education Foundation.

laparoscopic 5-mm curved scissors and a grasper/dissector. The dissection is continued medially and superiorly along the lateral edge of the vena cava. The right renal vein is the most inferior extent of the dissection. As one carefully dissects along the vena cava, the right adrenal vein is encountered. This vein is often short and sometimes large. Usually, the vein can be clipped with medium-large titanium clips, with at least two being placed on the vena cava side (Fig. 12-9). If there is not enough space for clips, then the vein can alternatively be divided using a cartridge of a 30- or 35-mm laparoscopic vascular stapler (EndoGIA, U.S. Surgical Corporation, Norwalk, CT, or Ethicon, Johnson & Johnson, Cincinnati, OH). A second adrenal vein of nearly equal length and girth is commonly encoun-

tered and should be carefully controlled as described. At the superior pole of the adrenal, small branches from the inferior phrenic vessels can usually be cauterized with the laparoscopic hook (Fig. 12-10). Again, tilting the bed into a head-up position permits all fluid to migrate downward. The lateral adrenal gland is then dissected from the perinephric fat using the same instruments. Meticulous dissection close to the gland prevents tearing of the lateral branches of the vena cava and other vessels from the retroperitoneum.

When a large mass is encountered, we prefer to dissect laterally and superiorly first and then continue caudally along the vena cava to reach the adrenal vein. Takeda and colleagues describe the use of an ultrasonic aspirator for better dissection of the perinephric fat around

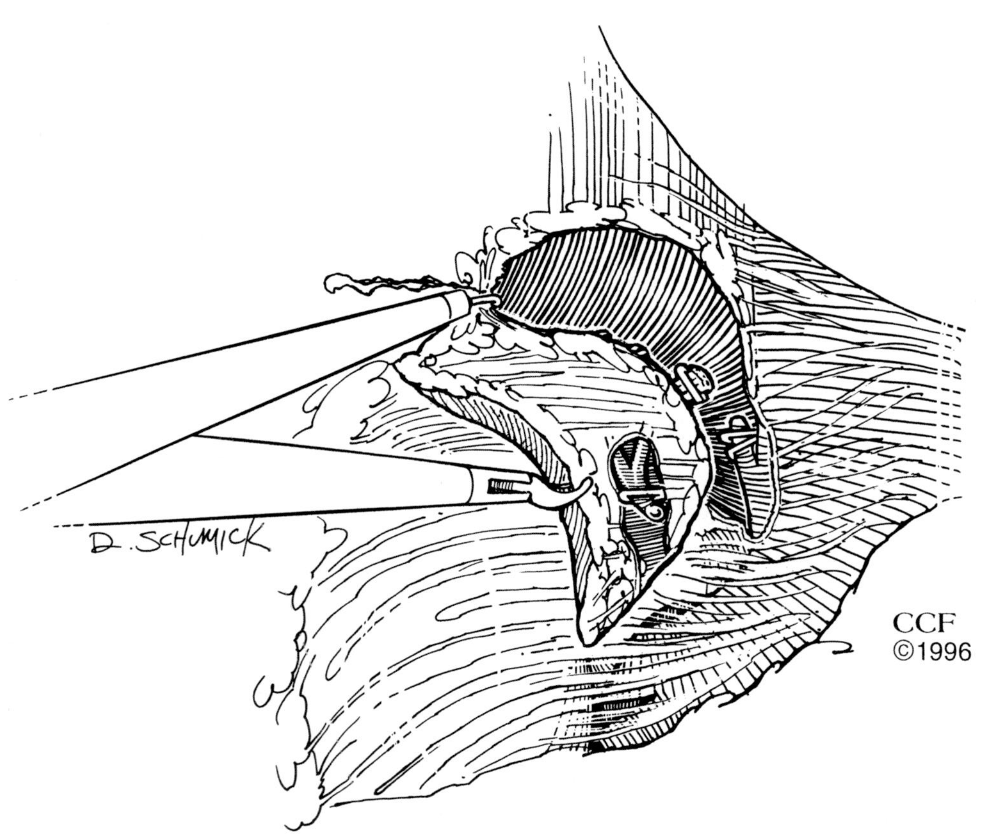

FIG. 12-10. Dissection of the superior extent of the right adrenal gland. © Cleveland Clinic Education Foundation.

the gland, particularly in patients with Cushing's syndrome (11). These authors also advocate using the argon beam coagulator for a right-sided adrenalectomy where the adrenal gland is embedded in the liver parenchyma. The argon beam facilitates partial hepatic resection and subsequent hemostasis.

Once the mass is completely mobilized, a sterile plastic bag with drawstrings is placed in the abdomen, the adrenal is placed in it, and it is removed through the initial incision, as previously described. All wounds are closed as described for the left adrenalectomy.

LAPAROSCOPIC BILATERAL ADRENALECTOMY

Bilateral laparoscopic adrenalectomy is infrequently required. When it is prescribed, we most often start with the patient in the lateral decubitus position with the left side up. Surgery on either side may be performed first; however, because it is easier on the left, with fewer chances of complications in the first half of the proposed procedure, we start on this side. The adrenalectomy is performed using the techniques described. After the procedure has been completed, the patient is repositioned and redraped for a right adrenalectomy. A 15- to 20-minute turnover time is often necessary. If one performs this operation in a supine patient with the trocars in the bilateral subcostal areas, this delay can be avoided; we initially attempted this but found the operation with the patient in the supine position to be more cumbersome. When the patient is in the lateral decubitus position, gravity does most of the retraction, which appears to result in a more smooth and effortless resection. In all of the operations we have performed in this manner, successfully performed bilateral laparoscopic adrenalectomy has been done in a reasonable amount of time. Fernandez-Cruz and colleagues have recommended helium pneumoperitoneum for bilateral laparoscopic adrenalectomy to prevent CO_2 retention (12). This has become less of a problem with improvements in surgical technique, decreased operative time, and mechanical hyperventilation.

POSTOPERATIVE CARE

The postoperative course is similar to that for laparoscopic cholecystectomy, except that some endocrine disorders necessitate additional clinical laboratory studies, steroid administration, or adjustments in antihypertensive medications. Nasogastric tubes are not necessary and are not routinely inserted in these patients. Oral fluids are started slowly on the day of surgery. If a Jackson-Pratt drain has been placed, it is removed the next morning. During the first 12 hours postoperatively, intramuscular narcotic injections or a narcotic pump may be necessary, but by the morning after surgery, nearly all patients take oral pain medication and a regular diet. Most patients are ambulatory on the evening of the procedure and are discharged on the second or third postoperative day.

CONTRAINDICATIONS

Our experience suggests that the absolute contraindications for laparoscopic adrenalectomy are few. We consider invasive adrenal carcinoma to be an absolute contraindication for the laparoscopic approach because of the possible extent and complexity of the operation required: en bloc resection of the kidney with the perinephric fat and spleen, extensive node dissection, and liver resection may be necessary. This operation is therefore formidable and not a desirable situation in which to use laparoscopic techniques at this time. A laparoscopic adrenalectomy can be included en bloc with a laparoscopic nephrectomy for certain indications such as renal cell carcinoma (13). Patients with malignant pheochromocytoma may have periaortic adenopathy. An open technique may be more desirable in these patients, particularly when a nuclear magnetic resonance or a metaiodobenzylguanidine nuclear scan shows that nodes are present in the periaortic chain or close to the bladder.

Another relative contraindication is a coagulopathy that is not adequately reversed preoperatively. One of our early complications occurred in a patient who was anticoagulated as a result of a mechanical mitral valve; a postoperative hematoma subsequently developed. The hematoma was evacuated laparoscopically without further incident, but we have since been meticulous in our workup and preoperative management to avoided this consequence. Major coagulation disorders are an absolute contraindication.

Other contraindications include previous trauma or surgery in the area, such as a nephrectomy or splenectomy. These may create dense adhesions that add to the difficulty of dissection and exposure in this space. A mass that is 10 cm or larger may also be considered a contraindication. The largest that we have resected is 14 cm, but such a mass makes dissection difficult and time-consuming. The time required for dissection depends in part on the surface area of the lesion. The exposure is also difficult because the space available in this area is limited. Frequently, large masses have unusual and numerous retroperitoneal feeding vessels that require tedious dissection and many clips to control. Only surgeons with extensive laparoscopic experience should attempt resection of larger adrenal masses.

RESULTS

From January 1992 to November 1995, we performed a total of 85 explorations and resections. Seventy-six were performed locally, and nine were done abroad. Of these, 75 were recently analyzed. Seventy-two adrenalectomies and three biopsies were done. Table 12-1 shows the indications for 67 of the procedures. The overall mean age was 44 years, and 60% of the patients (n = 43) were women.

Thirty-seven of the adrenalectomies were performed on the left, 31 on the right, and seven bilaterally. The mean operating time was 2.1 hours. The right side required more time, an average of 138 minutes compared to 102 minutes on the left. The time required for a bilateral adrenalectomy averaged approximately 45 minutes longer than the combined averages for the unilateral procedures alone. The indications for bilateral adrenalectomy

TABLE 12–1. *Indications for laparoscopic adrenalectomy in 67 of 72 patients*[a]

Indication	Patients (*n*)
Pheochromocytoma	19
Nonfunctional adenoma	11
Conn's syndrome	9
Cushing's adenoma	7
Cushing's disease	6
Paraneoplastic hypercortisolism	2
Metastasis	2
Macronodular hyperplasia	2
Carcinoma	2
Angiomyolipoma	2
Other	5

[a]Data were not available for the remaining five patients.

are listed on Table 12-2. The mean diameter of the lesions removed in this series was 4.1 cm (range, 1–14 cm). Overall, the mean postoperative stay was 3 days (range, 2–19 days). The mean number of postoperative narcotic injections was 5.5.

Conversion from laparoscopy to laparotomy was necessary in only two patients. One patient, who was thought to have a nonfunctioning adenoma on the left, was found to have a retroperitoneal sarcoma. In this case, a laparotomy was required to perform an en bloc resection of the sarcoma with the adrenal gland. The other conversion to an open technique occurred in the first patient in whom we attempted a minimally invasive adrenalectomy. The patient had a 15-cm angiomyolipoma. After the anterior surface was dissected, access to the posterior gland was difficult and vessels could not easily be controlled. This was partially related to our inexperience and to the fact that we attempted the procedure with the patient in the supine position.

TABLE 12–2. *Indications for bilateral laparoscopic adrenalectomy in 72 patients undergoing adrenalectomy*

Indication	Patients (*n*)
Malignant pheochromocytoma	2
Benign pheochromocytoma	1
Cushing's disease	2
Bilateral adenoma	1
Bilateral macronodular hyperplasia	1

Reoperations during the same admission were required in two patients and were accomplished laparoscopically. We evacuated a retroperitoneal hematoma in a patient who had been anticoagulated for a mitral valve prosthesis. The anticoagulation may have contributed to this patient's development of a large hematoma postoperatively. In one recent patient who was known to have asymptomatic gallstones preoperatively, acute cholecystitis developed on the fourth postoperative day, necessitating a laparoscopic cholecystectomy. The postoperative course following the cholecystectomy was uneventful. Other associated laparoscopic procedures are listed in Table 12-3.

Complications secondary to laparoscopic adrenalectomy are listed in Table 12-4. Of the 75 patients, 15% had perioperative complications and 15% had postoperative complications. Complications encountered in our last 30 patients who were not represented in the series presented include pulmonary edema 24 hours postoperatively and acute cholecystitis, as previously mentioned. In one patient, a small rim of approximately 1 mm of normal adrenal tissue was left behind as a result of a partially intrahepatic right adrenal gland. This procedure involved a well-circumscribed, nonfunctioning adenoma, which was removed *in toto* because of its location in the lateral portion of the gland. More than half of the patients had had previous abdominal surgery, but this did not interfere with the laparoscopic approach.

Patients with pheochromocytoma generally are considered separately in surgical studies.

TABLE 12–3. *Additional laparoscopic procedures performed during adrenalectomy in 72 patients*

Procedure	Patients (*n*)
Liver biopsy	5
Cholecystectomy	4
CBD exploration	1
Colorectal reanastomosis	1
Left ovarian cystectomy	1
Periaortic node dissection	1

CBD, common bile duct.

TABLE 12–4. *Type and number of complications occurring in 72 patients undergoing laparoscopic adrenalectomy*

Type of complication	Number
Perioperative	
Bleeding	1
Hypotension/hypertension	5
Postoperative	
Subdural hematoma	1
Urinary tract infection	1
Hematomas	2
Colonic pseudo-obstructions	1
Anemia	2

These tumors are generally larger: in our series, 6.3 cm versus 3.5 cm in patients who did not have pheochromocytoma ($p < .05$). Operative time was also longer, 2.5 hours versus 1.8 hours ($p < .05$). Almost 90% (seven of eight) of perioperative complications and 67% (six of nine) of postoperative complications were observed in the pheochromocytoma group. Associated multiple endocrine neoplasia (MEN) IIA syndrome was identified in six patients and MEN IIB in two patients. Metastases originating from medullary thyroid carcinoma were seen in 1 patient and metastases from the pheochromocytoma in 4 of 19 patients.

DISCUSSION

Our small series indicates that laparoscopic adrenalectomy is a safe, successful, and well-tolerated treatment for a range of endocrine disorders affecting the adrenal gland. This concept is supported worldwide (14–22). To study this, we retrospectively reviewed our open adrenalectomies performed over the past 10 years and compared them to our laparoscopic cases. Most often, the open technique was performed via the anterior route (82%), with the remainder being posterior (13%) or lateral (4%) approaches. The right adrenal was most often removed (67%). The indications for conventional adrenalectomy were primary hyperaldosteronism (33%), Cushing's adenoma (21%), pheochromocytoma (21%), nonsecreting adenoma (13%), and a variety of other pathologies (13%). In this analysis, there was no difference in operating time or adrenal dimensions. The estimated blood loss was less than 100 ml for the laparoscopic adrenalectomy versus approximately 200 ml for the open procedure; this difference was not statistically significant. The mean hospital stay for the conventional adrenalectomy patients was 9 days versus just more than 3 days for the laparoscopic group ($p <.01$). The total dose of narcotics used (500 mg versus 800 mg) and the time required for patient mobilization (1 day versus 3 days) were significantly lower in the laparoscopic group ($p <.01$).

Other studies have reported similar outcomes. Prinz compared conventional transabdominal and posterior adrenalectomy with the laparoscopic approach in lesions less than 10 cm (23). Although there were no differences in operating time for laparoscopic and anterior (open) adrenalectomy, the posterior approach required less time. The hospital stay was significantly shorter with laparoscopy (2.1 days) than with either conventional method (5 or 6 days). Another difference noted was the dramatic decrease in the number of meperidine doses used postoperatively by the laparoscopic patient group. A comparative study by Naito and colleagues also revealed a lower analgesia requirement in the laparoscopic group and a faster return to a normal diet and ambulation (24). These authors did document a longer operating time; however, the comparison was between their first six laparoscopic cases and their last 11 conventional cases. In the experience of Guazzoni and colleagues, the blood loss in laparoscopic surgery was less. In fact, in a comparative study of 40 patients, the three patients who received blood transfusions were in the open group; major complications also occurred only in the patients treated by laparotomy (6).

We, as well as others, believe that laparoscopic adrenalectomy is becoming the procedure of choice for hyperaldosteronism (25–27), Cushing's pituitary (1,2,28), and possibly pheochromocytoma (1,12,29). Bilateral laparoscopic adrenalectomy appears to facilitate the management of a failed transsphenoidal hypophysectomy for Cushing's disease with less discomfort and wound morbidity. Given this option, patients may be less reluctant to have a third or fourth surgical procedure performed for this disorder. Laparoscopic management of pheochromocytomas has also resulted in decreased discomfort and a reduced hospital stay, with an acceptable complication rate compared to historical controls.

Fletcher and colleagues have emphasized the need for adequate training and preparation to do these procedures and strongly advocate cadaver or animal experience before performing laparoscopic adrenalectomy in humans (30). We have used the pig model effectively to practice adrenal and vena cava dissection, as well as various extraction techniques (7).

CONCLUSION

The use of minimally invasive techniques to remove the adrenal gland has shown promise over the past several years. We believe that we have seen improvements in patient outcome with the development of this procedure, even though a majority of the comparisons were made in a retrospective manner. If the success and superior patient tolerance of this operation continue to be documented, the indications for adrenalectomy may slowly expand. Among other advantages, we may come to resect nonfunctioning adrenal masses when they are smaller than 5 to 6 cm or perhaps perform bilateral adrenalectomy with concomitant oophorectomy for advanced breast cancer instead of performing the chemotherapeutic organ ablation presently used.

REFERENCES

1. Gagner M, Lacroix A, Bolte E. Laparoscopic adrenalectomy in Cushing's syndrome and pheochromocytoma. *N Engl J Med* 1992;327(14):1003–1006.
2. Gagner M, Lacroix A, Prinz R, et al. Early experience with laparoscopic approach for adrenalectomy. *Surgery* 1993;114(6):1120–1125.
3. Gagner M, Lacroix A, Bolte E. Laparoscopic adrenalectomy. *Surg Endosc* 1993;7(2):122.
4. Higashihara E, Tanaka Y, Horie S, et al. A case report of laparoscopic adrenalectomy. *Jpn J Urol* 1992;83:1130.
5. Higashihara E, Tanaka Y, Nutahara, et al. Laparoscopic

adrenalectomy: technical review. *Jpn J Urol ESWL* 1992;5(2):150–153.

6. Guazzoni G, Montorsi F, Bocciardi A, et al. Transperitoneal laparoscopic versus open adrenalectomy for benign hyperfunctioning adrenal tumors: a comparative study. *J Urol* 1995;153(5):1597–1600.

7. Park A, Gagner M. A porcine model for laparoscopic adrenalectomy. *Surg Endosc* 1995;9(7):807–810.

8. Vaughan ED Jr. Adrenal surgery. In: Marshall FF, ed. *Atlas of urologic surgery*. Philadelphia: WB Saunders, 1991,131–156.

9. Prinz RA. Mobilization of the right lobe of the liver for right adrenalectomy. *Am J Surg* 1990;159(3):336–338.

10. Gagner M, Lacroix A, Bolte E, et al. Laparoscopic adrenalectomy: the importance of a flank approach in lateral decubitus position. *Surg Endosc* 1994;8:135–138.

11. Takeda M, Go H, Imai T, et al. Experience with 17 cases of laparoscopic adrenalectomy: use of ultrasonic aspirator and argon beam coagulator. *J Urol* 1994;152(3):902–905.

12. Fernandez-Cruz L, Saenz A, Taura P, et al. Pheochromocytoma: laparoscopic approach with CO_2 and helium pneumoperitoneum. *Endosc Surg Allied Technol* 1994;2 (6):300–304.

13. Rassweiler JJ, Henkel TO, Potempa DM, et al. The technique of transperitoneal laparoscopic nephrectomy, adrenalectomy, and nephroureterectomy. *Eur Urol* 1993;23(4):425–430.

14. Stanley DG. Laparoscopic adrenalectomy. *Int Surg* 1994;79(3):253–258.

15. Fernandez-Cruz L, Benarroch G, Torres E, et al. Laparoscopic approach to adrenal tumors. *J Laparoendosc Surg* 1993;3(6):541–546.

16. Costantino GN, Mukalian GG, Vincent GJ, et al. Laparoscopic adrenalectomy. *J Laparoendosc Surg* 1993;3 (3):309–311.

17. Guazzoni G, Montorsi F, Bergamaschi F, et al. Effectiveness and safety of laparoscopic adrenalectomy. *J Urol* 1994;152(5 pt 1):1375–1378.

18. Ono Y, Katoh N, Kinukawa T, et al. Laparoscopic nephrectomy, radical nephrectomy, and adrenalectomy: Nagoya experience. *J Urol* 1994;152(6 pt 1): 1962–1966.

19. Higashihara E, Tanaka Y, Horie S, et al. Laparoscopic adrenalectomy: the initial 3 cases. *J Urol* 1993;149(5): 973–976.

20. Peschel R, Janetschek G, Reissigl A, et al. Left-sided laparoscopic adrenalectomy. *Scand J Urol Nephrol* 1993;27(4):527–529.

21. Albala DM. Laparoscopic nephrectomy and adrenalectomy. *Semin Surg Oncol* 1994;10(6):417.

22. Fernandez-Cruz L, Saenz A, Benarroch G, et al. Technical aspects of adrenalectomy via operative laparoscopy. *Surg Endosc* 1994;8(11):1348–1351.

23. Prinz RA. A comparison of laparoscopic and open adrenalectomies. *Arch Surg* 1995;130(5):489–492.

24. Naito S, Uozomi J, Ichimaya H, et al. Laparoscopic adrenalectomy: comparison with open adrenalectomy. *Eur Urol* 1994;26(3):253–257.

25. Sardi A, McKinnon W. Laparoscopic adrenalectomy for primary aldosteronism. *JAMA* 1993;269(8):989–990.

26. Takeda M, Go H, Imai T, et al. Laparoscopic adrenalectomy for primary aldosteronism: report of initial ten cases. *Surgery* 1994;115(5):621–625.

27. Go H, Takeda M, Takahashi H, et al. Laparoscopic adrenalectomy for primary aldosteronism: a new operative method. *J Laparoendosc Surg* 1993;3(5):455–459.

28. Whittle DE, Schroeder D, Purchas SH, et al. Laparoscopic retroperitoneal left adrenalectomy in a patient with Cushing's syndrome. *Aust N Z J Surg* 1994;64(5): 375–376.

29. Meurisse M, Joris J, Hamoir E, et al. Laparoscopic adrenalectomy in pheochromocytoma and Cushing's syndrome: reflections about two cases reports. *Acta Chir Belg* 1994;94(6):301–306.

30. Fletcher DR, Beiles CB, Hardy KJ. Laparoscopic adrenalectomy. *Aust N Z J Surg* 1994;64(6):427–430.

Medical and Surgical Management of
Adrenal Diseases, edited by Joseph C. Cerny.
Lippincott Williams & Wilkins, Philadelphia © 1999.

13

Adrenal Surgery

Joseph C. Cerny

Department of Urology, Henry Ford Hospital, Detroit, Michigan 48202

Surgery of the adrenal gland has undergone dramatic change and improvement in the past 25 years. Major advances in adrenal imaging (see Chapter 3) have enabled precise preoperative delineation and localization of adrenal masses, metastases, and ectopic foci, allowing targeted operative procedures and minimizing the need for exploration. Laparoscopic adrenalectomy, with its reduced morbidity and other advantages, is increasingly applicable for most adrenal tumors. Sophisticated, efficient diagnostic algorithms permit early diagnosis and have demystified the spectrum of adrenal endocrinopathies. Significant improvements in preoperative preparation, anesthesia, and perioperative care have reduced the morbidity and mortality rates of adrenal surgery, such that overall operative mortality rate for surgical resection of pheochromocytoma (see Chapter 11), once a hazardous undertaking, is presently less than 2%.

PREOPERATIVE, PERIOPERATIVE CONSIDERATIONS

The successful operative management of a patient with an adrenal tumor represents the culmination of expertise of a team made up of endocrinologists, radiologists, anesthesiologists, urologic surgeons, and endocrine or general surgeons.

Preoperative preparation of patients with Cushing's syndrome (see Chapter 4), primary aldosteronism (see Chapter 5), and pheochromocytoma (see Chapter 11) is discussed within their respective chapters, as well as in Chapter 10. To summarize the essential factors in preparing patients for adrenal surgery, however, the following are necessary components of a successful surgical outcome (1):

1. Cushing's syndrome. Eradication of infection and control of abnormal glucose levels/diabetes are essential. Perioperative cortisone acetate, 100 mg intramuscularly (IM), is given the evening before and morning of surgery, as well as immediately postoperatively. Hydrocortisone intravenously (IV), 5 to 10 mg/h, is begun and cortisone acetate decreased from 75 mg IM every 8 hours on postoperative days 1 and 2, to every 12 hours on days 3 and 4. An equivalent of hydrocortisone, 300 mg per 24 hours, in the immediate postoperative period is then decreased to oral maintenance doses of hydrocortisone 25 mg twice daily and fludrocortisone 0.1 mg/d at the time of discharge. Replacement therapy may be necessary for many months, depending on the degree of contralateral adrenal gland suppression.

2. Primary aldosteronism. Hypertension and hypokalemia are usually corrected with spironolactone, 100 to 300 mg/d for 4 to 6 weeks. In refractory cases, usually those with a very large aldosterone-producing adenoma, potassium supplementation or specific antihypertensive therapy may be needed.

3. Pheochromocytoma. Alpha-adrenergic blockade with dibenzyline, 20 to 100

mg/d, is given for 1 to 2 weeks preoperatively. Volume expansion may be necessary. Beta-blockade is rarely needed unless cardiac arrhythmia persists, and only after alpha-blockade has been established. Preoperatively, the endocrinologist and anesthesiologist must work in close collaboration. Adequate intraoperative monitoring includes using central venous pressure, an intraarterial line, and electrocardiogram. There must be immediate intraoperative availability of beta-receptor antagonists and plasma volume expanders for cardiac arrhythmia or hypotension.

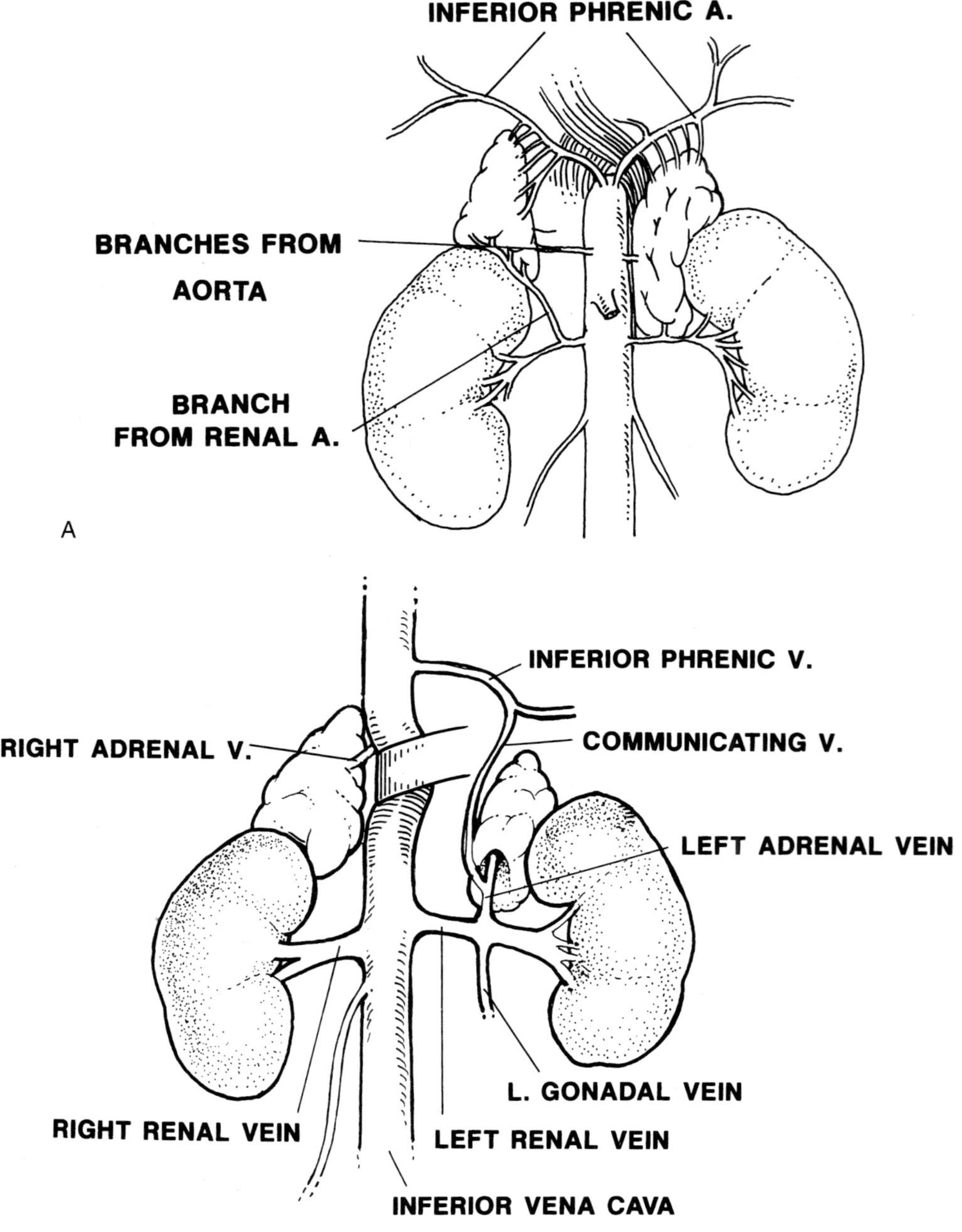

FIG. 13-1. Arterial supply **(A)** and venous drainage **(B)** of the adrenal glands.

SURGICAL ANATOMY

Surgery of the adrenal glands requires a fundamental knowledge of the anatomic relationships of these paired retroperitoneal structures. While contemporary imaging modalities such as CT, MRI, and isotope scanning permit precise preoperative localization of adrenal tumors, eliminating the need for bilateral exploration, successful, uncomplicated adrenal surgery demands a comprehensive understanding of the basic anatomic principles outlined in Chapter 1.

Technically important considerations include (a) the several origins of the adrenal arterial blood supply, significant during surgical mobilization of the gland (Fig. 13-1A), (b) the posterolateral entry of the right adrenal vein into the inferior vena cava, which necessitates meticulous dissection and ligation to avoid caval injury (see Fig. 13-1B), and (c) the multiple relationships of the adrenals to the diaphragm, pleura, and kidneys, as well as to the infradiaphragmatic great vessels and associated viscera, including the liver, spleen, and pancreas, contribute to the complexity of adrenal surgery (Figs. 13-2 and 13-3).

SURGICAL APPROACHES

The selection of an appropriate approach or incision for adrenal surgery depends in large part upon the diagnosis and type of adrenal pathology (Table 13-1). Individual patient considerations such as whether the tumor is small, large, or multifocal, the need for intraabdominal exploration, degree of confidence in preoperative localization studies, prior retroperitoneal or transabdominal surgery, patient habitus, and preference and experience of the operating surgeon, are also important factors in selecting the most suitable surgical option in a particular case.

Regardless of the surgical approach, there are common operative principles and considerations in all cases, whether by open or laparoscopic technique, which include the following technical caveats:

1. Adrenal exposure must be optimal to facilitate ready identification of small tumors.
2. The diseased adrenal gland is friable, and cannot be directly grasped lest fragmentation, bleeding, and intramedullary hematoma formation precludes recognition of pathology. Dissection is performed by grasping the periadrenal fat and fascia rather than the gland itself.
3. Adrenal mobilization is facilitated by clipping/ligating and dividing the superior and lateral arterioles and fascia early in the dissection, leaving attachments to

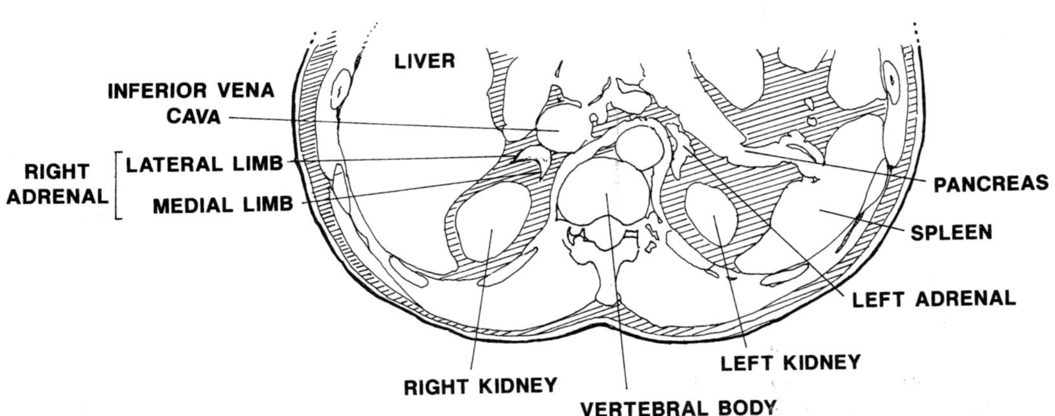

FIG. 13-2. Schematic representation of structures seen on computed tomography section at the level of the adrenal glands.

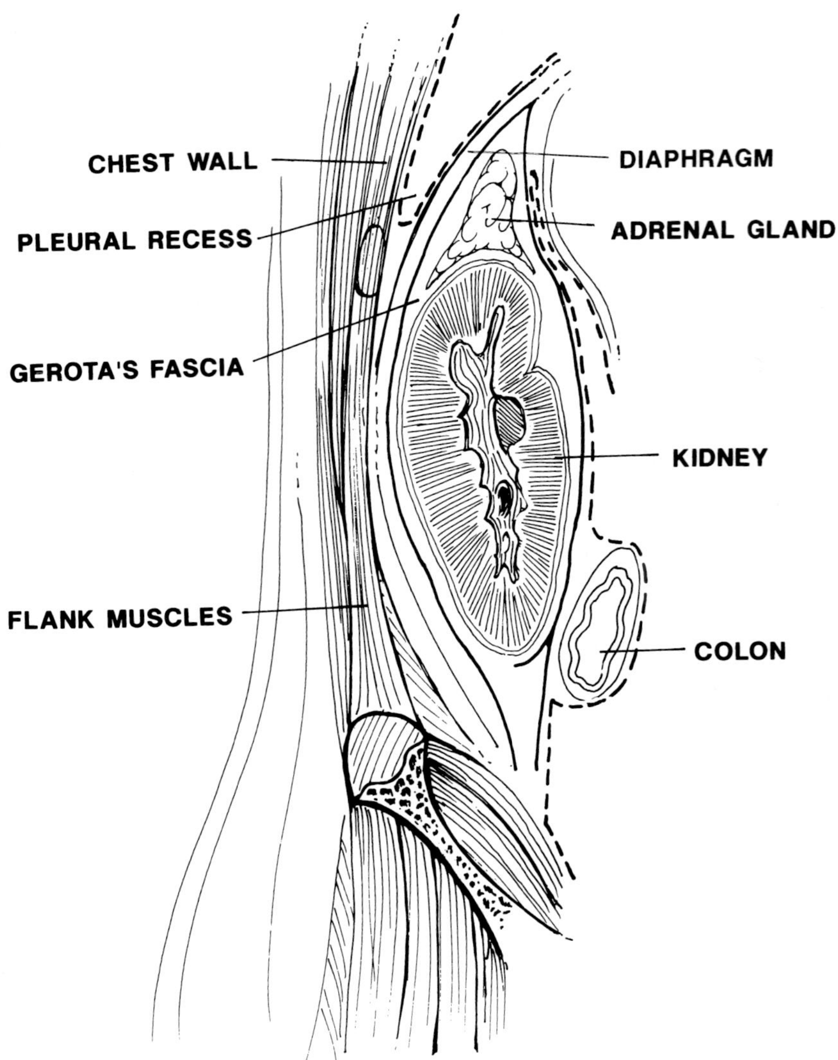

FIG. 13-3. Anatomic relationships demonstrated on sagittal section through the right adrenal gland and kidney. (Modified from William PL, Warwick R, Dyson M, et al., eds. *Gray's Anatomy*. Edinburgh: Churchill Livingstone, 1989.)

the kidney intact. Thus, gentle downward retraction of the kidney with the attached adrenal results in excellent exposure. Liberal use of surgical clips for the numerous arteriolar branches and fascial attachments achieves hemostasis and ready mobilization of the gland.

4. When operating upon the right adrenal, especially via a posterior or flank incision, gentle retraction, dissection, and ligation of the adrenal vein is necessary to avoid inferior vena caval injury and major hemorrhage.

5. In patients with pheochromocytoma, early ligation of the adrenal vein is necessary.

Posterior Approach

The traditional bilateral posterior approach for simultaneous exploration of both adrenals is no longer necessary, because precise preop-

TABLE 13–1. *Surgical options*

Disorder	Approach
Pheochromocytoma	Transabdominal (chevron)
	Thoracoabdominal
	Flank 11th rib
	Laparoscopy
Primary hyperaldosteronism	Laparoscopy
	Posterior (11th or 12th rib)
	Flank 11th rib
Cushing's adenoma	Laparoscopy
	Flank 11th rib
	Posterior (11th or 12th rib)
	Transabdominal ⎱ Large tumors
	Thoracoabdominal ⎰ Carcinoma
Cushing's disease	Laparoscopy
	Bilateral posterior
	Transabdominal
	Bilateral flank 11th rib
Bilateral hyperplasia	Laparoscopy
	Bilateral posterior
	Transabdominal
	Bilateral flank 11th rib
Bilateral adrenal ablation	Laparoscopy
	Bilateral posterior
Adrenal carcinoma	Transabdominal
	Thoracoabdominal
	Transthoracic
Neuroblastoma	Transabdominal
Adrenal incidentaloma	Laparoscopy
	Flank 11th rib
	Anterior (tumor >6 cm)

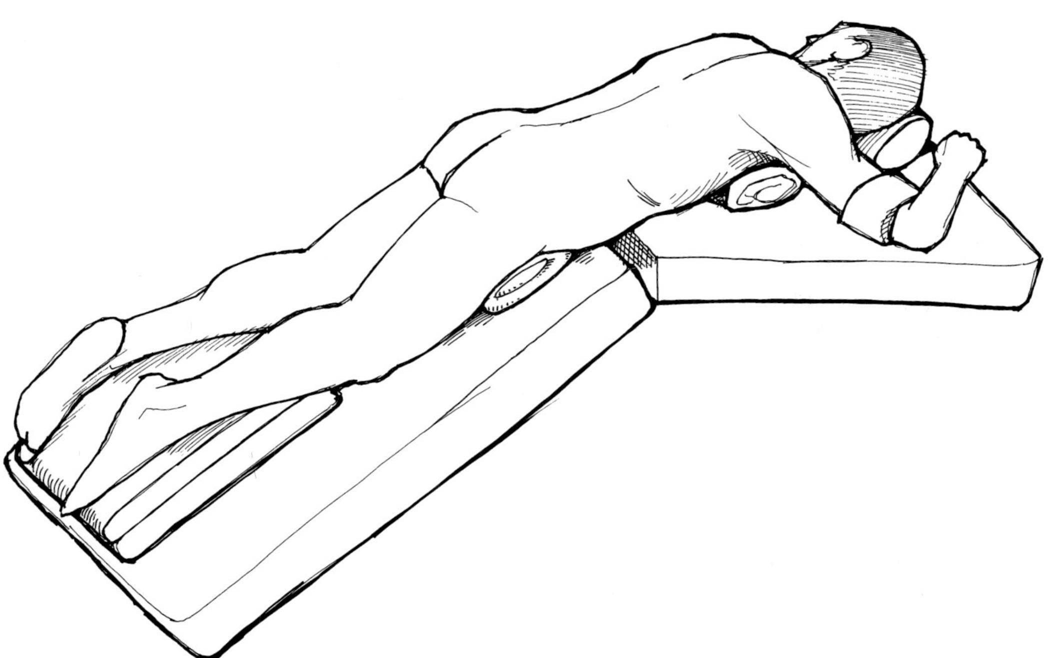

FIG. 13-4. Patient position for the posterior approach. (Modified from Hinman F. *Atlas of Urologic Surgery.* Philadelphia: WB Saunders, 1989:19;860.)

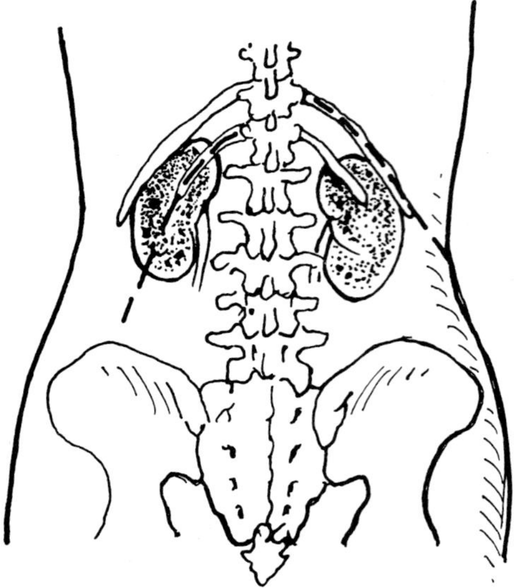

FIG. 13-5. Incision through the twelfth rib on the left side and the eleventh rib on the right. (Modified from Novick AC. Surgery for Primary Aldosteronism. In: Libertino JA, Novick AC, eds. Adrenal Surgery. *Urol Clin North Am* 1989;16:3,539.)

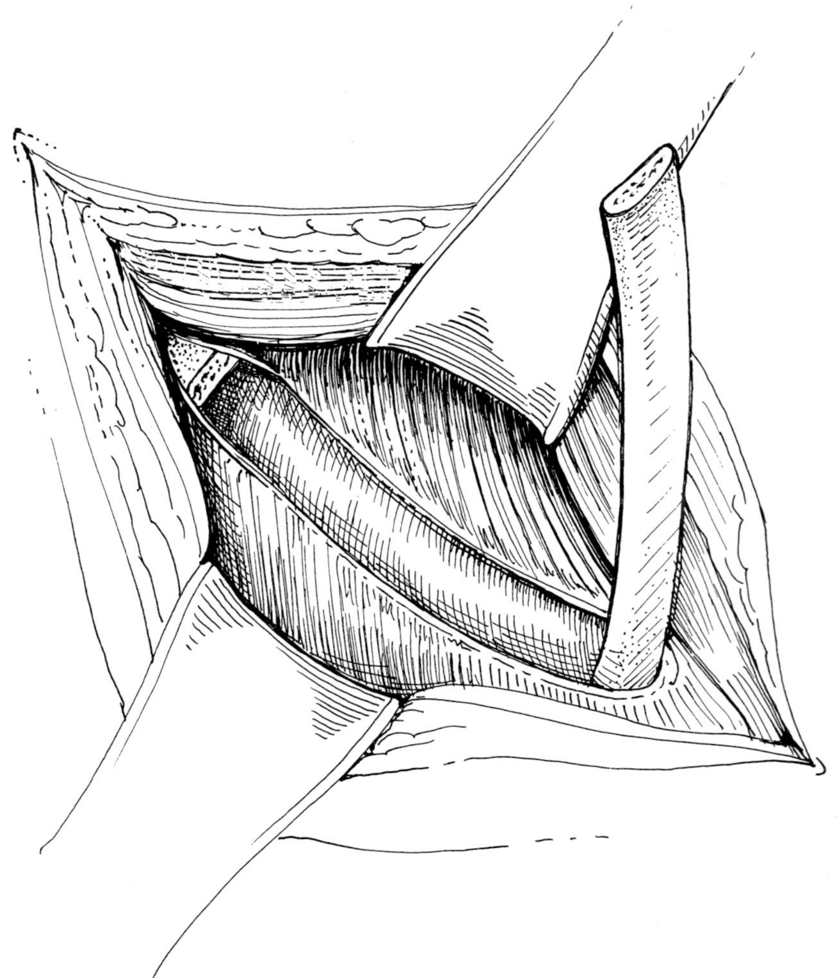

FIG. 13-6. Subperiosteal resection of left twelfth rib. (Modified from Bloom LS, Libertino J. Surgical management of Cushing's syndrome. In: Libertino JA, Novick AC, eds. Adrenal Surgery. *Urol Clin North Am* 1989;16:3,556.)

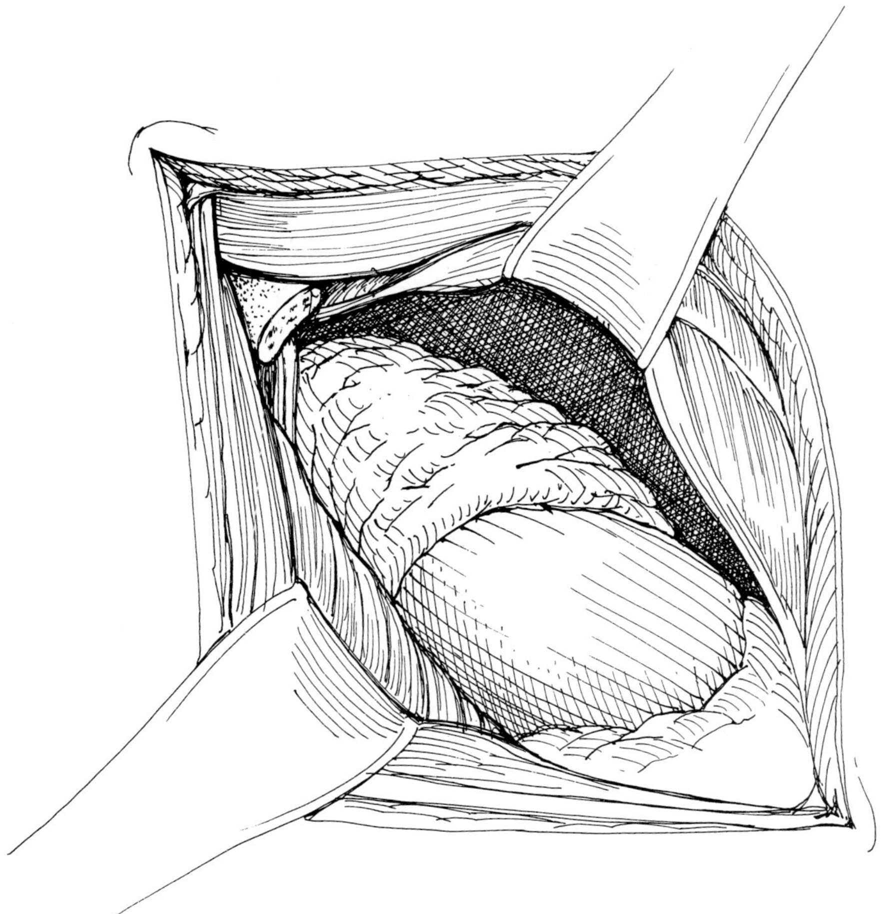

FIG. 13-7. Completion of incision and retraction of eleventh rib and diaphragm superiorly provides excellent adrenal exposure on the left. (Modified from Bloom LS, Libertino J. Surgical Management of Cushing's Syndrome. In: Libertino JA, Novick AC, eds. Adrenal Surgery. *Urol Clin North Am* 1989;16:3,556.)

erative localization of functioning adenomas in primary aldosteronism and Cushing's syndrome has become routine. Rarely, in patients with Cushing's disease who have failed to respond to transsphenoidal microsurgical removal of an adrenocorticotropic hormone–secreting pituitary adenoma, or pituitary irradiation, bilateral posterior excision of the hyperplastic adrenals may be necessary. In virtually all other clinical situations, the posterior approach is used for a unilateral incision, which permits direct access to either adrenal gland, has low morbidity, and is suitable for small, localized, benign adrenal tumors.

The patient is placed in the prone position with firm pillows or rolls supporting the shoulders and pelvis, avoiding compression of the chest and abdomen, and the operating table is flexed to 35 degrees (Fig. 13-4). The incision is made through the bed of the twelfth rib for exposure of the left adrenal and the bed of the eleventh rib for the more superiorly located right adrenal (Fig. 13-5). A variety of posterior incisions have been described; we prefer an oblique incision directly over the eleventh or twelfth rib, to the midaxillary line. The rib is resected subperiosteally in the usual manner, including as much of its medial extent as pos-

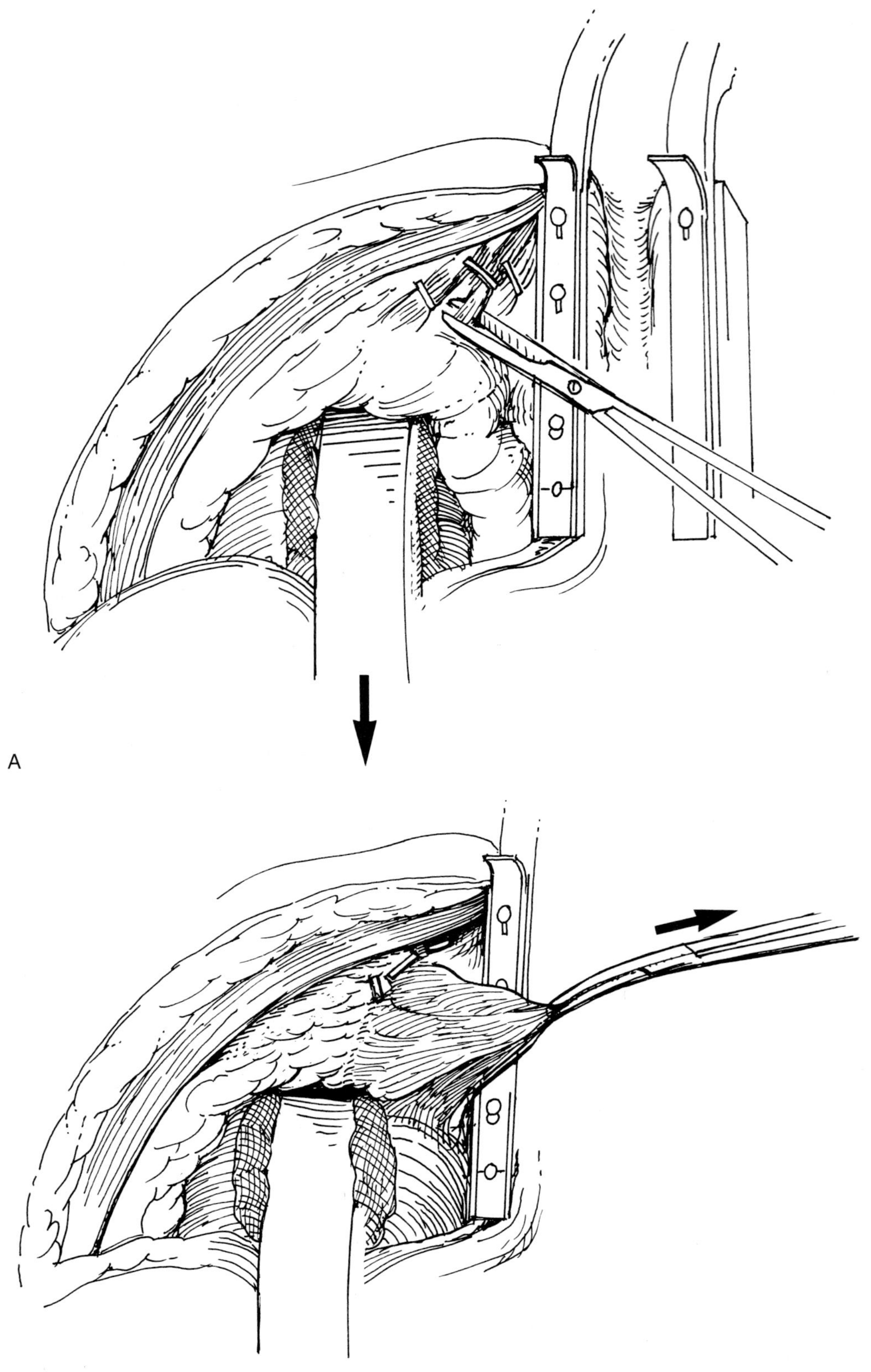

A

B

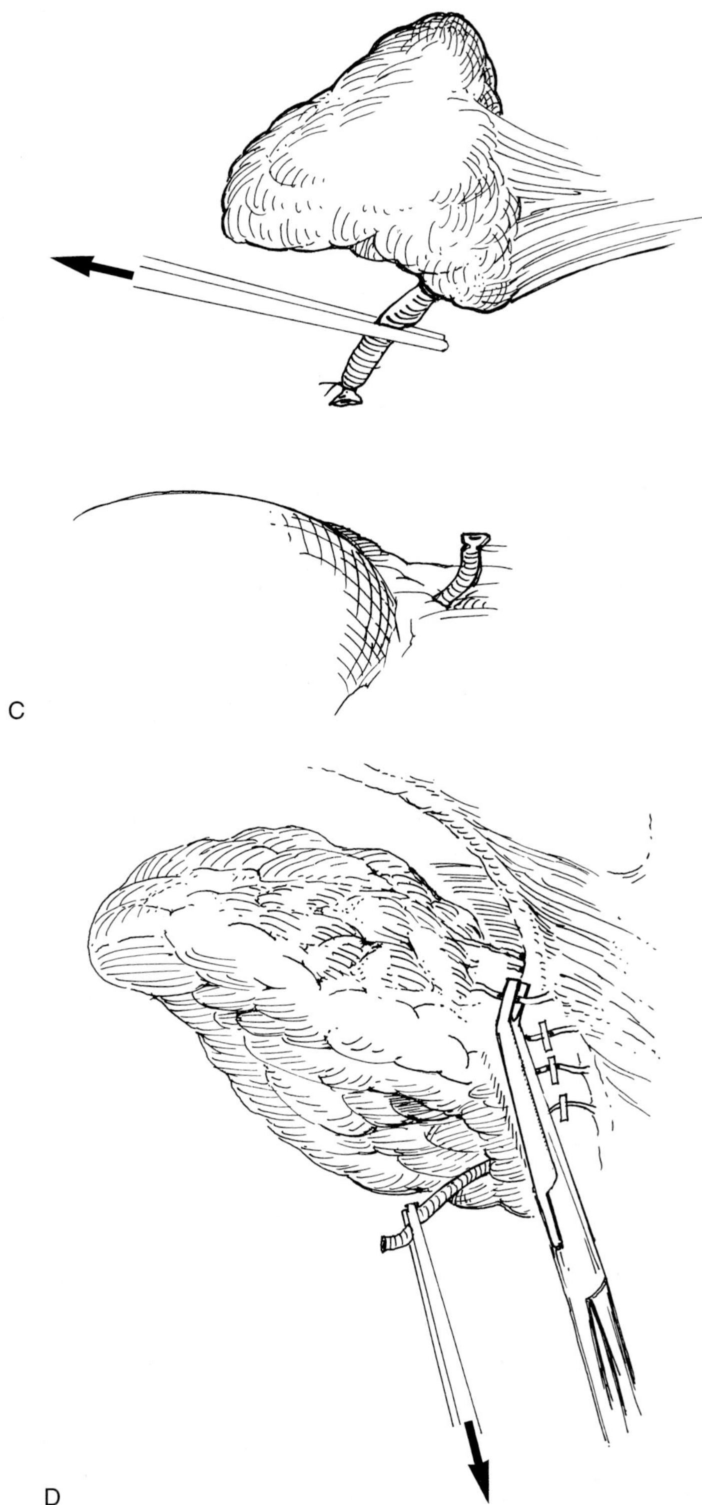

FIG. 13-8. Left adrenalectomy through a posterior incision. Key points, as described in text, include downward retraction of kidney, early division of the superior arterial branches and attachments, and atraumatic medial and lateral reflection of the gland during dissection. (Modified from Stewart BH. Bilateral Posterior Approach to the Adrenal Glands. In: Stewart BH, ed. *Operative Urology.* Baltimore, MD: Williams & Wilkins, 1975;96–97.)

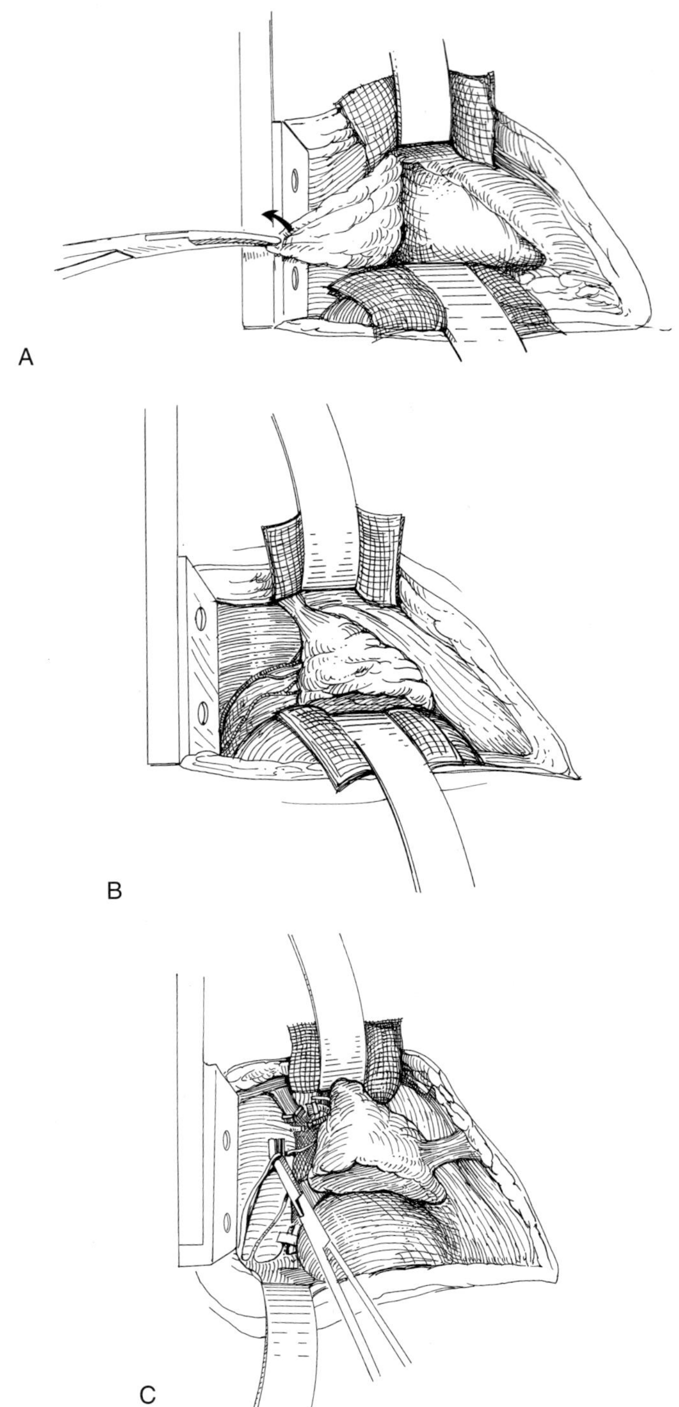

FIG. 13-9. Right adrenalectomy through a posterior incision. Care must be taken to avoid avulsion of the adrenal vein or injury to the inferior vena cava. (Modified from Stewart BH. Bilateral Posterior Approach to the Adrenal Glands. In: Stewart BH, ed. *Operative Urology*. Baltimore, MD: Williams & Wilkins, 1975;98–99.)

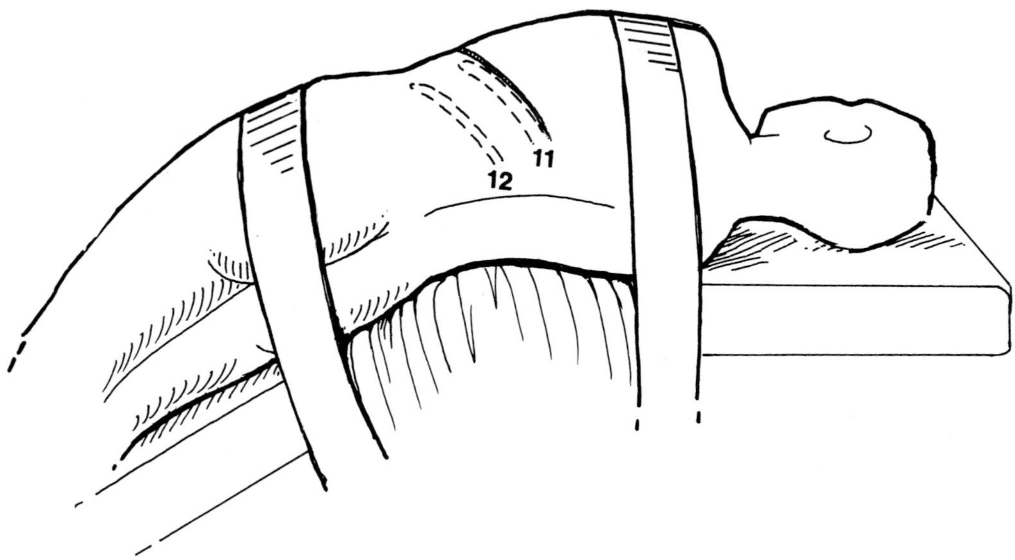

FIG. 13-10. Lateral eleventh or twelfth rib approach. (Modified from Bloom LS, Libertino J. Surgical Management of Cushing's Syndrome. In: Libertino JA, Novick AC, eds. Adrenal Surgery. *Urol Clin North Am* 1989;16:3,56.)

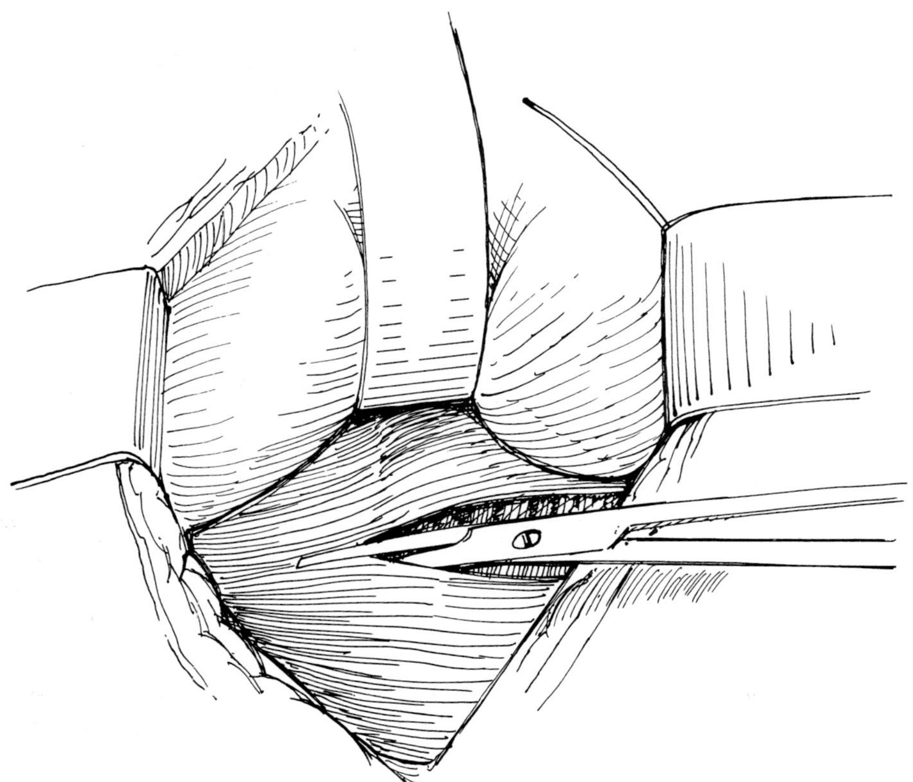

FIG. 13-11. The colon and peritoneum are mobilized medially and Gerota's fascia incised. (Modified from Hinman F. *Atlas of Urologic Surgery.* Philadelphia: WB Saunders, 1989:19;845.)

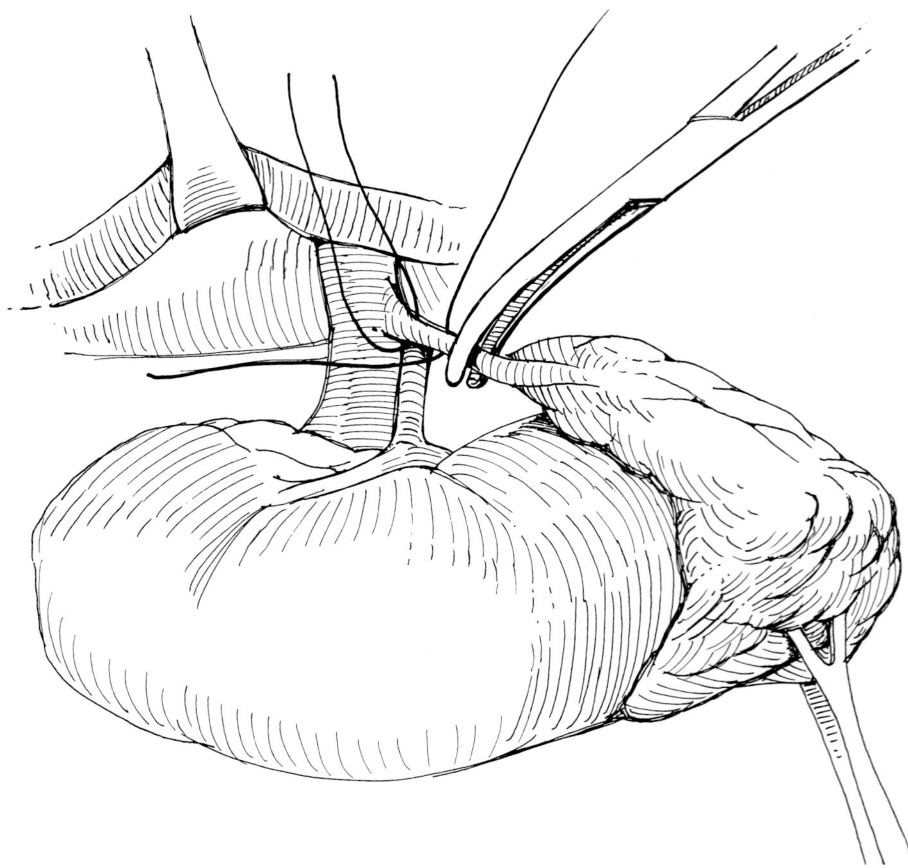

FIG. 13-12. Left total adrenalectomy through an eleventh rib flank incision. (Modified from Hinman F. *Atlas of Urologic Surgery*. Philadelphia: WB Saunders, 1989:19;846.)

sible (Fig. 13-6). Medial retraction of the sacrospinalis facilitates this step.

The diaphragm and pleura can be readily retracted superiorly when operating through the bed of the twelfth rib on the left. The eleventh rib incision on the right, however, results in more difficult pleural mobilization and retraction, and pleural entry is not uncommon. When this occurs, the pleural and diaphragmatic layers should be opened in the line of the incision. On either side, the retroperitoneal space is entered and Gerota's fascia incised, exposing the posterior surface of the kidney and adrenal (Fig. 13-7).

On the left side, apical adrenal vessels are clipped and divided. Attachments between the upper medial kidney and inferior adrenal gland are not interrupted at this time, and

downward retraction of the kidney results in descent and excellent exposure of the gland (Fig. 13-8A,B). Generous use of hemoclips facilitates dissection and division of vascular attachments of the lateral, medial, and anterior adrenal surface. The adrenal vein arising from the proximal left renal vein is ligated and divided, and the adrenal stump is used to retract the gland to aid dissection. The middle adrenal artery arising from the aorta and the inferior adrenal artery arising from the renal artery are ligated or clipped and divided (see Fig. 13-8C,D). During dissection, the gland is handled with care, grasping periadrenal tissue, to avoid fracture, bleeding, or an intramedullary hematoma, which could obscure identification of a small adenoma. Injury to the tail of the pancreas, which lies

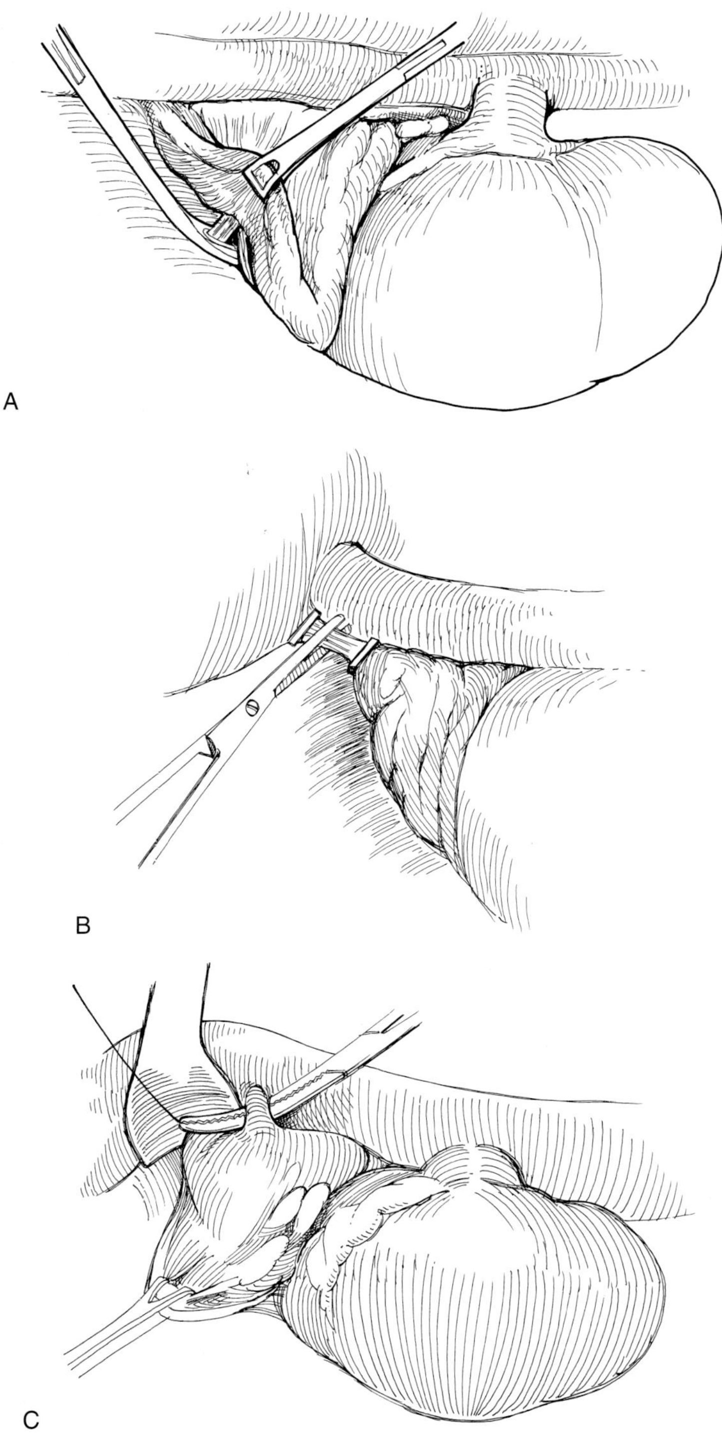

FIG. 13-13. Right total adrenalectomy dissection performed through an eleventh rib supracostal incision. Early ligation of the adrenal vein as it enters the posterolateral inferior vena cava is shown. (Modified from Hinman F. *Atlas of Urologic Surgery*. Philadelphia: WB Saunders, 1989:19;847–848.)

adjacent to the anteromedial aspect of the adrenal, must be avoided.

On the right side, the kidney and liver are gently retracted inferiorly and superiorly, respectively, to allow exposure of the adrenal (Fig. 13-9A). Adhesions of the adrenal to the liver, as well as apical vascular attachments, are divided between hemoclips. This allows further downward retraction of the adrenal and mobilization of its lateral and inferior aspect with vascular clips (see Fig. 13-9B). Gentle traction of the gland laterally demonstrates the adrenal vein entering the inferior vena cava. The vein is ligated and divided (see Fig. 13-9C). Any remaining vascular attachments are clipped, divided, and the gland removed. It must be emphasized again that retraction is always gentle, and dissection of the medial aspect of the right adrenal and its vein

meticulous, with precise ligation, because vena caval injury and bleeding can be most difficult to manage via a posterior incision (2). A modified right posterior incision that affords superior access to and exposure of the right adrenal vein and inferior vena cava has been described by Vaughan (3) and may be useful in patients with larger tumors in which a posterior approach is preferred.

In patients in whom a small solitary benign adenoma is unequivocally localized and peripheral in the gland, partial adrenalectomy may be appropriate (see Partial Adrenalectomy).

Following adrenalectomy, a standard closure is performed. No drains are necessary. In patients in whom the pleural cavity was entered and the diaphragm incised, airtight closure is accomplished in layers under positive pressure expansion. A chest tube is usually

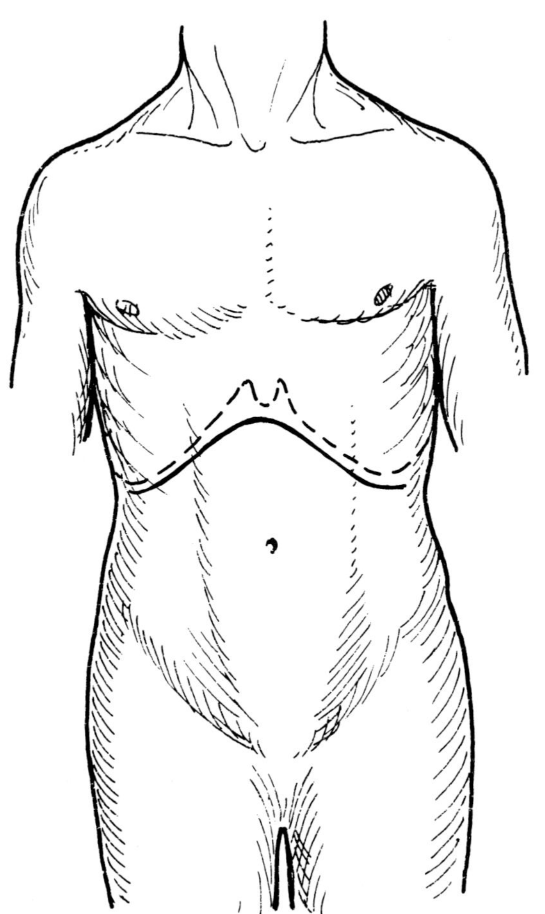

FIG. 13-14. Anterior transabdominal chevron incision is optimal for large adrenal masses, bilateral disease, or need for abdominal exploration. It may be modified for well localized unilateral adrenal tumors as necessary. (Modified from Bloom LS, Libertino J. Surgical Management of Cushing's Syndrome. In: Libertino JA, Novick AC, eds. Adrenal Surgery. *Urol Clin North Am* 1989; 16:3,557.)

not required. A chest film is obtained at the completion of the operation to confirm that the lung is normally expanded.

Flank Approach

The standard extrapleural, extraperitoneal flank incision through the bed of the eleventh or twelfth rib provides excellent unilateral adrenal exposure and is familiar to most urologic surgeons. It is suitable for unilateral adrenalectomy for small to moderate-sized (<6 cm) benign adrenal tumors. The flank position can be especially useful in patients who are markedly obese or who have undergone numerous intraabdominal procedures. In the flank position, the abdominal contents and retroperitoneal fat shift medially and away from the surgeon, resulting in the best possible exposure of the kidney and adrenal gland.

The patient is placed in the lateral position with the table broken and kidney rest elevated. The incision is made over the eleventh or twelfth rib, extending from the tip posteriorly (Fig. 13-10) and the rib resected. The pleura is dissected from the inner aspect of the rib, retracted upward with the diaphragm, and the retroperitoneal space entered.

On the left side, the colon and peritoneum are retracted medially, and Gerota's fascia is incised (Fig. 13-11). Care is taken to avoid pancreatic injury. The kidney is retracted inferiorly and the gland is mobilized in the usual fashion, using principles previously described, with early release of superior vascular attachments. The left adrenal vein is identified and ligated,

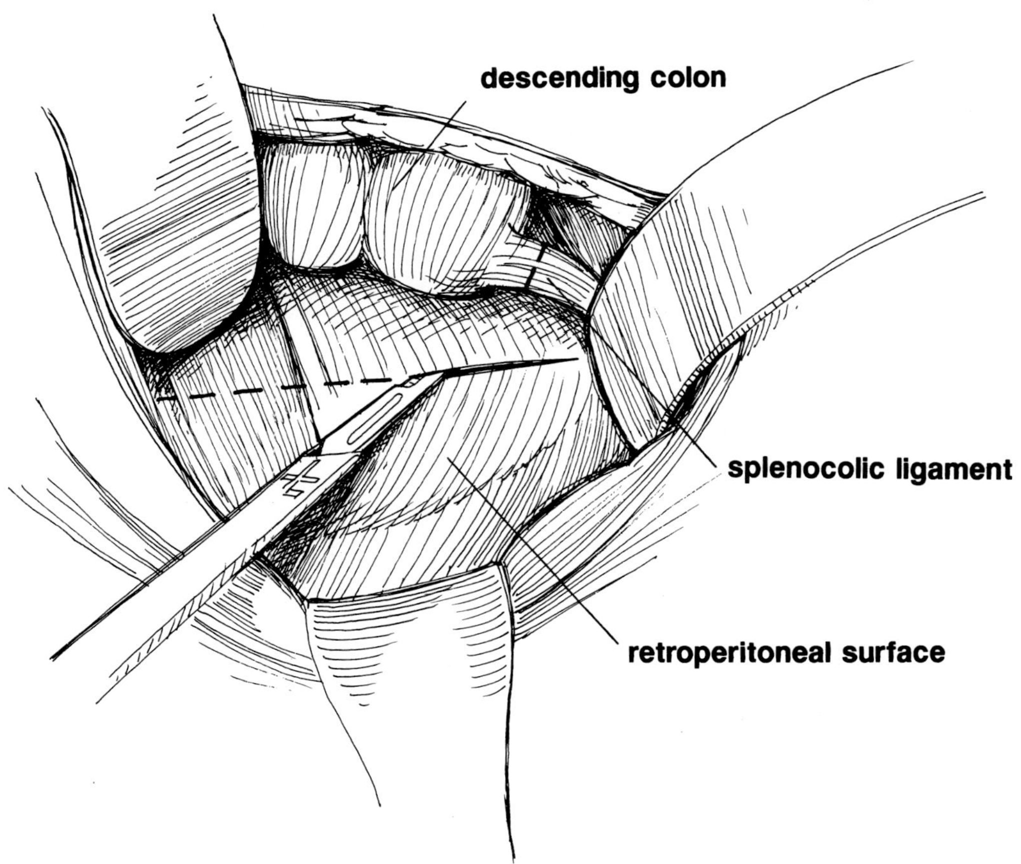

FIG. 13-15. On the left, incision of the peritoneum lateral to the descending colon and division of the splenocolic ligament provides access to the retroperitoneal space. (Modified from Hinman F. *Atlas of Urologic Surgery*. Philadelphia: WB Saunders, 1989:19;849.)

and the remaining vascular attachments are clipped and divided, completing the adrenalectomy (Fig. 13-12).

On the right, the colon and duodenum are reflected medially, and the liver is reflected upward. As noted, retracting the kidney downward facilitates clipping and dividing anterior, apical, and posterior vascular attachments (Fig. 13-13A,B). Gentle lateral retraction of the gland reveals small anterior vessels medially and inferiorly. These are clipped and divided, exposing the adrenal vein as it enters the posterolateral inferior vena cava. Ligation and division of the vein, as well as any remaining vascular branches, completes the adrenal excision (see Fig. 13-13C).

In patients in whom the pleural cavity was entered, airtight closure is accomplished in layers under positive pressure expension, chest tubes and drains are not necessary, and the flank incision is closed in the usual manner.

Anterior Transabdominal Approach

This approach is preferred for patients with pheochromocytoma in whom bilateral adrenal and complete intraabdominal exploration is necessary, for adrenal carcinoma and suspicious but equivocal large masses (>10 cm), and for adrenal surgery in children. With the patient in the supine position, our preference is the chevron incision (Fig. 13-14), which can be modified for well-localized unilateral adrenal tumors as necessary. The rectus muscles and sheath and the lateral obliques are incised, the peritoneal cavity is entered, and careful intraabdominal palpation is carried out.

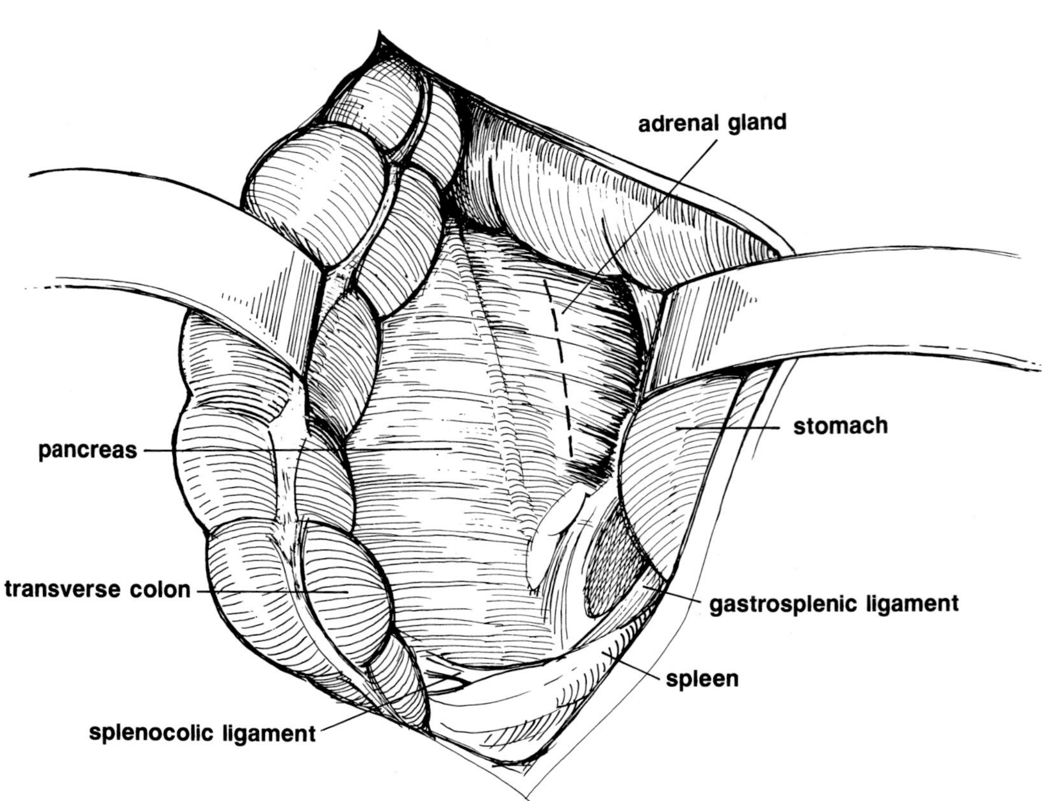

FIG. 13-16. Alternatively, the left retroperitoneal space and adrenal can be approached by dividing the omentocolic ligament and entering through the lesser sac. (Modified from Hinman F. *Atlas of Urologic Surgery.* Philadelphia: WB Saunders, 1989:19;854.)

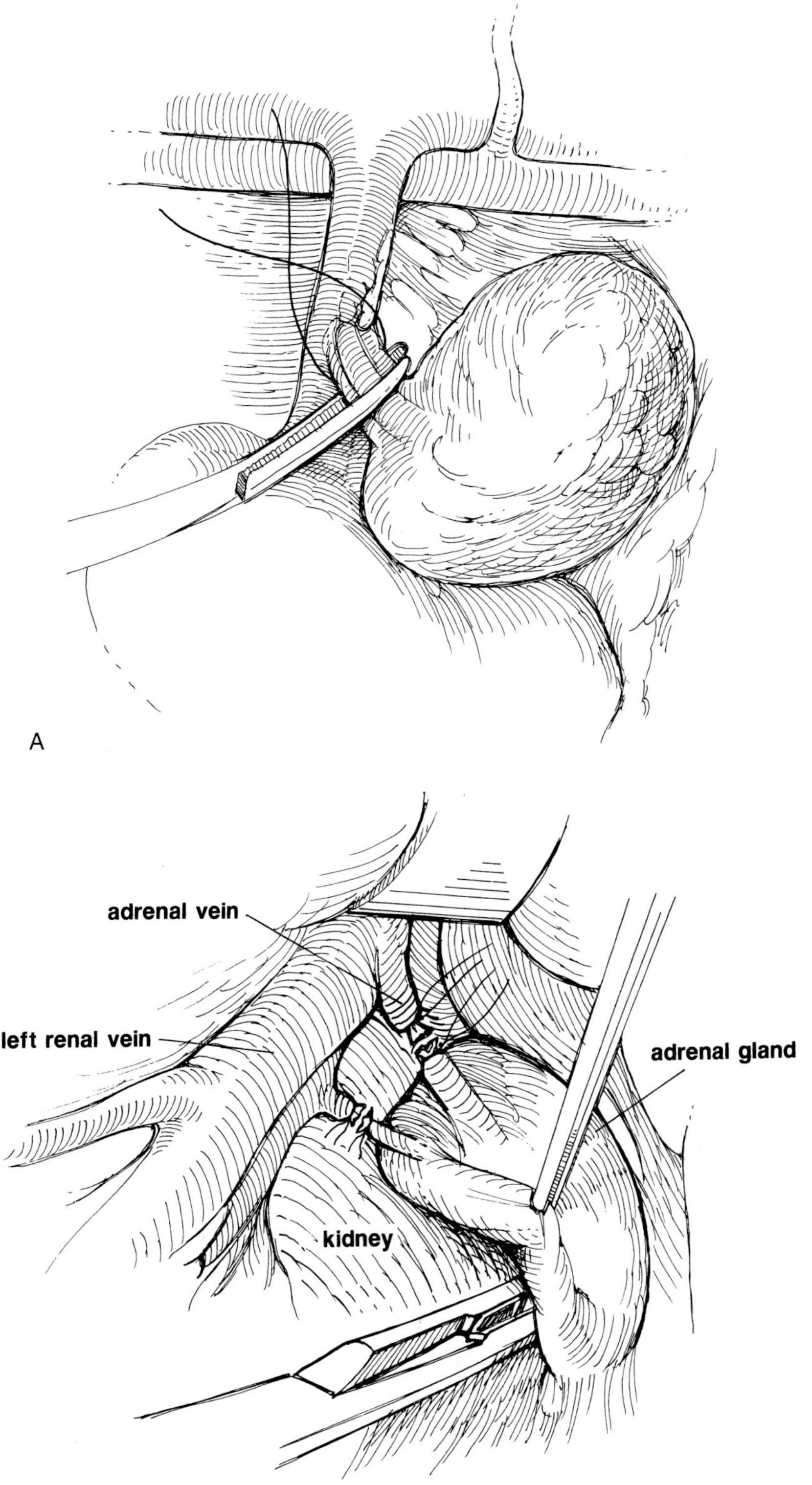

FIG. 13-17. This approach readily facilitates left adrenalectomy for pheochromocytoma **(A)**, or other adrenal pathology, such as adenoma and hyperplasia **(B)**. (Modified from Hinman F. *Atlas of Urologic Surgery*. Philadelphia: WB Saunders, 1989:19;850,854.)

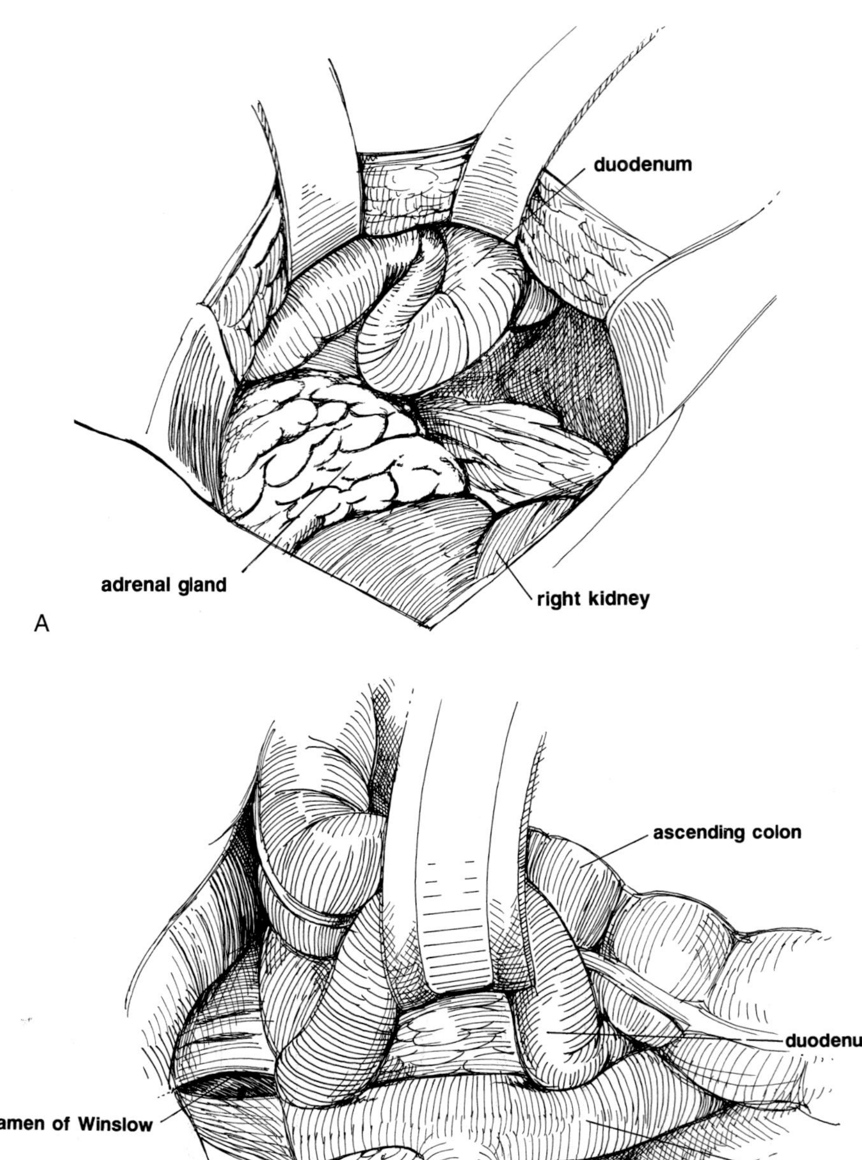

FIG. 13-18. Right adrenal exposure is accomplished by performing the Kocher maneuver and mobilizing the hepatic flexure of the colon **(A)**, as well as exposing the inferior vena cava, renal vein, and suprarenal space **(B)**. (Modified from Hinman F. *Atlas of Urologic Surgery*. Philadelphia: WB Saunders, 1989:19;855–856.)

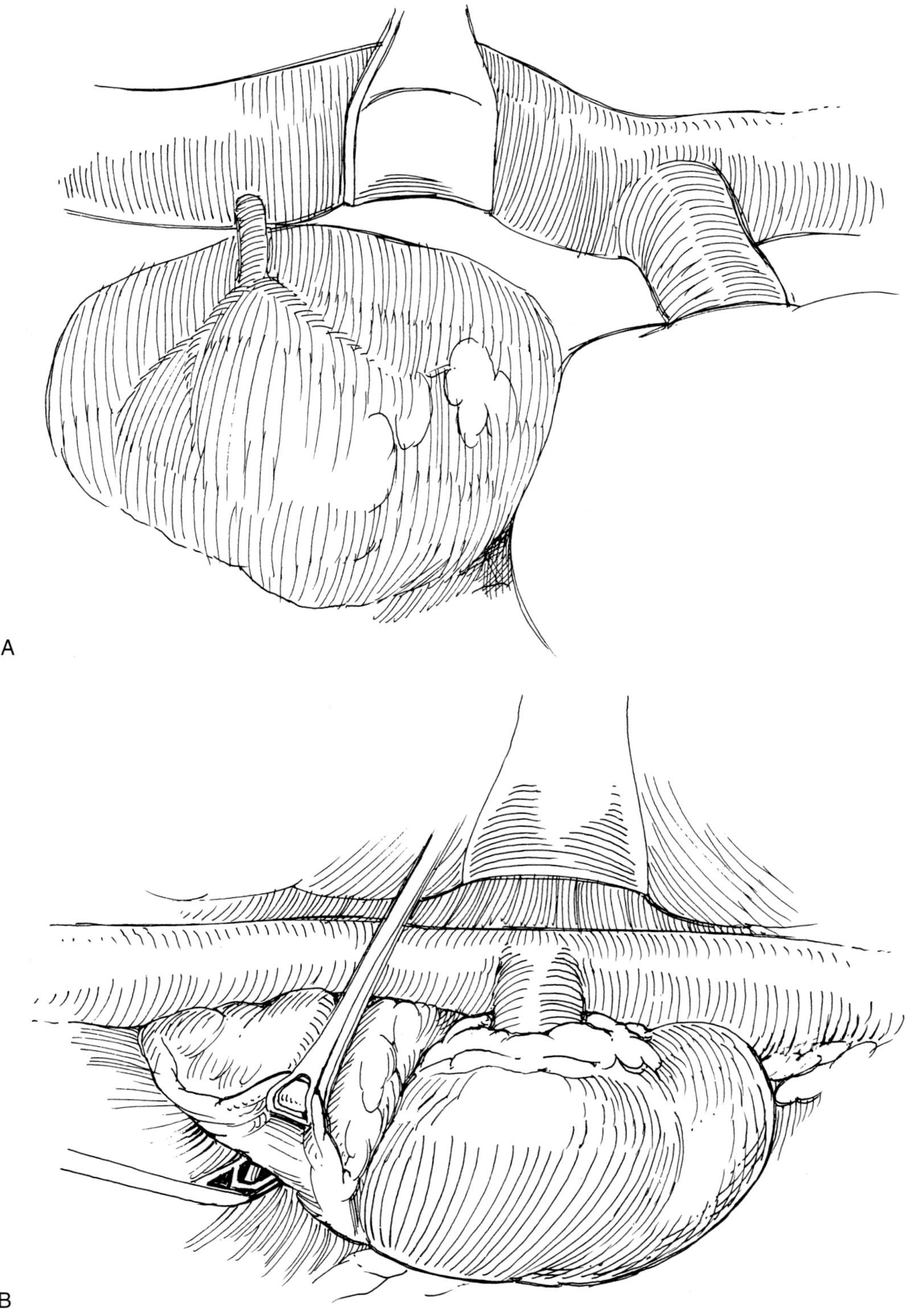

A

B

FIG. 13-19. The exposure obtained permits early control of the adrenal vein for pheochromocytoma **(A)** or adrenalectomy for other indications **(B)**. (Modified from Hinman F. *Atlas of Urologic Surgery*. Philadelphia: WB Saunders, 1989:19;853,856.)

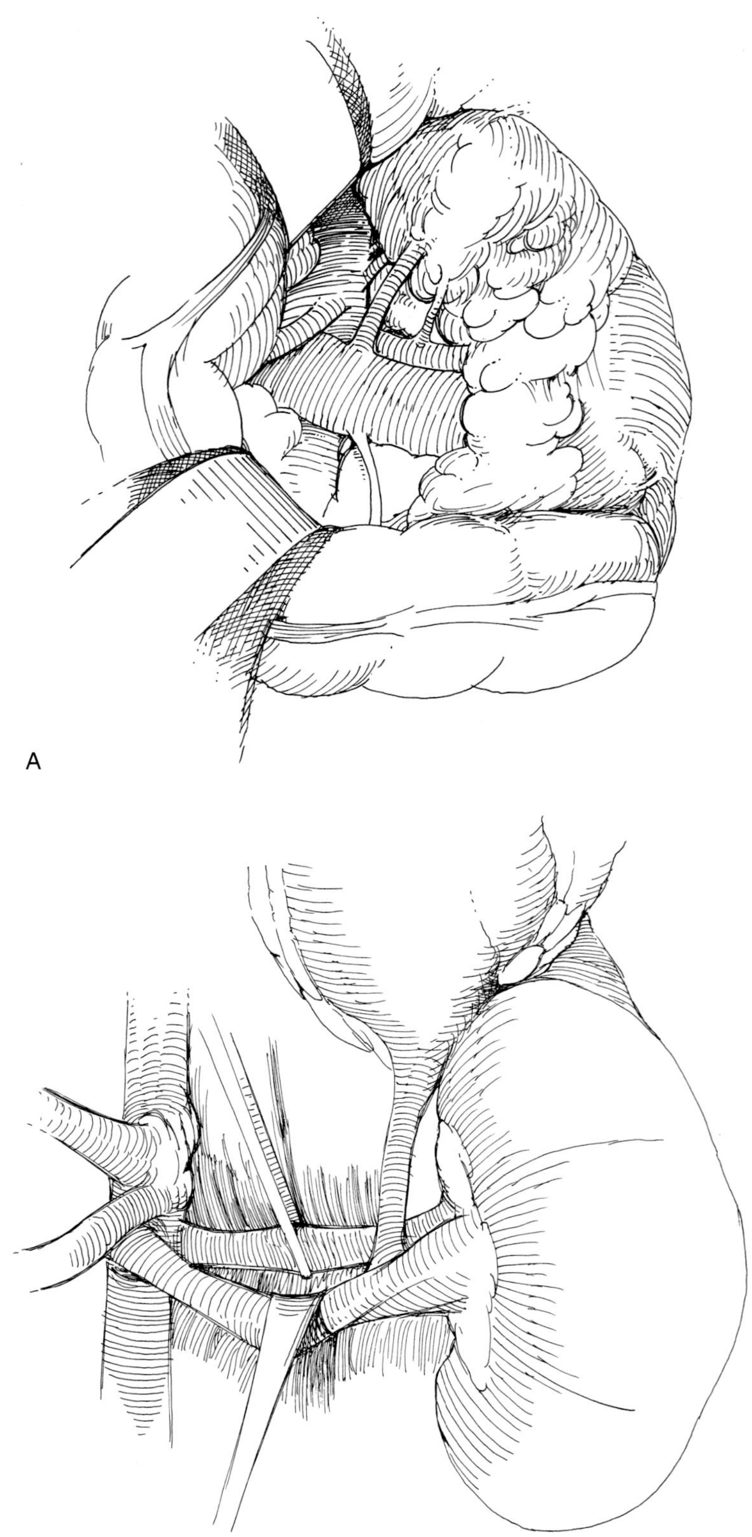

A

B

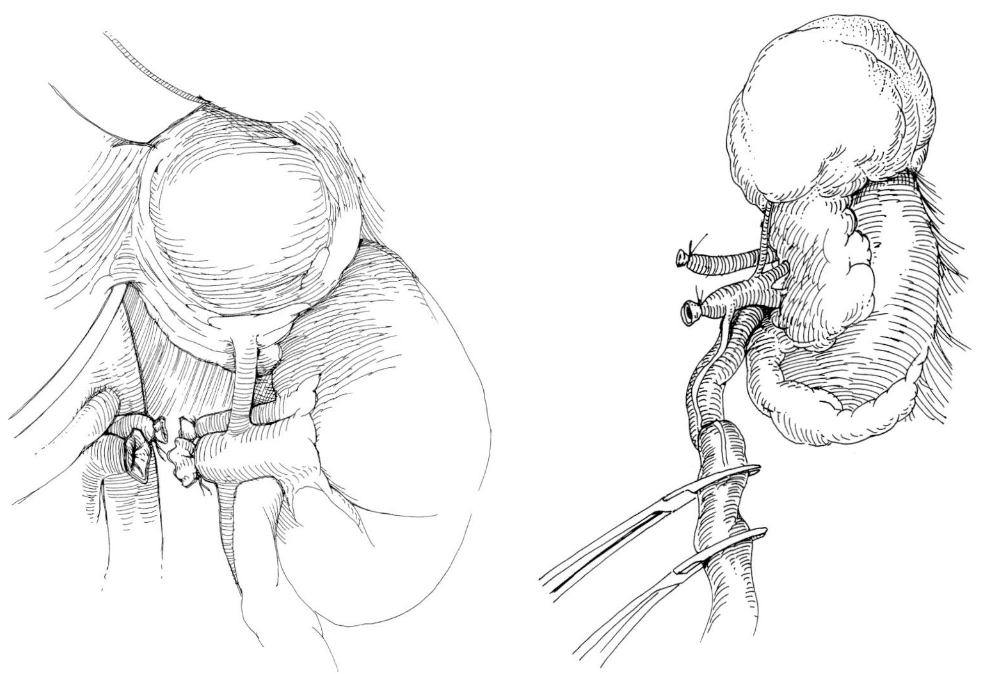

C

D

FIG. 13-20. In patients with large, extensive adrenal cortical carcinoma, regional lymphadenectomy **(A)** or nephroadrenalectomy **(B-D)**, as well as partial pancreatectomy, may be necessary to remove all neoplasm. The transabdominal approach as shown here on the left, as well as a thoracoabdominal incision, is best suited to large adrenal masses. (**A** and **D** modified from Stewart BH. Operations Upon the Adrenal Glands. In: Stewart BH, ed. *Operative Urology.* Baltimore, MD: Williams & Wilkins, 1975. **B** and **C** modified from Hinman F. *Atlas of Urologic Surgery.* Philadelphia: WB Saunders, 1989:19;857.)

On the left, incision of the retroperitoneum lateral to the descending colon and division of the splenocolic ligament provide access to the retroperitoneal space (Fig. 13-15). Alternatively, the left retroperitoneal space and adrenal can be approached by dividing the omentocolic ligament and entering through the lesser sac (Fig. 13-16). Gerota's fascia is incised, the kidney exposed, and the entry of the left adrenal vein into the renal vein dissected. Following gentle downward retraction of the kidney, with division of the splenorenal ligament, the adrenal gland is mobilized in the usual manner beginning cephalad and lateral. Care is taken to avoid injury to the tail of the pancreas where it overlies the medial aspect of the adrenal; the vein and remaining vascular attachments are ligated and divided, and adrenalectomy is completed (Fig. 13-17A,B).

On the right, adrenal exposure is achieved by performing the Kocher maneuver and mobilizing the hepatic flexure of the colon (Fig. 13-18A), as well as by exposing the inferior vena cava, renal vein, and suprarenal space (see Fig. 13-18B). This exposure allows early control of the adrenal vein for pheochromocytoma (Fig. 13-19A) or adrenalectomy for other indications (see Fig. 13-19B).

In patients with large extensive adrenal cortical carcinoma, the transabdominal chevron incision, as well as a thoracoabdominal incision, allows regional lymphadenectomy (Fig. 13-20A) and exposure for nephroadrenalectomy (Fig. 13-20B–D), as shown on the left.

Thoracoabdominal Approach

This approach is particularly useful in patients with a very large, invasive adrenal corti-

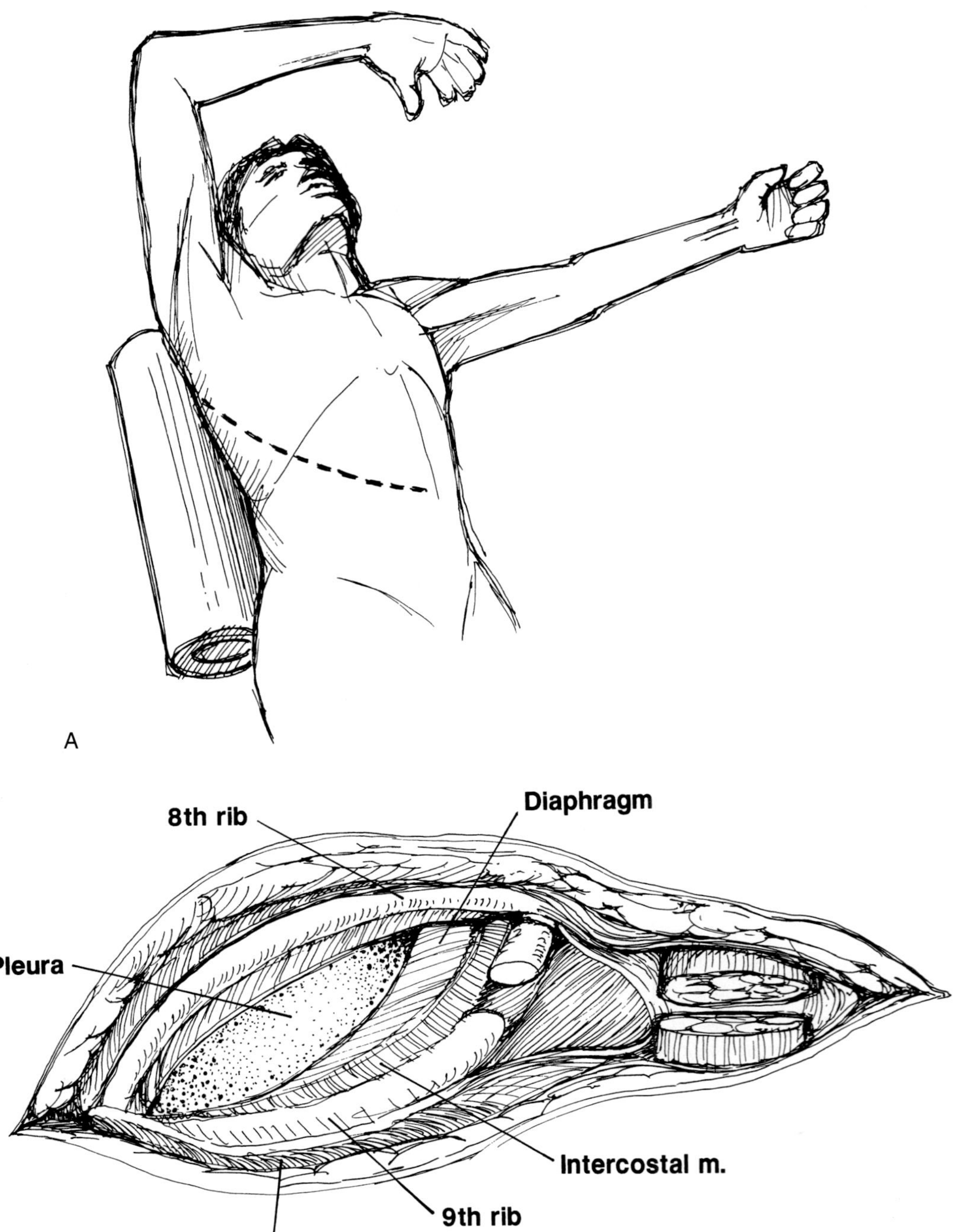
A
8th rib
Diaphragm
Pleura
Intercostal m.
9th rib
External oblique m.
B

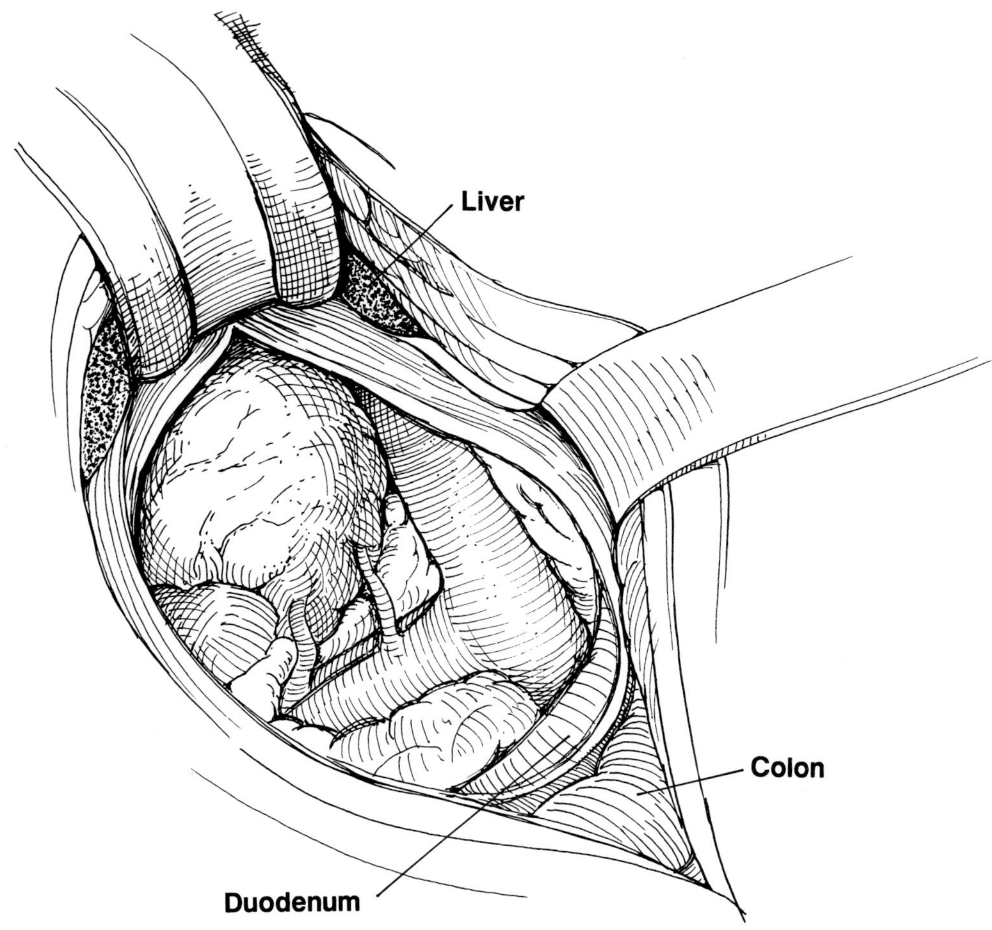

FIG. 13-21. Thoracoabdominal approach to the right adrenal gland. The patient is positioned obliquely with a large roll, and arm is raised and suspended. The incision extends from the eighth or ninth intercostal space to the abdominal midline **(A)**. After the intercostal muscles have been divided, the diaphragm and pleura are seen, and the diaphragm incised. Upward retraction of the liver and mobilization of the colonic hepatic flexure and duodenum provide excellent exposure for large, right adrenal masses **(B, C)**. (Modified from Guz B, Straffon R, Novick A. Operative Approaches to the Adrenal Gland. In: Libertino JA, Novick AC, eds. Adrenal Surgery. *Urol Clin North Am* 1989:16;3,532.)

cal carcinoma, in which radical adrenalectomy and wide excision of all neoplasm afford the only opportunity for cure. The exposure obtained with a thoracoabdominal incision facilitates regional lymphadenectomy, en bloc excision of the adrenal and kidney, as well as splenectomy and partial pancreatectomy when necessary to eradicate all evident extension of the carcinoma. The approach is also well suited for excision of a large right adrenal pheochromocytoma while permitting palpation of the retroperitoneum and intraabdominal contents.

The patient is placed in a 40-degree semioblique position. With the patient supported by a roll beneath the flank and with the patient's arm raised and resting on a Mayo stand or suspended from the anesthesia screen, the surgeon extends the incision from the eighth or ninth intercostal space and across the costal margin to the abdominal midline, as show on the right in Figure 13-21A. After the latissimus dorsi, external oblique, and rectus muscles have been divided, the intercostal muscles are incised in the direction of the incision and the costal margin is divided, exposing the pleura and diaphragm (see Fig. 13-21B). The pleural and peritoneal cavities are entered by circumferentially dividing the diaphragm, retracting the liver upward and the duodenum and hepatic flexure of the colon medially. The excellent suprarenal exposure obtained with a right thoracoabdominal approach is shown in Figure 13-21C.

The creation and closure of this incision is time-consuming, and there may be increased postoperative pulmonary morbidity. Nevertheless, in properly selected patients with extremely large or invasive adrenal neoplasms, the thoracoabdominal incision is often the best choice.

PARTIAL ADRENALECTOMY

Partial adrenalectomy may be considered in young patients with bilateral benign adrenal tumors (e.g., pheochromocytoma, adenoma) in whom the prospect of lifelong steroid replacement following bilateral total adrenalectomy entails potential morbidity and unpleasant sequelae. In the rare patient with a solitary adrenal gland and functioning tumor, enucleation or partial adrenalectomy is useful.

The indications for adrenal-sparing surgery in patients with a unilateral tumor and normal contralateral gland are not well defined. We have performed partial adrenalectomy in seven patients with aldosterone-producing adenomas who were followed up for more than 10 years with no evidence of recurrent hyperaldosteronism. Other reports of partial adrenalectomy in primary aldosteronism, both by open and laparoscopic surgery, have shown no evidence of recurrence (4–6).

When partial adrenalectomy may be indicated, as for a benign, peripheral adenoma, mobilization of the gland is performed so as to

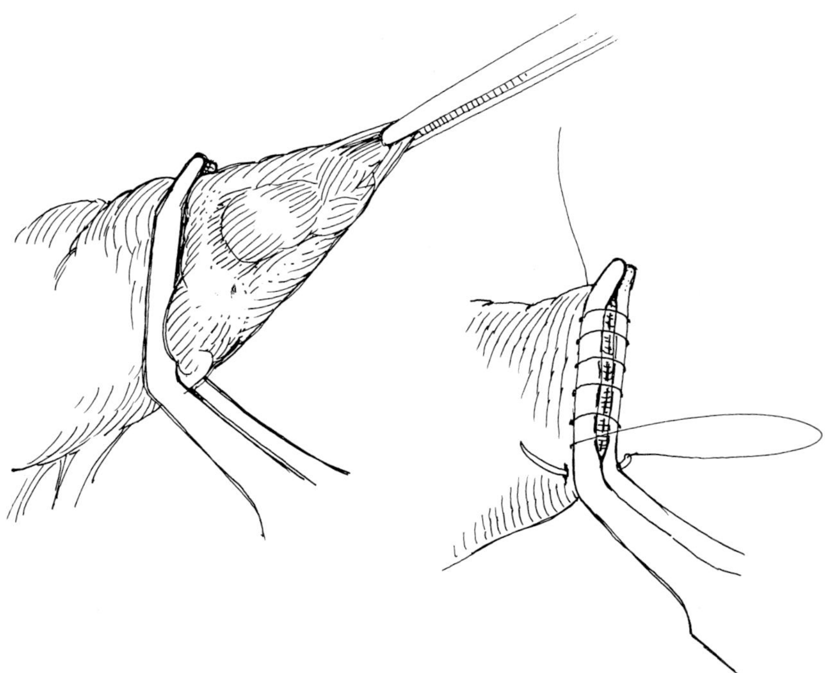

FIG. 13-22. When partial adrenalectomy is indicated, as for a small peripheral benign adenoma, excision using a Satinsky clamp with oversewing is an effective technique. Other techniques including stapling have been used. (Modified from Hinman F. *Atlas of Urologic Surgery*. Philadelphia: WB Saunders, 1989:19;846.)

preserve the vein and as many arterioles as possible. A Satinsky clamp is placed as shown in Figure 13-22, and the adenomatous portion of the gland is excised and the clamp oversewn. Other techniques for partial adrenalectomy use stay sutures rather than a clamp, excision of the diseased segment, and interrupted sutures for adrenal closure and hemostasis.

LAPAROSCOPIC ADRENALECTOMY

Indications for, technique, and results of laparoscopic adrenalectomy are discussed in Chapter 12. As more studies of patients undergoing laparoscopic versus open adrenalectomy become available for analysis, it is apparent that the laparoscopic approach is preferred in most cases of small (<6 cm) benign adrenal neoplasms (7–16). Significant benefits in the laparoscopic group include reduced length of hospitalization, lessened analgesic pain requirements, shortened convalescence, and more rapid return to normal diet and resumption of employment. The cure rate following laparoscopic adrenal surgery is equal to that of open surgical techniques, blood loss is less, and there is reduced morbidity. Surgical operating time for the laparoscopic approach is at least 50% longer than for open surgery in most series; however, once the learning curve of at least 10 cases has been surmounted, differences become less striking, less than 20 minutes in one report. Partial adrenalectomy has been performed by laparoscopy. Laparoscopic adrenalectomy should not be undertaken for masses greater than 6 cm, in which there is a question of multifocality, or in cases of adrenal cortical carcinoma in which necessary en bloc resection cannot be adequately accomplished.

It is also important that the availability of the minimally invasive technique not encourage expansion of indications for excision of incidentally found, nonfunctioning adrenal masses (e.g., <3 cm in size, with no change in size or shape on serial CT or MRI scan).

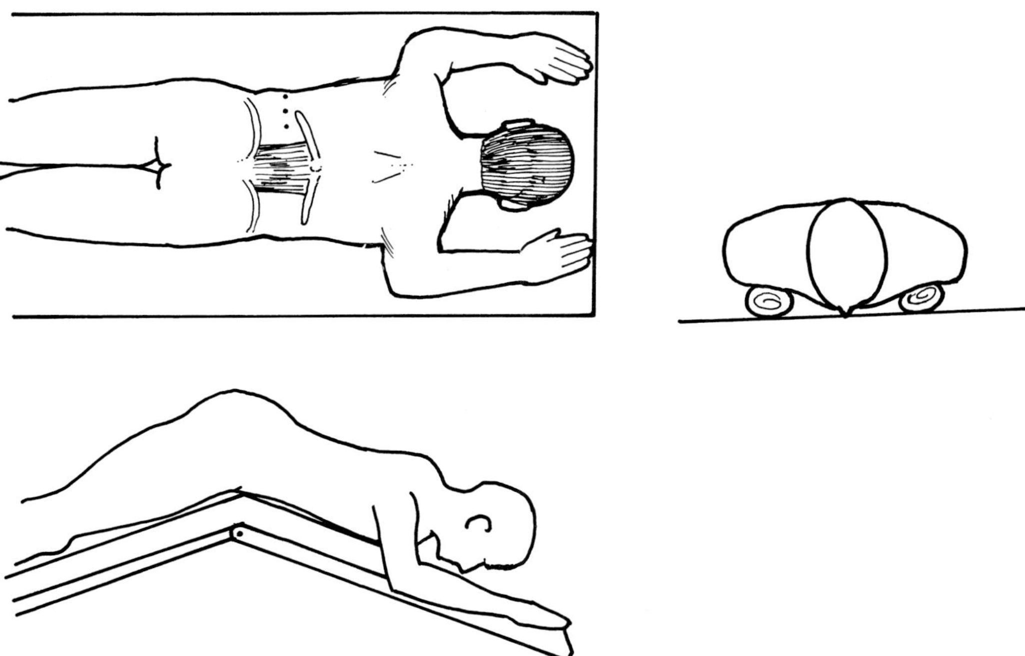

FIG. 13-23. Patient position and trocar location for posterior retroperitoneal laparoscopic adrenalectomy. (Modified from Van Heerden JA. Endocrine Surgery. *J Am Coll Surg* 1998:186;141.)

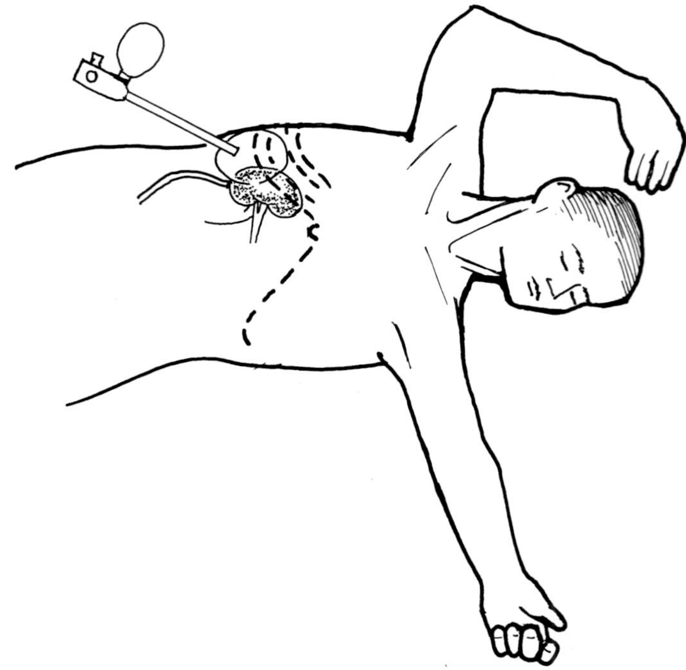

FIG. 13-24. Patient placed in the lateral decubitus position for right retroperitoneal adrenalectomy. Balloon dilation enlarges the working space. (Modified from Van Heerden JA: Endocrine Surgery. *J Am Coll Surg* 1998;186:141.)

The transperitoneal approach is most commonly used for laparoscopic adrenalectomy. The posterior retroperitoneal approach (Fig. 13-23) and lateral retroperitoneal approach (Fig. 13-24) are also advocated, although resulting in a more limited working space. Balloon dilation of the retroperitoneal space has been used in some cases (17).

REFERENCES

1. Malhotra V, ed. *Anesthesia for renal and genitourinary surgery*. New York: McGraw Hill, 1995.
2. Libertino JA. Surgery of adrenal disorders. *Surg Clin North Am* 1988;68:1027–1056.
3. Vaughan ED Jr, Phillips H. Modified posterior approach for right adrenalectomy. *Surg Gynecol Obstet* 1987;165:453–455.
4. Nakada T, Kubota Y, Sasagawa I, et al. Therapeutic outcome of primary aldosteronism: adrenalectomy versus enucleation of aldosterone-producing adenoma. *J Urol* 1995;153:1775–1780.
5. Clark L. What's new in endocrine surgery. *J Am Coll Surg* 1997;184:130–131.
6. Janetschek G, Lhotta K, Gasser R, et al. Adrenal-sparing laparoscopic surgery for aldosterone producing adenoma. *J Endourol* 1997;11:145–148.
7. Gagner M, LaCroix A, Bolte E. Laparoscopic adrenalec-

tomy in Cushing's syndrome and pheochromocytoma [letter to the editor]. *N Engl J Med* 1992;327:1033.
8. Go H, Takeda M, Takahashi H, et al. Laparoscopic adrenalectomy for primary aldosteronism: a new operative method. *J Laparoendosc Surg* 1993;3:455.
9. Suzuki K, Kageyama S, Ueda D, et al. Laparoscopic adrenalectomy: clinical experience with 12 cases. *J Urol* 1993;150:1099–1102.
10. Takeda M, Go H, Imai T, et al. Laparoscopic adrenalectomy for primary aldosteronism: report of initial 10 cases. *Surgery* 1994;115:621–625.
11. Naito S, Uozumi J, Shimura H, et al. Laparoscopic adrenalectomy: review of 14 cases and comparison with open adrenalectomy. *J Endourol* 1995;9:491–495.
12. Brunt L, Doherty G, Norton J, et al. Laparoscopic adrenalectomy compared to open adrenalectomy for benign adrenal neoplasms. *J Am Coll Surg* 1996;183:1–10.
13. Prinz R. Laparoscopic adrenalectomy [editorial]. *J Am Coll Surg* 1996;183:71–73.
14. Winfield H, Hamilton B, Bravo E, Novick A. Laparoscopic adrenalectomy: the preferred choice? A comparison to open adrenalectomy. *J Urol* 1998;160:325–329.
15. Janetschek G, Finkenstedt G, Gesser R, et al. Laparoscopic surgery for pheochromocytoma: adrenalectomy, partial resection, excision of paragangliomas. *J Urol* 1998;160:330–334.
16. Gagner M, et al. Laparoscopic adrenalectomy lessons learned from 100 consecutive procedures. *Trans Am Surg Assoc* 1997;115:28–37.
17. Van Heerden J. Endocrine surgery. *J Am Coll Surg* 1998;186:141–147.

Subject Index